NOTES ON
OBSTETRICS
AND
GYNAECOLOGY

.al

Commissioning Editor: Ellen Green
Project Development Manager: Colin Arthur
Designer: Erik Bigland
Project Manager: Nancy Arnott

NOTES ON
OBSTETRICS
AND
GYNAECOLOGY

Gordon M. Stirrat MA MD FRCOG
Emeritus Professor of Obstetrics and Gynaecology
University of Bristol

Martin S. Mills MD MRCOG
Consultant Obstetrician and Gynaecologist
St. Michael's Hospital, Bristol

Timothy J. Draycott MD MRCOG
Consultant Obstetrician and Gynaecologist
Southmead Hospital, Bristol

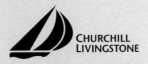
CHURCHILL
LIVINGSTONE

EDINBURGH LONDON NEW YORK OXFORD PHILADELPHIA
ST LOUIS TORONTO 2003

CHURCHILL LIVINGSTONE
An imprint of Elsevier Science Limited

ISBN 0 443 07223 X

British Library Cataloguing in Publication Data
A catalogue record for this book is available from the British Library

Library of Congress Cataloging in Publication Data
A catalog record for this book is available from the Library of Congress

Note
Medical knowledge is constantly changing. Standard safety precautions must
be followed, but as new research and clinical experience broaden our
knowledge, changes in treatment and drug therapy may become necessary or
appropriate. Readers are advised to check the most current product
information provided by the manufacturer of each drug to be administered
to verify the recommended dose, the method and duration of administration,
and contraindications. It is the responsibility of the practitioner, relying on
experience and knowledge of the patient, to determine dosages and the best
treatment for each individual patient. Neither the Publisher nor the
author/editor/contributor assumes any liability for any injury and/or damage
to persons or property arising from this publication.
The Publisher

The
publisher's
policy is to use
**paper manufactured
from sustainable forests**

Printed in China

PREFACE

Although this is the first of the series with this title, this book is, in fact, the fifth edition of what was previously, 'Aids to Obstetrics and Gynaecology'. Our aim is the same—to provide an authoritative and comprehensive synoptic guide to the practice of obstetrics and gynaecology. It is primarily aimed at candidates for the MRCOG but prior experience has shown that medical students, DRCOG candidates, nurses and midwives may find it valuable.

Yet again, the content and style have been extensively revised. Recent RCOG, NICE and other expert guidelines and recommendations have been incorporated. It is as up to date and accurate as we can make it. It is acknowledged that new knowledge will appear during its lifetime and the text should, therefore, be read with a properly critical attitude.

Reading the list of contents confirms that no other single specialty has the scope and variety of ours. We are also at the front-line of all of the major ethical issues. It remains a great privilege to be entrusted with the clinical management of women who have the right to expect the highest standards of care.

The first edition, under the authorship of GMS, was published in 1982. Twenty years and four editions later, it is entirely appropriate that two co-authors, younger colleagues at the peak of their profession, join him in this endeavour. In 1907 Henry Brook Adams wrote 'a teacher affects eternity: he can never tell where his influence stops'. For us, as practitioners and teachers, there can be no greater reward than to think that we too might influence those seeking knowledge as we have benefited from the wisdom of great teachers and mentors.

Bristol 2003   GMS, MSM, TJD

CONTENTS

SECTION 2
GYNAECOLOGY

SECTION ONE
OBSTETRICS

1. Obstetric care

Obstetric care has four phases:

- Pre-conception (p. 5)
- Antenatal (p. 6)
- Intrapartum (p. 136)
- Postnatal (p. 185)

Its objectives are:

- *Risk assessment*—to assess risk of harm to mother and baby.
- *Counselling*—to advise on the nature and extent of any perceived risks, and how to minimise or eradicate them.
- *Education*—to provide information on normal pregnancy and childbirth and give some guidance about pregnancy problems and possible interventions.
- *Treatment*—to treat any condition that might affect, or be affected by, the pregnancy.
- *Satisfaction*—to make the pregnancy and delivery as fulfilling yet as safe as possible.

RISK AND PREGNANCY

Risk is the probability that a particular event will occur.

- An 'at risk' pregnancy is one in which the probability of an adverse outcome in the mother and/or baby is greater than that for pregnant women in general.

Factors associated with risk of a particular event are 'risk markers'. For the terms 'high risk' and 'low risk' to be useful, the probability, nature and extent of specific risks must be considered:

- A high risk of one particular outcome does not necessarily imply a high risk of other adverse outcomes.
- A low risk of a serious condition with a bad outcome should be given more weight than a high risk of a lesser problem, which has minor effects.
- Perception of risk varies among individuals.

A guide to the extent of particular risks in pregnancy (e.g. pre-term birth, intrauterine growth restriction, congenital malformation or perinatal death) can be obtained from:

- History and examination for presence of risk markers
- *Screening tests*—offered to all pregnant women (see p. 6)
- *Diagnostic tests*—for those in whom a screening test is positive, or who have clinical signs and symptoms.

For a screening test to be of value it must:

- Predict the great majority of those who have the condition (*high positive predictive power*)
- Exclude those who do not have the condition (*high negative predictive power*).

All screening tests have some *false-positive and false-negative* results.

- The clinical value of a test depends on the balance between false-positive and false-negative results and the severity of the condition.
- A test that is of value when the incidence of a condition is high will be of poorer predictive value in another population with a low incidence of the same condition.

Interventions

Diagnostic and therapeutic interventions have their own intrinsic risk.

On some occasions an intervention may cause the harm one is trying to prevent.

An intervention without proven benefit cannot be justified on the basis that it will 'do no harm'.

RISK MARKERS ASSOCIATED WITH RISK OF ADVERSE OUTCOME TO BABY AND/OR MOTHER

The nature and extent of the risks are discussed in the text.

Physical factors
- Height <1.54 m
- Obesity—body mass index (BMI) >30 kg/m^2
- Underweight—BMI <20 kg/m^2

Social factors
- Teenage pregnancy
- Maternal age >35, increasing further from 38 then 40 years
- High parity and low interpregnancy interval
- Poor socioeconomic conditions
- Alcohol intake >80 g/day
- Substance abuse

Genetic factors
- Family history of diabetes in first-degree relative
- Family or personal history of inheritable diseases e.g. haemoglobinopathy, thrombophilia, etc.
- Congenital malformations in mother, family or previous child

Past medical history
- Maternal medical disorder
- Maternal prescribed medication
- Previous surgery
- Previous anaesthetic complications

Obstetric/gynaecological factors
- History of subfertility or recurrent miscarriage
- Previous gynaecological surgery e.g. myomectomy, cone biopsy, pelvic floor repair
- Presence of sizeable fibroids
- Previous pre-term delivery or low birthweight infant
- Previous baby >4 kg
- Previous placental abruption or third stage abnormality
- Previous caesarean section
- Previous stillbirth or neonatal death
- Previous third degree tear
- Elevated serum α-fetoprotein (AFP) in absence of NTD (see p. 43)
- Multiple pregnancy

PRE-CONCEPTION CARE

It is important that care begins before pregnancy because:
- Many women enter pregnancy poorly nourished, smoking heavily and in a less than optimal state of health.
- The most critical phase of fetal development is complete before the first visit to an antenatal clinic, and adverse factors have already begun to produce their effects.

Pre-conception clinics allow:
- Women with chronic diseases (e.g. diabetes) to become pregnant in as healthy a condition as possible
- Dietary advice to be offered to those above or below ideal body weight
- Encouragement to give up smoking and reduce alcohol ingestion
- Advice to be given to those who are anxious, have had problems in a previous pregnancy, or who have a personal or family history of a congenitally malformed child
- Supplements such as folic acid to be prescribed
- Rubella immunisation to be offered if the woman is susceptible
- Baseline measures of weight and blood pressure to be obtained

Much of this care is the proper responsibility of the primary health care team; however, obstetricians, physicians and clinical geneticists should be prepared to provide the benefit of their expertise.

ANTENATAL CARE

Antenatal care is a screening system that aims to assess and obviate risk of harm to mother and baby.

Traditional patterns of care were established over 50 years ago; their primary objective was to reduce maternal mortality and morbidity.

Few of the measures used routinely today are of proven benefit.

'Proof' is not easy, given the difficulty in determining what outcomes should be measured let alone measuring them!

BOOKING CLINIC

Assessment of risk begins when the woman is seen by her midwife or general practitioner (GP) early in pregnancy (best within the first 8 weeks).

The first hospital booking visit should take place around 12 and not later than 16 weeks' gestation.

ROUTINE BOOKING ASSESSMENT

Administrative details, including age, marital status and gravidity, are recorded.

An accurate menstrual history is important to assess gestational age.

History
• Medical and surgical; obstetric; family; social, smoking, alcohol and drug ingestion; inoculation risk (see p. 115)

Examination
• Weight; height; blood pressure; urinalysis for protein, blood and glucose
• General—chest, heart, breasts, etc.
• Abdominal—fundal height (if palpable), presence of any abnormal masses or tenderness,
• Pelvic—routine vaginal examination is unnecessary;
• Cervical smear if none within past 5 years
• Ultrasound scan (see p. 8)

Investigations
• FBC and check for haemoglobinopathy when indicated (see p. 94); ABO and Rh group and check for antibodies; Rubella immunity; VDRL

- Biochemical screening for Down syndrome (see p. 35) at 15 weeks' (optional); hepatitis B status; HIV status (with consent—see p. 114)
- Screen for toxoplasmosis if at high risk (see p. 118)
- Mid-stream urine (MSU) for culture and sensitivity
- Chest X-ray (if at high risk of tuberculosis)

The appropriate pattern of antenatal care and place of delivery is determined based on maternal choice and the presence of risk markers (see above).

The policy must be continually reappraised during pregnancy.

Women at low risk of pregnancy problems can be cared for and delivered by their own midwife and GP.

Among the criteria for booking in a GP or midwifery unit isolated from a maternity hospital or for home confinement are:

- Second, third or fourth pregnancy; under 35 years of age
- No medical, psychological or obstetric contraindications
- No recognised fetal risk (e.g. growth restriction; rhesus or other antibodies)

Individual cases can be discussed with the mother by the midwife, the GP and the hospital team.

CONTINUING ANTENATAL CARE

The traditional pattern of care involved the woman being seen by a midwife and/or doctor every 4 weeks to 28 weeks, every 2 weeks from 28 to 36 weeks, and weekly thereafter (approx 13 visits).

This has not been proven to be necessary in women at low risk of developing complications for whom community care may be appropriate, as follows:

- 8–12 weeks—booking visit, dating scan and routine blood tests
- 15–16 weeks—serum screening for aneuploidy
- 20 weeks—anomaly scan
- 26–28 weeks—to check fetal growth
- 36 weeks—to check presentation
- 40 weeks—pre-delivery assessment
- 41 weeks—to hospital if not delivered

Any additional visits should have a clearly specified objective, e.g. risk markers now present.

ROUTINE ASSESSMENTS

Every visit:

- Carry out urinalysis.
- Measure blood pressure.

- Exclude peripheral oedema.
- Measure and record fundal height (in centimetres above symphysis pubis).

Every visit in third trimester:

- Assess fetal lie and presentation.
- Check presence of fetal heart.
- Record patient awareness of fetal movement.

At 28 and 34 weeks (as a minimum):

- Carry out full blood count.
- Test for Rh-D antibodies in Rh negative women, and other antibodies if necessary.
- Administer prophylactic anti-D gammaglobulin in non-sensitised Rh negative women at 28 and 34 weeks.

The presence (or development) of adverse features demands closer attention than the routine assessments listed above and the introduction of more sophisticated methods of assessment of maternal and fetal welfare (see pp. 54–57).

Among the risk markers that can arise during pregnancy are:

- Vaginal bleeding
- Hypertension
- Proteinuria
- Persistent glycosuria
- Urinary tract or other infections
- Oligohydramnios
- Polyhydramnios
- Marked reduction in fetal movements in last trimester
- Fetal growth restriction (FGR: p. 57)
- Malpresentations (after 34 weeks)

ULTRASOUND IN ANTENATAL CARE

Among the clinical situations in which ultrasonic imaging is most useful are:

- Assessment of vaginal bleeding and/or abdominal pain in early pregnancy. This can be done most efficiently and effectively within an organised early-pregnancy problem clinic (see p. 16).
- Accurate ascertainment of gestational age—menstrual history can be unreliable in up to 45% of women.
- Allowing more exact interpretation of serum AFP levels.
- Detection of multiple pregnancy and determination of zygosity (see below).
- Examination of the fetus for severe congenital anomaly as part of a screening programme (see below) or when the individual risk is high; and before amniocentesis or chorionic villus sampling.

- To check fetal size and liquor volume when the uterus is small or large for dates.
- Monitoring fetal growth in high-risk pregnancies (see p. 51). The addition of Doppler ultrasound assessment of fetal umbilical artery waveforms can be useful in this circumstance *but not as routine in low-risk pregnancies.*
- Ascertaining the placental site and identifying the source of some antepartum haemorrhages (APH).
- Determination of fetal presentation if it is unclear by palpation.
- Discovering fetal attitude in malpresentations.
- More confident timing of any obstetric intervention (e.g. for postmaturity).

ROUTINE ULTRASOUND SCANS?

Although a policy of routine scanning has not been shown significantly to affect pregnancy outcome, it is generally considered to be of clinical value. Each centre must have a clear policy.

If it is offered, the suggested optimal programme is:

- *A first scan at around 12 weeks'* can confirm continuing pregnancy and gestational age (allows better counselling for, and accurate timing of, Down's screening tests at 15 weeks); exclude such major anomalies as anencephaly (allows safer termination of pregnancy); and determine zygosity in a multiple pregnancy.
- Fetal nuchal translucency at 10 to 14 weeks of gestation can be used to screen for fetal trisomies (sensitivity approx 80%; false positive 6–11%).
- *A second scan at 20 weeks' gestation* has the best predictive value in the detection of serious malformations (earlier scanning is more likely to miss serious cardiac anomalies).
- No further scanning is indicated in the absence of any risk markers.

Scans must be performed (or supervised) only by fully trained personnel (see below).

SAFETY OF ULTRASOUND

There is no good evidence that ultrasound is anything but safe for mother, baby and operator (see 'further reading'). However, the following must be considered:

- The skill of the operator is of prime importance.
- The main danger of obstetric ultrasound is misdiagnosis.
- Misleading information will lead to wrong management decisions.

OTHER ASPECTS OF CARE

This is an important time to provide health education and advice on, for example, diet, dental care, smoking (avoid it), coitus (no association with adverse pregnancy outcome), substance abuse and maternity benefits.

Preparation for labour and breast-feeding should begin well in advance.

FURTHER READING

Chamberlain G and Steer P (ed) 2001 Turnbull's Obstetrics (3rd edition). Churchill Livingstone, Edinburgh

Enkin M, Kierse M J N C, Neilson J, Crowther C, Duley L, Hodnett E, Hofmeyr J (eds) 2000 Guide to effective care in pregnancy and childbirth (3rd edition). Oxford University Press, Oxford

James D K, Steer PJ, Weiner CP, Gonik B (eds); 1999 High Risk Pregnancy—Management Options (2nd edition). Saunders, London

RCOG 1995 Report of Joint Working Group on Organisational Standards for Maternity Services. RCOG, London

RCOG 1997 Report of RCOG Working Party. Ultrasound Screening for Fetal Abnormalities. RCOG, London

RCOG 1999 Use of Anti-D Immunoglobulin Prophylaxis. Green Top Clinical Guideline No. 22. RCOG, London

RCOG 2000 Routine Ultrasound Screening in Pregnancy. Protocol, Standards and Training. RCOG, London

2. Maternal adaptation to pregnancy

The conceptus (morula) reaches the uterus 4–5 days after fertilisation and becomes the blastocyst. Implantation begins at about day 7, and it is complete by day 14. The fetal circulation becomes established by day 21–28.

Maternal adaptation to pregnancy involves fundamental physiological changes in *every* system in the body; some of these changes are unique to pregnancy.

These changes, which start early in the pregnancy, *must* occur if it is to progress normally. Many pregnancy complications (even those that only become apparent in the third trimester) are determined because physiological adaptation does not occur.

Probably the most important single adaptation is to the vascular endothelium, particularly in the placental bed.

Some of the most important adaptations are briefly described. For fuller discussion see 'Further Reading'.

SYSTEM OF COMMUNICATION BETWEEN MOTHER AND FETUS

Maternal adaptation depends on signals passing between the embryo/fetus and the mother. Most of the signals emanate from the trophoblast mediated by, for example:

- *Cell-adhesion molecules* (many of which act as growth factors or their receptors) and *cytokines*. These act locally on the decidua
- A large number of *hormones* for local and distant effects (e.g. oestrogens, progesterone, human chorionic gonadotrophin)

HAEMODYNAMIC CHANGES IN PREGNANCY

Heart rate increases by about 15 bpm (typically rising from 70 bpm to 85 bpm) within 2 weeks of fertilisation.

Cardiac output (CO) increases by up to 40% by 20 weeks' and remains at that level thereafter. This is due to the increase in heart rate and stroke volume. Most of the increase occurs in the first trimester starting early in pregnancy.

Vascular resistance (VR)—A fall from 60–70 to about 10 dynes/s/cm^{-5} occurs within 2–3 weeks of fertilisation. Among the factors producing this change are increases in endothelial:

- vasodilatory prostacyclin (prostaglandin I$_2$; PGI$_2$) relative to vasoconstrictive thromboxane A$_2$ (TXA$_2$)
- nitric oxide (NO)—a potent vasodilator and inhibitor of platelet activation
- inducible NO synthase (iNOS). It is also produced by the placenta, possibly as a mechanism for controlling feto-placental perfusion pressure.

VR falls to a nadir in mid-pregnancy and gradually rises thereafter.

A systemic effect of the above is that *blood pressure* (BP = CO × VR) falls slightly (diastolic more than systolic):

- 80–90% of the change in BP occurs within 5 weeks of fertilisation.
- Mean arterial pressure (MAP) continues to decrease to 23–24 weeks' gestation and slowly rises thereafter.

For measurement of blood pressure in pregnancy see page 58.

HAEMATOLOGICAL SYSTEM

Plasma volume increases gradually by up to 40% or about 1250 ml in first and 1500 ml in subsequent pregnancies to its maximum at 30 weeks'. It remains at this level until delivery.

Red cell mass increases by 25%, consequently *haematocrit* tends to fall because this increase is relatively less than that of plasma volume.

Fibrinogen levels increase along with some other *clotting factors* (see below).

HAEMOSTASIS AND FIBRINOLYSIS

Small vessel injury leads to platelet adherence and activation. Two interlinked processes then take place:

- Growth and other factors are released, which modify endothelial cells.
- Haemostatic factors (e.g. TXA$_2$, β-thromboglobulin) are released, triggering the coagulation cascade that ends in the production of stable fibrin clot.

Large vessel injury is much more dependent on the coagulation cascade.

Normal pregnancy is associated with major changes in the coagulation and fibrinolytic systems, but the clotting and bleeding times are unchanged.

Coagulation system in pregnancy

There is a gradual increase in *factors V, VIII, X and von Willebrand's factor Ag. Fibrinogen* levels increase from 2.5–4 g/l to about 6 g/l in late pregnancy. Placental separation is a potent activator of clotting.

Endogenous anticoagulants

Protein C (with its co-factor *protein S*) cleaves factor Va and VIIIa, thus inhibiting the conversion of factor X to Xa and prothrombin to thrombin. Activated *protein C* resistance is increased by the third trimester of pregnancy due to raised levels of factors Vc and VIIIc and a reduction in *protein S*.

Fibrinolysis

Fibrin is gradually broken down into *fibrin degradation products* by *plasmin*, which is produced by the action of a complex of plasma and tissue activators on *plasminogen*. Fibrinolytic activity in plasma decreases during pregnancy despite elevated levels of fibrinogen and plasminogen. This is probably due to:

- Reduced levels and impaired release of fibrinolytic activators from endothelium
- High levels of plasmin inhibitors such as α_1-antitrypsin and α_2-macroglobulin in the placenta.

Fibrinolytic activity returns to normal within 15 minutes of delivery of the placenta.

IMMUNE SYSTEM

The major factors protecting the semi-allogeneic (foreign) fetus and placenta from maternal immune attack are:

- The absence of class I (HLA A, B, C) and class II (HLA DP, DQ, DR) major histocompatibility complex (MHC) antigens from villous trophoblast
- The presence on extravillous trophoblast of non-classical MHC antigens to which T cells cannot respond. Protective responses may occur to minor trophoblast antigens.
- Possible suppression of local immune responses by non-specific suppressor cells and other factors in the maternal decidua
- Potential damage from complement activation via the alternative pathway is inhibited by complement regulatory proteins on the trophoblast.

The placenta acts as a barrier, preventing the passage of maternal cells to the fetus. IgG, but not IgM, is actively transported. This provides passive immunity to the fetus, but it can also cause pathology (e.g. Rhesus haemolytic disease and allo-immune thrombocytopenia).

ADRENAL GLAND

Among the physiological changes that occur in pregnancy are:

- Aldosterone levels rise within days of conception due to an increase in angiotensin II. This reaction is necessary in pregnancy to conserve sodium (see below).
- Plasma cortisol levels, both bound and free, are elevated with loss of the normal diurnal variation. This increase is due to a slight rise in adrenocorticotrophic hormone (ACTH) as a result of placental secretion.
- Deoxycorticosterone (DOC) shows the largest increase of all adrenal steroids, starting by 8 weeks' gestation. DOC is not suppressible by dexamethasone during pregnancy. It may be intimately involved with parturition.
- Plasma testosterone rises secondary to the rise in sex hormone-binding globulin, although unbound testosterone is unchanged.
- The catecholamines adrenaline and noradrenaline do not change in pregnancy.

PITUITARY GLAND

Changes in prolactin levels during and after pregnancy:

- Prolactin secretion from the anterior pituitary increases throughout pregnancy in response to oestrogen stimulation.
- By term, the plasma concentration has increased ten- to twenty-fold.
- Basal concentrations fall rapidly after delivery but remain above the normal range in lactating women.
- Suckling induces a prompt release and levels rise five- to ten-fold.
- Its main role in pregnancy is trophic action on the breast. After delivery it initiates and maintains lactation, and prevents ovulation (a contraceptive function).

THYROID GLAND

The pregnant woman remains functionally euthyroid. The main physiological changes in pregnancy are:

- Renal clearance of iodide doubles in the first trimester and then remains stable.
- The level of thyroid-hormone-binding proteins (globulin, pre-albumin and albumin) more than doubles due to an oestrogen effect on the liver.
- Although total triiodothyronine (T_3) and thyroxine (T_4) levels rise markedly, the levels of free hormones fall gradually (but remain within normal limits) as pregnancy progresses.
- Basal metabolic rate (BMR) increases by up to 30% by the third trimester. This is necessary because of the requirements of the uterus and fetus (75% of the change) and increased maternal respiratory and cardiac effort (25% of the change).
- Thyroid stimulating hormone (TSH) levels are unchanged in pregnancy.

URINARY SYSTEM AND WATER BALANCE

The *renal tracts* begin to dilate and kidneys enlarge by 10 weeks of pregnancy (right more than left):

- Renal parenchymal volume increases by 70% by the beginning of the third trimester.
- Pregnancy effects persist for 12–16 weeks after delivery.

Ureteric dilatation ends at the pelvic brim. The dilatation is not due to loss of tone, indeed tone is increased in the upper ureter.

Renal blood flow increases by about 75% in pregnancy with a resulting increase in *glomerular filtration rate* (GFR).

- 24-hour creatinine clearance rises by 45% by 9 weeks'.
- There is a gradual decrease to non-pregnant levels during the third trimester.

Total body water increases by 6–8 l and *plasma osmolality* falls. The passage of normal urine volumes in the face of these changes is unique to pregnancy. This is due to a resetting of the osmoreceptors and the maintenance of arginine vasopressin (AVP) secretion.

The retention of sodium despite the changes in body water is probably the most energy costly process faced by the pregnant woman.

FURTHER READING

de Swiet M, Chamberlain G, Bennett P 2001 Basic Science in Obstetrics and Gynaecology. Churchill Livingstone, Edinburgh
Chamberlain GVP, Broughton-Pipkin F (eds) 1998 Clinical Physiology in Obstetrics (3rd edition). Blackwell Scientific, Oxford

3. Problems in early pregnancy

EARLY PREGNANCY CLINIC

Problems in early pregnancy, and some other gynaecological emergencies, are best dealt with in a specific clinic, the main elements of which are:

• Direct daily access by general practitioners (GPs)
• Staffed by nurses, medical staff and radiographers trained in transvaginal ultrasound
• Same day β-hCG testing available
• Immediate admission possible when necessary with access to theatre during working hours.

In order to minimise the chances of evacuation of a live embryo in error the Royal College of Obstetrics and Gynaecology (RCOG) recommends the following as a written protocol in each unit:

• Two transvaginal scans at least 7 days apart are required before the death of an embryo can be confirmed.
• Only those adequately trained and experienced in ultrasound should carry out the examinations.
• The following features need to be recorded:
  • number of sacs
  • crown–rump length (CRL)
  • mean gestation sac diameter
  • presence or absence of heart
  • findings suggestive of ectopic pregnancy (e.g. tubal mass, or fluid in pouch of Douglas)
  • presence of any haematoma
  • presence of a yolk sac
  • appearance of ovaries
  • presence of an embryo

MISCARRIAGE

Definition
Expulsion of products of conception before viability. In the UK a miscarriage is a pregnancy loss prior to 24 completed weeks gestation. In most medical textbooks miscarriage is termed as abortion, although this can be very easily misinterpreted by patients.

It is a common and distressing complication of pregnancy, occurring in at least 20% of pregnancies.

Causes and associations
- No demonstrable cause—this is the commonest situation
- Chromosome anomalies may cause up to 25% of all miscarriages, particularly trisomy, XO and triploidy
- Anembryonic pregnancy ('blighted ovum'); abnormality of placental development
- Multiple pregnancy
- Thrombophilias, including antiphospholipid antibodies and Activated Protein C Resistance (Factor V Leiden mutation), are a potentially treatable cause for miscarriage.
- Uterine, e.g. congenital or acquired cervical incompetence; congenital uterine anomalies (classically occur in mid-trimester)
- Polycystic ovary syndrome (PCOS; see p. 213)
- Infections, e.g. rubella, cytomegalovirus, or any acute pyrexial illness or condition causing peritonitis.

CATEGORIES OF MISCARRIAGE

These are defined by the clinical and ultrasound findings:

Threatened—Bleeding and pain with closed cervical os. Now also used to mean a history of bleeding with a viable pregnancy seen on ultrasound scan.

Inevitable—Bleeding and pain with an open cervical os.

Incomplete—Miscarriage history with an open os and products of conception (POCs) seen on scan.

Septic—A complication of an incomplete miscarriage where the remaining POCs become infected by ascending organisms. Septic complications are more common where there has been instrumentation of the uterus.

Complete—A history of pain and bleeding; often POCs are seen, followed by a diminution as the POCs are completely expelled. The ultrasound scan shows an empty uterus.

Missed—An ultrasound diagnosis of a non-viable pregnancy in the absence of vaginal bleeding or pain. If a sac develops to >20 mm diameter without a fetal pole or a fetal pole of >5 mm is seen without a fetal heart, then these are termed a blighted ovum and a missed abortion, respectively.

MANAGEMENT

Treatment aims to reduce the potential complications of miscarriage, i.e. prolonged pain and bleeding, sepsis and rhesus iso-sensitisation.

Conservative

Expectant management avoids a surgical procedure and, therefore, an anaesthetic. It may be appropriate for women with an incomplete miscarriage where the retained POCs were less than 50 mm in diameter on transvaginal ultrasound.

Conservative management is less useful for a blighted ovum, as bleeding appears to be heavier and more prolonged than with surgical management; 60% of women with a blighted ovum treated conservatively require an evacuation of retained products of conception (RPC) at some stage.

Medical

Medical management (misoprostol +/− mifepristone) reduces the requirement for surgery by 50%, but is associated with greater analgesia requirements and more vaginal bleeding.

Surgical

An evacuation of the retained products of conception (ERPC) is still the most common form of treatment for miscarriage, including incomplete, missed abortions and blighted ova.

The cervix is dilated and the retained POCs removed using a suction curette.

Complications include:

- Perforation of the uterus either with the dilator or the curette, infection and incomplete emptying of the cavity, in up to 6% of cases
- Potential anaesthetic complications.

From 1997 to 1999, there were two maternal deaths following miscarriage (one of these a hydatidiform mole), two after termination of pregnancy and five *direct* deaths from sepsis associated with miscarriage. (See 'Further reading')

RECURRENT MISCARRIAGE

Definition

Three or more consecutive miscarriages.

Incidence

Less than 1% of women of reproductive age.

CLINICAL MANAGEMENT OF RECURRENT MISCARRIAGE

- Even after three consecutive losses the spontaneous chance of a successful pregnancy is over 60%.

- The success of all 'treatments' needs to be viewed with the spontaneous success rate in mind.
- When the woman with a history of repeated miscarriages becomes pregnant, she requires careful antenatal supervision.

Table 3.1   Clinical management of recurrent miscarriage

Associated factor	Investigation and diagnosis	Treatment	Comment
Anatomical disorders			
Uterine abnormalities	Hysterosalpingogram (HSG) or vaginal ultrasound	A septum can be divided by utriculoplasty or vaginally using an operating hysteroscope	Abdominal operation can cause infertility
Fibroids	Hysterosalpingogram (HSG) or vaginal ultrasound	Myomectomy	True role of fibroids unclear
Asherman's syndrome (intrauterine synechiae)	Hysteroscopy	Division of synechiae	Usually caused by multiple curettage
Cervical incompetence, congenital or acquired	HSG or vaginal ultrasound	Cervical cerclage	True diagnosis difficult and benefit from treatment uncertain
Genetic disorders			
Recurrent aneuploidy	Fetal karyotyping	None— occurs as a chance event or related to maternal age	Sporadic genetic disorders recurring consecutively by chance may explain many recurrent miscarriages
Parental balanced translocation	Parental karyotypes	Genetic counselling (see p. 46)	Accounts for 4% of cases
Molecular mutations	DNA analysis may be available in the future		Speculative

Table 3.1 (Cont'd)

Associated factor	Investigation and diagnosis	Treatment	Comment
Endocrine factors			
Inadequate luteal phase	Luteal phase <10 days; progesterone levels <15 nmol/L in five consecutive cycles; endometrial biopsy(?)	Clomiphene, progesterone or hCG (empirical treatment not justified)	Reported incidence varies between 3 and 60%
Polycystic ovary disease associated with increased luteinising hormone (LH)	See p. 213	See p. 215	Role in recurrent losses becoming clearer
Thyroid function	Not justified	Not justified	Not a cause
Diabetes	Not justified	Not justified	Not a cause

Reproductive tract infections
Few data exist to support infection as a cause of recurrent pregnancy loss. Well-designed studies are necessary.

Immunological causes			
Anti-cardiolipin (ACA) syndrome	Check APTT* routinely in all cases; carry out more detailed auto-immune screen and check specifically for anti-cardiolipin antibodies and lupus inhibitor if indicated (see p. 81)	Low-dose aspirin and/or steroids for women with ACA syndrome (see p. 81); *not* justified empirically	Tends to be associated with secondary recurrent miscarriage
Disorders of materno-fetal immune status	None routinely	The benefit of immuno-therapy is not proven	Scientific basis for investigation and therapy not strong
Psychological causes	?	'Tender loving care'	Evidence for this is no better and no worse than for several other 'causes'

*APTT: activated partial thromboplastin time

ECTOPIC PREGNANCY

Definition
The implantation of a pregnancy outside the uterine cavity.

Incidence
- The estimated incidence in the UK from 1994 to 1996 was 11 in 1000 pregnancies.
- Women in age range 25–34 years comprise about 65% of ectopics.
- After one ectopic the risk of recurrence is between 10 and 20%.

Maternal risk
- Ectopic pregnancy caused 13 *direct* maternal deaths between 1997 and 1999 or 12% of the total. The number shows an increase and the rate has not declined since 1994 to 1996. It remains the commonest cause of first-trimester deaths.
- The risk of death was 4 in 10 000 ectopics.
- 'Substandard care' contributed to 65% of the deaths. The most common problem was failure to suspect an ectopic pregnancy, particularly, but not solely, in A&E departments.

TUBAL PREGNANCY

Tubal pregnancies account for 95% of ectopic pregnancies.

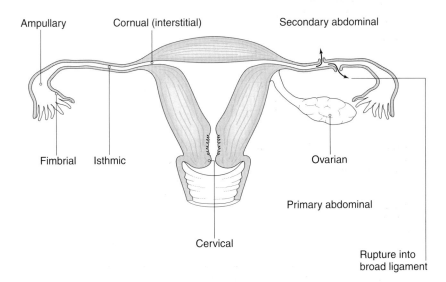

Fig 3.1

Risk factors include:

- A history of infertility
- Pelvic inflammatory disease
- Pelvic operations (particularly tubal surgery)
- Presence of an intrauterine device
- Previous tubal pregnancy
- Assisted conception (particularly IVF if tubes are patent and damaged)

There has also been a tendency to postpone pregnancy to the age range of greatest risk.

Antibodies to *Chlamydia trachomatis* can be found in up to 80%, and to *N. gonococcus* in up to 30%, of women with ectopic pregnancy (compared with 40% and 4%, respectively, for intrauterine pregnancy).

Symptoms and signs

The following 'classical' symptoms and signs are not always present:

- Amenorrhoea
- Unilateral lower abdominal pain
- Slight vaginal bleeding arising after the onset of the pain
- Shoulder tip pain due to irritation of the diaphragm by blood leaking from the ectopic
- Slight enlargement of the uterus, with cervical excitation and tenderness
- A small tender mass may be palpable to one side of the uterus.

Diagnosis

Non-rupture of a tubal pregnancy has a positive association with future fertility. Early diagnosis and conservative surgical management are, therefore, important. Problems with diagnosis:

- The diagnosis is not made in 20–25% of cases.
- Even when it is made, the presentation-to-treatment interval is over 48 hours in 40–50%, and over 1 week in 20–25%.

When a woman of reproductive age presents with unexplained abdominal pain, with or without vaginal bleeding, do not allow her home until ectopic pregnancy has been excluded.

Differential diagnosis

- *Threatened or incomplete miscarriage.* In the former there is no pain and in the latter pain tends to follow vaginal bleeding.
- *Bleeding corpus luteum*—laparoscopy is required to make this differentiation.
- *Accident to an ovarian cyst*—there is usually no menstrual delay; transvaginal scan and/or laparoscopy is indicated.
- *Pelvic inflammation*—the systemic reaction is more profound and the signs are usually bilateral.

- The majority of women who died from ruptured ectopic pregnancies from 1997 to 1999 had gastrointestinal or urinary symptoms.

Appropriate intervention must be based on index of suspicion—'think ectopic'.

Management of non-acute situation
This applies to women in a clinically stable condition with no evidence of intra-abdominal bleeding.

Transvaginal ultrasound—If carried out by properly trained and experienced personnel, it may:

- Demonstrate an intrauterine pregnancy with no other pelvic pathology (in normal pregnancy a heartbeat can be detected 17 days after the missed period)
- Visualise an ectopic pregnancy, or complex cystic adnexal masses
- Show free fluid (blood) in abdomen.

β-hCG *estimations* using monoclonal antibody tests (which can detect β-hCG at a level of 1 IU/l):

- Where there is a positive pregnancy test and an empty uterus, a β-hCG test can provide a useful threshold for laparoscopy.
- Where the β-hCG is <1500 IU/l the pregnancy can be managed conservatively, but >1500 IU/l an intrauterine pregnancy should be seen on scan and should raise suspicion of an ectopic if not seen. A laparoscopy is indicated.
- The rate of rise of β-hCG is not sufficiently predictive to allow it to be used in clinical practice.

A serum progesterone level of 25 ng/ml or more indicates a normal intrauterine pregnancy; a level below 15 ng/ml suggests an abnormal pregnancy, but it cannot discriminate between a failing intrauterine pregnancy and an ectopic.

Laparoscopy—This is the gold standard for diagnosis and is indicated if the index of suspicion is high. However, very early tubal pregnancies (3–4% of total) can still be missed at laparoscopy.

Management of acute situation
- If the patient is shocked, laparotomy must be undertaken as quickly as possible.
- The priorities are to stop haemorrhage and prevent further bleeding.
- Conservative surgery is less likely to be possible under these circumstances.

Surgical approach if tube unruptured
The RCOG recommendations are that:

- Surgical treatment is to be preferred for most ectopic pregnancies.
- Laparoscopy is superior to a laparotomy in terms of recovery from surgery, subsequent rates of intrauterine pregnancy and recurrent

ectopic, but it is associated with a higher risk of persisting trophoblastic tissue in the treatment episode.

- Salpingectomy is to be preferred to salpingotomy when the contralateral tube is healthy, as it is associated with a lower rate of persisting trophoblast and subsequent repeat ectopic with a similar intrauterine pregnancy rate.
- Salpingotomy is reasonable when there is only one tube, but it is associated with a 20% rate of further ectopic. Whenever possible, patients should be counselled about this before surgery.
- In selected cases, methotrexate is an effective alternative to salpingotomy. It is best indicated for early, small ectopic pregnancies with low β-hCG levels.
- Non-sensitised Rh-D negative women should receive anti-D immunoglobulin (see p. 96)

Laparotomy
Conservative surgery should be attempted whenever possible. *Routine salpingectomy is to be deprecated.*

Procedures:

- Try to milk the pregnancy from the tube, or
- Perform a linear salpingostomy along the anti-mesenteric border. The tubal incision can be left open or closed in one or two layers by 6/0 sutures.

CORNUAL (INTERSTITIAL) PREGNANCY

- Although rare, cornual pregnancy can have serious consequences because it is difficult to diagnose early and, when it ruptures, it is associated with profuse intraperitoneal bleeding.
- Surgical removal is difficult so injection of methotrexate into the sac laparoscopically or under ultrasound guidance should be considered (see above).

OVARIAN PREGNANCY

To make a diagnosis of primary ovarian pregnancy the following three features must be present:

- The fallopian tube must be intact
- The gestation sac must occupy the anatomical site of the ovary
- Ovarian tissue must be demonstrable histologically in the specimen.

ABDOMINAL PREGNANCY

- Both primary and secondary abdominal pregnancies are rare events.
- The fetus may very rarely develop fully and survive, but the woman usually presents as an acute abdominal emergency in the second trimester.

- It may be possible to make a prospective correct diagnosis if the following features are borne in mind:
  - There is often a history of an episode of abdominal pain and slight vaginal bleeding early in pregnancy, which settled.
  - Maternal serum AFP may be elevated.
  - The ultrasound scan shows oligohydramnios and no clear uterine outline around the sac. There is also a separate mass related to the gestation sac (this is the uterus).
- When laparotomy is carried out it may not be possible or advisable to remove the placenta because it is likely to be fixed to the abdominal viscera.

CERVICAL PREGNANCY

- Cervical pregnancy is rare but may cause profuse vaginal bleeding. It was associated with 1 maternal death from 1997 to 1999.
- Hysterectomy may be necessary.
- Injection of methotrexate into the sac is an alternative, if the diagnosis is made early enough.

GESTATIONAL TROPHOBLASTIC DISEASE (GTD)

HYDATIDIFORM MOLE (HM)

Molar pregnancies occur in about 1 in 1200 pregnancies. There are two types of hydatidiform mole

Complete mole (CHM)
The conceptus consists solely of hyperplastic, hydropic chorionic villi; no fetus is present. Characteristics of a CHM are as follows:

- It usually results from fertilisation of an ovum that then loses its nucleus. The haploid sperm duplicates its own chromosomes by meiosis. The result is that:
  - The chromosome complement is usually homozygous 46XX derived solely from the father (androgenetic)
  - Only one pair of paternal HLA antigens is expressed.
- About 10% of CHM are heterozygous—usually 46XY but sometimes 46XX. They arise from fertilisation of an anucleate egg by two sperm.
- CHM uniquely combine paternal nuclear DNA with maternal mitochondrial DNA.
- Women with CHM have an increased incidence of balanced translocations and this could explain the loss of the ovum nucleus.

Partial mole (PHM)
There is focal hyperplasia of trophoblast with varying degrees of hydropic villous degeneration; a fetus is present. Characteristics are as follows:

- Chromosomal abnormalities (particularly triploidy-69, XXX or XXY) are often found.
- The source of the extra set of chromosomes may be double fertilisation (dispermy) or failure of the first paternal meiotic division.

Risk markers for HM
- *Age*—increased for CHM (but not PHM) at extremes of reproductive life (>30 years and <15 years of age).
- *Ethnicity*—the traditionally reported excess in South-East Asia has decreased and may have been explained by reliance on hospital- rather than population-based data, and greater incidence of pregnancy in young and older women.
- *Previous HM*—The box outlines risk in the next pregnancy.
- *Previous multiple pregnancy*—twinning and HM may both represent different defects in gametogenesis or fertilisation.

Number of previous HM	Risk in next pregnancy
1	1:75
2#	1:65

#These women still have a 75% chance of a next successful pregnancy.

Symptoms
Most symptoms are related to excessive production of β-hCG:

- Amenorrhoea combined with exaggerated pregnancy symptoms (e.g. hyperemesis gravidarum).
- There may be irregular vaginal bleeding that may contain vesicles; many present as incomplete miscarriages.
- Pre-eclampsia may develop unusually early.
- Hyperthyroidism develops in about 5% of women with CHM.
- Rarely, massive trophoblastic embolisation may cause respiratory distress requiring prompt treatment (see Further reading).

Signs
- The uterus may be large for dates.
- Ovaries may be palpably enlarged due to presence of theca-lutein cysts.

Diagnosis
- β-hCG can be markedly raised in serum and urine, but most patients have values within the normal range for pregnancy.
- *Ultrasound scan*—the characteristic 'snow-storm' appearance is not pathognomonic. In CHM, fetal parts are absent. PHM and missed miscarriage can be confused with one another.

Management

- In the rare event of a twin pregnancy with a viable fetus and a molar pregnancy, the pregnancy can be allowed to proceed.
- Surgical evacuation of molar pregnancies is advisable. Routine repeat evacuation after the diagnosis of a molar pregnancy is not warranted.
- Registration of any molar pregnancy is essential (see below).
- The combined oral contraceptive pill and hormone replacement therapy are safe to use after β-hCG levels have returned to normal.

Women should be advised not to conceive until the β-hCG level has been normal for 6 months or follow-up has been completed (whichever is the sooner).

INVASIVE MOLE (IM)

- There is local invasion of the myometrium, and it is, therefore, much less readily removed by evacuation. The tumour may perforate the uterus. Vaginal metastases may also occur, but more distant spread is uncommon.
- This is a histological diagnosis usually made after hysterectomy that has become necessary because vaginal bleeding has continued and β-hCG levels have remained raised after initial attempts to empty the uterus.
- There is usually a good response to chemotherapy.

PLACENTAL SITE TROPHOBLASTIC TUMOUR (PSTT)

- This is a rare form that appears to arise from placental bed trophoblast rather than the usual villous origin for HM, etc.
- Most cases follow within 3 years of miscarriage or term pregnancy.
- PSTT can be associated with hypertension and the nephrotic syndrome.
- The response to chemotherapy is poor, and hysterectomy is indicated (unless metastasis is advanced).

GESTATIONAL CHORIOCARCINOMA

- This is a highly malignant tumour characterised by disordered growth of syncytio- and cytotrophoblast and invasion of the myometrium causing necrosis and haemorrhage. Metastasis is common.
- It usually arises within 2 years of the causal pregnancy.

Incidence
About 1 in 20 000–40 000 pregnancies in Western countries, increasing to about 1 in 13 000 pregnancies in the Far East.

Risk markers for choriocarcinoma

- Age—as for CHM.
- Obstetric history—only about 1 in 30 hydatidiform moles develop into choriocarcinoma. However, the risk of subsequent choriocarcinoma is 1000 times greater after a mole than after a normal pregnancy. Thus, as many cases follow moles as follow other pregnancies.
- Heterozygous CHM have a greater malignant potential than do homozygous CHM.
- ABO blood group—the risk of choriocarcinoma is increased when the woman and her partner have different ABO groups. Groups B and AB patients have a less good prognosis.
- HLA compatibility between partners may be associated with increased risk of developing choriocarcinoma.

Pathology

- Local extension is frequent but ovarian spread is uncommon.
- The predominant route of spread is vascular. Lymphatic spread is rare.
- Pulmonary metastases occur in about 70% of cases. They may have a 'cannon-ball' or 'snow-storm' appearance or appear intravascular on chest X-ray.
- Haemoptysis is a common symptom.

STAGING OF GTD

Stage	Disease development
0	Molar pregnancy
I	Persistently elevated β-hCg titres (i.e. 6 months or more after evacuation) and tumour confined to body of uterus
II	Pelvic and/or vaginal metastasis
III	Pulmonary metastasis
IV	All other distant metastases

A prognostic scoring system can be used in Stages I–IV to determine the appropriate treatment for each patient. (For details see Further reading.) It is based on:

- The extent of the tumour burden (e.g. β-hCG level), and number, site and size of metastases
- Patient characteristics (e.g. risk increases with age and parity)
- The nature of, and the interval since, the antecedent pregnancy: the risk is highest for a term pregnancy and lowest for a hydatidiform mole. The longer the interval, the higher the risk.
- The patient's ability to respond immunologically (e.g. a well-developed lymphocytic infiltrate around the tumour is a favourable feature)

- ABO blood groups of both partners
- Poor response to previous chemotherapy.

MANAGEMENT OF GTD

Stage 0
- Once a firm diagnosis is made the mole needs to be removed, preferably by suction evacuation and curettage.
- This may need to be repeated if:
  - irregular bleeding persists, or
  - β-hCG levels are still elevated 6 weeks after initial evacuation.

Hysterectomy can be carried out in older women whose family is complete.

- In the UK, patients should be registered with one of the three reference laboratories—London, Sheffield and Dundee.
- Follow-up—serum β-hCG estimations should be carried out weekly until levels are normal (<5 IU/l). If that happens within 6 weeks, tests are continued monthly for 6 months.
- If serum β-hCG levels take longer than 8 weeks to become normal, follow up monthly for 1 year and then 3-monthly during the second year.
- The patient may begin to try to become pregnant 6 months after β-hCG values have become, and remain, normal.
- A barrier method of contraception should be used until β-hCG levels are normal; then oral contraception can be used.
- There may be a higher incidence of subsequent choriocarcinoma if the 'pill' is started before β-hCG levels fall.
- β-hCG levels should be checked 3 weeks after the end of any pregnancy subsequent to a molar pregnancy.

Stages I–IV
- The disease progresses in <10% of affected women. Among the indications that chemotherapy may be necessary are:
  - β-hCG levels remain markedly elevated 6 weeks after evacuation.
  - β-hCG levels remain the same for 3 successive months or begin to rise again.
  - Persistent or recurrent uterine bleeding with raised β-hCG levels.
- Management of Stages I–IV should be confined to specialised centres (see Further reading).

Results of therapy
Remission can be expected in all women adequately treated in Stages I–III and in up to 70% of women with Stage IV disease.

Subsequent pregnancies
- A normal outcome can be expected.
- The incidence of congenital malformation does not seem to be increased in women who have received chemotherapy.

FURTHER READING

Cahill D. 2001 Managing 1st Trimester Miscarriage. British Medical Journal 322:1315

Chamberlain G, Steer P (ed) 2001 Turnbull's Obstetrics (3rd Edition). Churchill Livingstone, Edinburgh

James D K, Steer P J, Weiner C P, Gonik B (eds) 1999 High risk pregnancy—Management Options (2nd Edition). Saunders, London

RCOG The management of Gestational Trophoblastic Disease. RCOG Green Top Guideline. www.rcog.org.uk

RCOG Why Mothers Die?—Report of the Confidential Enquiry into Maternal Deaths (1997–9) RCOG Press, London

RCOG The management of tubal pregnancies. RCOG Greentop Guideline. www.rcog.org.uk

4. Congenital abnormalities

Malformation
- A primary error in normal development of an organ or tissue.

Disruption
- A secondary malformation resulting from damage to a previously normal organ or tissue.
- About 15% of newborns have a single minor malformation.
- Major congenital malformations constitute 10% of miscarriages, 3% of all deliveries, under 2% of live births, and about 30% of all stillbirths, neonatal deaths and infant deaths.
- The incidence is more than doubled in multiple pregnancy (especially in monozygotic twins).
- Perinatal mortality due to malformations is around 2.5 in 1000 births.
- Thirty percent of all children born alive with major malformations die within 5 years.
- The information box gives the approximate birth incidence of major malformations.

Deformation
- An alteration in shape or position due to inappropriate mechanical forces.
- The most significant deformations are congenital dislocation of the hip (CDH) and talipes equinovarus.
- They can have intrinsic or extrinsic causes and can be associated with:
  - Neuromuscular or connective tissue disorders
  - CNS malformation (intrinsic)
  - Oligohydramnios, malpresentations, uterine anomalies and multiple pregnancy (extrinsic).
- About 2% of newborns are affected; one third of these have multiple deformations.

Major malformations: approximate incidence in 1000 births			
CNS	10	Limbs	2
CVS	8	Others	6
Renal tract	4	Total	30

AETIOLOGY

The most important causes of congenital defects and their approximate incidence are given in the information box.

Cause	Incidence (%)
'Multifactorial'	20
Single-gene disorders	7–8
Chromosomal	6
Infections	2
Maternal illness (e.g. epilepsy, diabetes)	3
Drugs, radiation, alcohol	1–2

GENETICS

Major increases in knowledge have occurred in this field over the last decade and will continue. Scientists, doctors and society in general have hardly begun to consider the ethical and practical implications of this information explosion.

Cytogenetics

The normal human karyotype has 46 chromosomes: 22 pairs of autosomes, and 2 sex chromosomes—XX in the normal female and XY in the normal male.

Each chromosome has:

- A *centromere*—the narrow waist that may be near the middle (metacentric), close to one end (acrocentric), or in an intermediate position (submetacentric)
- A long arm (q) and a short arm (p)
- A *telomere* at the tip of each arm.

Mitosis

A process by which all somatic cells divide.

It involves splitting of each of the 46 chromosomes to provide a full identical (diploid) complement for both daughter cells.

It is divided into five stages:

- *Interphase*—the period between successive cell divisions.
- *Prophase*—the chromatids split longitudinally into pairs of chromatids connected at the centromere.
- *Metaphase*—movement of the chromatids occurs towards the equator of the cell.
- *Anaphase*—the centromeres divide, and the paired chromatids separate.

- *Telophase*—the cytoplasm divides, the chromosomes unwind, and two genetically identical daughter cells are formed.

Meiosis
A process by which all germ cells (gametes) divide and during which the chromosome of the daughter cells is halved (haploid).

Two sequential cell divisions are involved:

- First division—interchange or cross-over of chromosomal material can take place during prophase of the first division; daughter cells inherit chromatid pairs still attached at the centromere.
- Second division—chromatids separate.

Summary
- The somatic cell produces, by mitosis, two diploid cells, each containing 46 chromosomes.
- The germ cell produces, by meiosis, four haploid gametes, each with 23 chromosomes.
- Gametogenesis is discussed on page 229.

CHROMOSOMAL DISORDERS

- Ninety-five percent of gametes with chromosome abnormalities are not viable.
- They affect at least 7% of all conceptions and 6 in 1000 of all livebirths.
- They are present in 60% of first-trimester miscarriages, 5% of second-trimester miscarriages, and 4–5% of stillbirths.
- Abnormalities can be numerical or structural.

NUMERICAL ABERRATIONS

Aneuploidy
An abnormality in number of chromosomes, usually by mutation.

- It can arise during meiosis or mitosis.
- It is usually due to the failure of paired chromosomes to separate at anaphase (non-disjunction), or their delayed movement at the same stage (anaphase lag).
- Two cells are produced: one with an extra copy of a chromosome (trisomy), the other with that chromosome missing (monosomy).
- *Polyploidy*—the number of chromosomes is an exact multiple of the haploid, but greater than the diploid number, e.g. triploidy (69XXY is the most common), or tetraploidy (4n)

STRUCTURAL ABERRATIONS

Due to chromosome breakage and inappropriate rejoining of the broken ends.

Translocation

There are three types of translocation of fragments between chromosomes:

- *Reciprocal*, in which the chromosomal material distal to breaks in two chromosomes is exchanged
- *Robertsonian*, in which breaks in two acrocentric chromosomes (most commonly numbers 13 and 14) occur near the centromere with cross-fusion of the products
- *Insertional*, in which three breaks occur in one or two chromosomes (often inherited).

A *balanced translocation* exists when the genome contains the correct amount of genetic matter. There is usually no outward manifestation.

Parental karyotyping is essential. If one parent has a balanced translocation the theoretical outlook for any offspring is:

- 1:4 have the same balanced translocation
- 1:4 have normal chromosomes
- 1:2 have an unbalanced translocation (although many of these will result in miscarriage or stillbirth).

For *unbalanced translocations:*

- The origin rather than the new site is of greater importance.
- If the chromosomal anomaly is large enough to be seen under the microscope, it is likely to involve enough chromatin to cause major problems.
- Malformations are usual, and mental retardation invariable.
- Parental karyotyping will identify a balanced rearrangement in the parent.

Deletion

This is loss of any part of a chromosome:

- Substantial losses are nearly always lethal.
- A *ring chromosome can* result if both arms of a chromosome break, the terminal ends are lost, and the two proximal sticky ends unite.

Duplication

Two copies of a chromosome segment are present.

- It is more common than deletion but generally less harmful

Inversion

Two breaks occur in one chromosome with inversion of 180° of the segment between breaks.

- It does not usually produce a clinical abnormality but can give rise to unbalanced gametes.

Isochromosome

This is deletion of one and duplication of the other chromosome

- The commonest in live births is that of the long arm of X, which is a cause of Turner's syndrome (p. 209)

OTHER ABERRATIONS

Mosaic—an individual with two or more cell lines derived from a single zygote.

Chimaera—two cell lines are derived from two separate zygotes. It can arise by:

- Early fusion of dizygotic twin zygotes
- Double fertilisation of the egg and a polar body
- Exchange of haemopoietic cells *in utero* between dizygotic twins.

AUTOSOMAL ABNORMALITIES

DOWN'S SYNDROME

- The overall incidence is about 1 in 650 live births
- Between 65 and 80% of affected fetuses miscarry or are stillborn.
- Genetic abnormalities are listed in the box.

Genetic abnormalities in Down's syndrome	
Trisomy 21 (due to non-disjunction)	95%
Translocation 14:21	2%
Other translocations	2%
Mosaicism	1%

- The maternal risk of trisomy 21 is age related: 1 in 1500 at 20 years rising to 1 in 37 at 44 years.
- The risk of recurrence of Down's syndrome due to trisomy 21 is approximately three times the age-related risk.
- The risk of translocation 14:21 recurring is about 1 in 10 if the mother has a balanced translocation; 1 in 50 if the father has it.

Effects of Down's syndrome

- Newborn babies are often 'small for dates' and hypotonic.
- Facies are characteristically 'mongoloid'.
- Mean IQ is 40–50 (moderate disability) with a range of 20 (severe) to 70 (mild). Most have an IQ of less than 50.
- Associated complications include congenital heart disease (40%): duodenal atresia (<10%) and leukaemia (1%).
- Men are infertile; women are subfertile.
- Many develop Alzheimer's disease in later life.

Biochemical screening for Down's syndrome

- Even if all pregnant women aged 35 years or over elected to have an amniocentesis, this would result in a detection rate for Down's syndrome of 35% for an amniocentesis rate of 7.5%.
- Detection rates are increased by measuring α-fetoprotein (AFP), unconjugated oestriol (E_3), and β-hCG at 15–19 weeks and calculating a maternal age specific related risk of Down's syndrome. Detection rates are best at 15–17 weeks. AFP and E_3 tend to be reduced and β-hCG increased in affected pregnancies. Accurate assessment of gestational age is essential.
- At a risk cut-off level of 1 in 200, biochemical screening raises the detection level to 60% with an amniocentesis rate of 5% and a 4.5% false-positive rate. A higher cut-off level (e.g. 1 in 300) increases the detection level at the expense of a higher false-positive rate.

Ultrasound screening for Down's syndrome

Markers—the following have been reported to be sonographic markers for aneuploidy:

- choroid plexus cysts
- ventriculomegaly
- echogenic bowel

- abnormal head shape
- cleft lip
- echogenic foci in heart
- dilated renal pelvis

- short femur/humerus
- talipes
- 'sandal gap' between great and second toe
- clinodactyly (marked curving of any finger—most common in the little finger)
- persistently clenched hand
- two vessel cord

The presence of more than one marker increases the risk of aneuploidy.

Nuchal translucency is increased skin thickness on the posterior aspect of the fetal neck due to fetal oedema. Increasing evidence exists between increased nuchal translucency and a risk of Down's syndrome. Measurements at 10–14 weeks combined with the crown–rump length and adjustments for maternal age give a sensitivity of 84–86% with a false-positive rate of 6–11%. It is also a marker for congenital cardiac anomalies.

Concerns

- The anxiety induced by a false positive diagnosis must not be underestimated.
- Mothers must be enabled to make a properly informed choice to 'opt in' to the programme.
- The programme must be adequately resourced to include counselling for those found to be at 'high risk'.

TRISOMY 13 (PATAU'S) AND 18 (EDWARDS') SYNDROMES

- Also maternal age-related: due to non-disjunction.

- Both are universally lethal, usually in the neonatal period.
- Cleft lip and palate, renal and other malformations (e.g. holoprosencephaly in t13) and fetal growth restriction (FGR) are usual.
- Recurrence risk is probably low.

TRIPLOIDY

- Survival to livebirth is rare with subsequent neonatal death associated with severe FGR and multiple malformations.
- Elongation of second digit and syndactyly (fusion) of third/fourth digit is characteristic.

SEX CHROMOSOME DISORDERS

- These conditions have a much better outlook than was originally thought (for further discussion see p. 209).
- Antenatal detection does not necessarily warrant termination of pregnancy.
- About 5% XO females will have periods and a few may be fertile.

Table 4.1 Sex chromosome disorders

Defect	Incidence compared with livebirths	Average IQ	Association with maternal age
XO	1:3000 (1:100 conceptions)	100	Incidence falls as age rises
XXX	1:1000	Possible slight reduction	Increased × 2–3 when maternal age >40
XXY	1:700	100	Increased × 2–3 when maternal age >40
XYY	1:700	100	None

COMMON SINGLE GENE DISORDERS

AUTOSOMAL DOMINANT CONDITIONS

- These are often mild (e.g. polydactyly—additional fingers), have various degrees of manifestation or, if severe, arise during adulthood (e.g. polycystic kidneys) or at the end of the reproductive period (e.g. Huntington's chorea).
- The combined incidence of all dominants is 7 in 1000 live births.

- Fifty percent of the offspring of an affected individual will be affected.
- Counselling is complicated by variable expression and incomplete penetrance, which cause the various degrees of manifestation.
- The commonest dominant condition is *familial hypercholesterolaemia* (up to 1 in 250 of the population).

Myotonic dystrophy (MD)
Caused by a gene defect on chromosome 19q.

- It is important because of its incidence (approx. 1 in 5000), variability of expression with increased severity in each subsequent generation, increased subfertility and anaesthetic risks in those affected.
- If a mother has symptomatic MD the condition may present *in utero* with reduced fetal movement, polyhydramnios and pre-term delivery of a baby who has contractures, hypotonia and respiratory and feeding difficulties.
- A direct and specific DNA test is available for pre-pregnancy and prenatal testing if:
  - there is a family history of MD
  - either parent is affected
  - a previous child had congenital MD.

Huntington's chorea
Caused by a gene defect on chromosome 4p.

- Although rare, its effects are devastating and there is no treatment.
- The symptoms of involuntary movement, depression and dementia usually commence between 30 and 60 years of age.
- DNA testing is available for diagnosis in symptomatic cases.
- Its use for prenatal testing is highly controversial because of the major implications of a positive test for a presymptomatic parent.

Prenatal testing
Can be offered for many other dominant conditions by DNA analysis from chorionic villus sampling (CVS).

- In most cases, at present, this relies on linked polymorphic DNA markers, which require prior family studies (e.g. adult polycystic kidneys, familial retinoblastoma or Marfan's syndrome).
- Diagnosis by direct mutation detection is increasingly possible (e.g. peroneal muscular atrophy, retinitis pigmentosa (some families) or familial polyposis coli).

AUTOSOMAL RECESSIVE CONDITIONS
- The gene must be inherited from both parents.
- The effects are usually severe.

- Fifty percent of offspring of affected individuals will be carriers.
- Consanguinous couples have an increased risk depending on closeness of relationship and family history (FH).
  - If there is no significant FH the risk in offspring of first cousins is 5% (c.f. 2% background risk).
  - Offer prenatal diagnosis if both partners are carriers or carrier status cannot be determined

Cystic Fibrosis (CF)

The commonest recessive condition in the UK. See Table 4.2 for testing for CF.

- 1 in 22 persons are carriers (heterozygotes).
- 1 in 500 couples are at a 1 in 4 risk of having an affected child.
- The CF gene is located on chromosome 7 (region 7q32).
- One mutation (ΔF508) causes 70% of all faulty CF genes in the UK.
- Adults with CF are often subfertile (males may be sterile), although an increasing number of women are surviving to an age at which pregnancy is possible.

Presentation of CF

- The fetus or neonate may have meconium ileus or peritoneal calcification.
- CF typically presents in childhood with failure to thrive, recurrent chest infection and malabsorption.
- The risk of pre-term delivery and maternal and perinatal mortality may be increased.
- Affected mothers are at risk from cardiorespiratory failure—regular antenatal assessment is necessary. Women with severe respiratory impairment should be strongly advised to avoid pregnancy.

OTHER RECESSIVE DISORDERS

- Most serious disorders are very rare (<1 in 40 000) and carrier frequency is low (<1 in 100).
- For parents with a previously affected child the recurrence risk is 1 in 4.
- Prenatal diagnosis is by CVS—biochemical analysis for metabolic disorders; DNA analysis is available for an increasing number of others (consult geneticist).
- DNA studies on parents and affected child are first required to discover how informative testing will be.
- In different racial groups some recessive conditions are more frequent and prenatal testing is as for CF (Table 4.2) for example:
  - Thalassaemias in Asian, African and Mediterranean populations
  - Sickle cell disease in Afro-Caribbean population
  - Tay–Sachs in Ashkenazi Jews.

Table 4.2 Testing for cystic fibrosis (CF)

Index Pregnancy	One affected parent	Couple with previous CF child	Family history or one parent with CF child by different partner	Fetus with meconium ileus or peritoneal calcification
Risk of CF	1/44	1/4	Risk depends on closeness of relationship	Diagnostic tests needed
Pre-pregnancy	Screen *both* parents for DNA mutations	Screen DNA from affected child and both parents	Screen DNA from both parents.	
Antenatal	Offer CVS at 11 weeks only if partner has a CF mutation (because risk of CF in fetus now 1/2)	Offer CVS at 11 weeks if both parents carry a mutation otherwise discuss with genetecist	Offer CVS if both parents carry a mutation (risk now 1/4)	Obtain DNA from CVS: if both parents carry a mutation diagnosis confirmed: check alkaline phospatase in 16–19 wk amniocentesis if only 1 or 0 mutations found

CVS, chorionic villus sampling

Thalassaemias
Autosomal recessively inherited defects in the rate of synthesis of one or more globin chains:

- Alpha-thalassaemia is due to the deletion of structural DNA genes affecting the α-Hb chains.
- HbF contains α-chains, therefore, the fetus can be affected to an extent varying from anaemia to hydrops.
- Beta-thalassaemia is due to a messenger RNA abnormality causing defective production of β-Hb chains:
  - β^+ disease—reduced production of β-chains
  - β^0 disease—no β-chains
- In β^0 and β^+ disease homozygotes are affected severely, (thalassaemia major) from which up to 100 000 children die world-wide each year.
- In high risk population screen before pregnancy by full blood count, film and Hb electrophoresis.

- If both parents are carriers for same type check blood for DNA mutations.
- If both parents carry the mutation, offer CVS for DNA testing or check globin chain synthesis by fetal blood sampling (see p. 49).
- If each parent carries a different mutation, discuss with clinical genetics and a haematologist for likely clinical significance.
- If previous child affected, offer CVS as above.

Sickle-cell disease
This is due to structural alterations in one of the globin chains.

- There are more than 80 α-chains and 180 β-chain variants; the most important clinically are HbS and HbC.
- HbS/S is commonest and most troublesome in tropical Africa (heterozygote frequency 20–40%). It is also present among African-Americans (heterozygote frequency 9%), in the Middle East, India and the Mediterranean littoral.
- HbS/C affects West Indian black populations particularly severely.
- The high world-wide frequency of the sickle-cell and thalassaemia genes probably occurs because heterozygotes are protected against falciparum malaria.
- Screen for carrier status by 'sickle test' in Afro-Carribean population.
- Direct DNA testing is available for fetus—the sickle cell mutation alters a 'restriction enzyme chopping site' in the β-globin gene.

Phenylketonuria (PKU)
- The gene defect is on chromosome 12q. Carrier detection and prenatal diagnosis in affected families is now possible using direct DNA testing.
- Routine neonatal screening is still mandatory.
- A mother with PKU has about an 8% chance of having an affected child.
- She must receive a phenylalanine-free diet from before conception, otherwise the risk of spontaneous abortion, infant death or severe mental retardation is high, even if the child has not inherited the disorder.

X-LINKED RECESSIVE DISORDERS

- An initial guide to carrier status is based on family studies plus clinical, biochemical or haematological tests.
- More definitive information is obtained from DNA studies. In most cases this is by analysis of indirect linked markers, but an increasing number of individual gene mutations are being discovered, which can be analysed directly.
- Prenatal diagnosis should be considered only after full evaluation of carrier status by a clinical geneticist and by prior consideration of what can/should be done with the information.

Duchenne/Becker muscular dystrophies (DMD/BMD)

- Boys with DMD may present with delayed onset of walking (i.e. after 18 months) with progressive muscular weakness and death from cardio-respiratory failure by 25 years of age. BMD is milder, progressing to wheelchair use by 45 years of age.
- 1 in 3000 males are born with a mutation in the dystrophin gene at *Xp21* resulting in either DMD or BMD.
- 1 in 2000 women are carriers—a few may have mild symptoms (or very rarely the full disease due to X–autosome translocation or as a monozygous twin).
- Fresh mutation accounts for 1 in 3 boys with DMD (i.e. 2 in 3 mothers are carriers): a higher proportion of BMD mothers are carriers.

Pre-pregnancy screening for DMD/BMD

- Indicated if previously affected son or family history of DMD or BMD.
- Direct DNA testing is possible in the 70% of families with a readily detectable dystrophin gene mutation. Indirect DNA testing is used for the remaining 30%.
- If the male partner is affected, check his DNA for deletion in dystrophin gene. Prenatal testing is not indicated—no son will be affected but all daughters will be carriers.

Pre-natal diagnosis of DMD/BMD

- Offer CVS if dystrophin gene deletion found in above. Otherwise discuss with geneticist.
- Ethical debate continues about investigation and reporting of carrier state in female fetus.

FRAGILE X-ASSOCIATED MENTAL RETARDATION

- The second commonest genetic cause of mental retardation (after Down's syndrome).
- Due to mutation in *FraX* gene at tip of X chromosome.
- Incidence is 1 in 2500 males.
- About 1 in 3 female carriers have mental retardation (usually milder than in affected males).
- Prenatal DNA testing is now possible.
- Antenatal screening cannot yet be justified and needs further study.
- Referral to clinical geneticist is essential in presence of FH of condition.

Other X-Linked recessive disorders—e.g. *Haemophilia A* (factor VIII deficiency affecting 1/5000 males) or *Haemophilia B* (factor IX deficiency affecting 1/30000 males)—should be approached as above.

MULTIFACTORIAL DISORDERS

The most significant conditions within this group are neural tube defects, many congenital heart lesions, facial clefts, diaphragmatic herniae and gut atresias.

NEURAL TUBE DEFECTS (NTD)
- Anencephaly and spina bifida comprise 95% of NTDs and encephalocoele the remaining 5%.
- The incidence is inversely related to socioeconomic status and shows marked geographical variation (ranging from 3 in 1000 births in SE England to 8–10 in 1000 in Ireland).
- It has dropped steadily over the past 20 years—this is not entirely accounted for by antenatal screening programmes.
- In the UK the recurrence risk after one affected child is 1 in 25, rising to 1 in 10 after two or more. An affected parent has a 1 in 25 risk of producing a child with a NTD.

Screening for NTD
- This has relied on a cut-off level for maternal serum AFP of around 2.5 multiples of the normal median (MoM) at 15–18 weeks' gestation that detects 90% of anencephaly, 80% of open spina bifida, but will include 3% of unaffected singleton pregnancies.
- Increasingly, high-resolution ultrasonography is used to screen for NTD. Detection rates approaching 100% have been reported. The average detection rate in the UK is around 80–90%.

Prevention of NTD
- The risk of NTD may be reduced if multivitamin tablets, which include folic acid (400 µg daily), are taken from at least 1 month before conception to about 10 weeks of pregnancy.
- Following a previously affected pregnancy 4 or 5 mg folic acid should be taken.

AFP and other fetal problems
- High serum AFP levels may be associated with conditions such as exomphalos, congenital nephrosis, posterior urethral valves, Turner's syndrome and trisomy 13.
- High serum AFP alone predicts an increased risk of a variety of obstetric problems, including FGR and perinatal death, particularly if oligohydramnios is present.

CONGENITAL HEART LESIONS
- The overall incidence has inexplicably increased over the past 15 years and is now about 8 in 1000 births.

Table 4.3 Congenital heart lesions: incidence and recurrence rate

Defect	Birth incidence	Recurrence risk for sibs	Recurrence risk for offspring
Ventricular septal defect	1/400	1 in 25	1 in 25
Atrial septal defect	1/1000	1 in 33	1 in 33
Tetralogy of Fallot	1/1000	1 in 33	1 in 25
Coarctation of aorta	1/1600	1 in 50	1 in 50
Aortic stenosis	1/2000	1 in 50	1 in 33
Transposition of the great vessels	1/16000	1 in 50	unknown

- The incidence and recurrence risks for various types of congenital heart defects are given in Table 4.3.
- Prenatal diagnosis of some of the most serious of the defects is possible using high-resolution ultrasound imaging and fetal echocardiography at 20 weeks' gestation (see p. 48).

FACIAL CLEFTS

- Cleft lip and/or palate occurs in 1 in 1000 births.
- Most cases are multifactorial, but it is associated with over 150 rare single-gene traits or chromosomal abnormalities (e.g. trisomy 13).
- Surgical repair with good results is usual.
- Recurrence risks for the multifactorial lesions are:
  - Child with unilateral cleft lip in normal parents: 1 in 50
  - Child with bilateral cleft lips and palate in normal parents: 1 in 20
- Isolated cleft palate is distinct. It affects 1 in 2500 births, with a recurrence risk of 1 in 50 for sibs and offspring.

ANTERIOR ABDOMINAL WALL DEFECTS

These occur in about 1 in 6000 pregnancies, and the two main forms are:

- *Exomphalos*—the umbilical cord is involved and is attached to the apex of the sac, which may contain liver and/or intestines. Associated chromosomal anomalies occur in 30% and cardiac lesions in 10%.
- *Gastroschisis*—the umbilical cord is not involved and there is no sac. Associated gut atresias and cardiac lesions (but not chromosome abnormalities) occur in up to 20%.

- Prenatal diagnosis by ultrasound is possible.
- Maternal serum AFP may be elevated.

Chromosomal anomalies should be excluded if exomphalos is suspected.

Vaginal delivery should be aimed for except for obstetric indications.

Isolated defects are often correctable surgically.

Body stalk anomalies form a third, less common defect. They are associated with major lower body deformities.

GASTROINTESTINAL ANOMALIES

Among those with multifactorial inheritance patterns are:

Hirschsprung's disease
Affects 1 in 8000 newborn with a 3-to-l male excess.

Table 4.4   Recurrence risk of Hirschsprung's disease

	Sibs	*Offspring*
Affected male	1 in 25	<1 in 100
Affected female	1 in 8	<1 in 100

Pyloric stenosis
Incidence is 1 in 200 in males and 1 in 1000 in females.

- The greatest risk of recurrence is in male relatives of an affected female (1 in 6).
- The lowest risk is for female relatives of an affected male (1 in 50).
- The risks for the other two possible combinations are intermediate.

Oesophageal atresia/tracheo-oesophageal fistulae
Affects 1 in 3000 newborns.

- May be associated with cardiac defects.
- Can be suspected prenatally by persistent absence of stomach bubble on ultrasound.

Gut atresias
Affects 1 in 330 newborns and may occur at any level of the intestine.

- Can be diagnosed prenatally by ultrasound.

Diaphragmatic hernia
Occurs in 1 in 2000 to 1 in 5000 births.

- The incidence of associated anomalies may be as high as 60% overall.

OTHER MALFORMATIONS

Obstructive uropathies

Dilatation of whole or part of urinary tract is most commonly due to *urethral valves.*

- This affects males 20 times more often than females.
- The prognosis depends on the time of onset and severity of the obstruction.
- The dilated urinary tract can be observed ultrasonically in the fetus.
- The role of fetal therapy is discussed on p. 50.

GENETIC COUNSELLING AND PRENATAL DIAGNOSIS

Ethical issues

Knowledge about and techniques for studying fetal development in general and genetics in particular are advancing rapidly.

This increases our responsibility to consider the ethical issues raised. 'What *can* we do?' must be balanced by 'What *ought* we to do?'.

Among the ethical dilemmas are:

- General population screening for defective genes (e.g. the cystic fibrosis gene).
- Testing of pre-implantation embryos after assisted conception.
- More aggressive prenatal screening for conditions causing varying degrees of disability (e.g. Down's syndrome).
- False-positive rates inherent in all screening programmes.

Genetic counselling is the imparting of knowledge and advice about inherited conditions. This involves:

- Complete history from or about the affected individual (proband).
- Construction of pedigree.
- Physical examination of proband with particular reference to dysmorphic features.
- Accurate diagnosis—among the indications for chromosome analysis are:
  - Family history of chromosomal aberration
  - Multiple congenital anomalies
  - Unexplained short stature in female
  - Unexplained stillbirth
  - Dysmorphic features
  - Ambiguous genitalia
  - Unexplained mental retardation
  - Recurrent miscarriage

- Some forms of cancer associated with chromosomal rearrangements
- Neuroblastoma, leukaemia, retinoblastoma, Wilm's tumour
- Non-directive counselling.
- Follow-up.

Prenatal diagnosis
- Can be justified if the condition:
  - Is severe in its effects
  - Has a high genetic risk
  - Has a poor prognosis or is untreatable.
- The test must be reliable, and must be preceded by counselling.
- Tests for those anomalies which can be diagnosed antenatally can be applied:
  - As a *screening test* in a whole population to define a subgroup at particular risk with whom diagnostic procedures can be discussed.
  - As *diagnostic tests* in a group of women at high risk of a particular problem, such as a previous personal or family history of chromosomal disorders or inborn errors of metabolism: women with 'positive' screening tests.
- The basis of diagnosis is either:
  - The search for characteristic intracellular defects in fetal tissue obtained by invasive procedures (see below), or
  - The visualisation of morphological defects by ultrasound.

DIAGNOSTIC TECHNIQUES
Ultrasonography
- This has become the main diagnostic technique for prenatal diagnosis of congenital anomalies by allowing:
  - Direct visualisation of the defect (e.g. anencephaly).
  - Detection of markers of chromosomal defects.
  - Accurate direction of instruments during invasive procedures.
- The best time for routine examination is 18 to 22 weeks.
- Detailed ultrasound requires great interpretative skill from the operator if unacceptable levels of false-positive and false-negative diagnosis are to be avoided.
- Some of the more sophisticated techniques should be carried out in regional centres with the appropriate expertise.
- The following table highlights some specific points. For more detailed discussion see 'Further reading'.

Chorionic villus (CV) biopsy
- CV biopsy (or chorionic villus sampling; CVS) obtains fetal tissue from the chorion under ultrasound guidance.
- One technique uses a transcervical approach between 8 and 12 weeks. The second, and now more popular, transabdominal route

Table 4.5   Ultrasonography in prenatal diagnosis

Condition	Ultrasonic examination	Comment
Spina bifida	Bi-parietal diameter (BPD) and head circumference reduced; ventriculomegaly; scalloping of frontal bones ('lemon sign'); anterior curve of cerebellar hemispheres ('banana sign') or absent cerebellum (all at 16–18 weeks)	Reliable when examined by experienced personnel. The presence of some of these signs indicates need for more detailed examination.
Congenital heart defects	'Four chamber' view of heart at transverse section of thorax	Optimum time for examination: 18–22 weeks
	Echocardiography for individual women at high risk	For specialised centres only: 18–22 weeks
Down's syndrome	Ratio of bi-parietal to occipito-frontal diameter to detect brachycephaly	Of no value in population screening
	Nuchal skin thickness	May occur in normal fetuses; varies with attitude of fetal head; can be produced artificially by angle of transducer
	Short femur (using Increased BPD: femur length ratio as index)	May be useful as ancillary screening method at 16 weeks

can be used from 8 weeks to term. Most centres defer CVS until after 11 weeks due to reports of possible limb reduction deformities following early CVS.
- The additional procedure-related risk of miscarriage is about 1–2%.
- Its potential advantages are:
  - It can be carried out in the first trimester.
  - The tissue is ideal for DNA analysis and gene probing (see below).
  - Initial chromosome analysis can be ready in about 48 hours (full cultures still take 2–3 weeks).
- However, the genetic composition of the chorion (trophoblast) is not necessarily the same as that of the fetus. For example, mosaicism and some rare trisomies confined to the trophoblast occur in about 1% of cases.
- Chromosomal aberrations found after CVS must, therefore, be assessed carefully.

Amniocentesis

This is best carried out at 15–18 weeks' gestation. The culture failure rate is <1%. The average time for culture is 10–12 days.

Indications:

- Maternal request based on age related risk or screening test.
- Previous infant affected by a condition diagnosable antenatally.
- Family or personal history of diagnosable condition.

Risks:

- Miscarriage—the excess procedure-related risk is between 0.5 and 1%. It is related to experience and use of ultrasound guidance.

Precautions:

- Always use ultrasound to continuously observe the needle during the procedure.
- Give anti-D immunoglobulin 50 μg in all antibody-negative, Rh-D-negative women. More can be given to cover any serious feto-maternal transfusion (see p. 96)

Fetal blood sampling (cordocentesis)
- The sample is taken under ultrasonic guidance from the area of the insertion of the cord into the placenta.
- It must be carried out only in specialist centres.
- Among the indications are red-cell iso-immunisation (see p. 96); non-immune hydrops (see p. 130); exclusion of fetal infection (see p. 109); and rapid karyotyping in some cases of FGR (see p. 57).
- Anti-D immunoglobulin (100 μg, or more if Kleihauer indicates it) should be given to Rh-D-negative women carrying Rh-D-positive fetuses.
- The risk of fetal loss is about 1%.

Embryo biopsy
- IVF and embryo culture allow sampling of one or two cells at the 8 to 16-cell stage.
- DNA analysis of a single cell and/or karyotyping of cultured cells could be used for diagnosis of genetic defect in women at high risk of a serious disorder.
- Only normal embryos should be reimplanted.
- This is potentially more acceptable for some couples than later prenatal diagnostic methods.
- It could ultimately allow 'gene therapy' in some cases.
- However, even if the embryos are 'normal' the rate of successful pregnancies will be 25–30% in the best centres.

FETAL THERAPY

- This can be achieved indirectly *via* the mother (e.g. digoxin or flecainide for fetal cardiac arrythmias) or directly to the fetus, as listed in the information box.

Therapy direct to the fetus

Medical
Intravascular infusions or injections by cordocentesis for
- Transfusion to correct anaemia e.g. for iso-immunisation
- Platelet infusion injection for allo-immune thrombocytopenia (see p. 99)
- Drug injection, e.g. to treat fetal hypothyroidism or cardiac failure

Surgical
Ultrasound-guided techniques can be used to:
- Drain pleural effusions or ascites
- Insert pleuro-amniotic shunts for non-immune hydrops or chylothorax
- Insert vesico-amniotic shunts to relieve obstructive uropathies. No consensus exists about criteria for this. In selected cases decompression may restore amniotic fluid volume and prevent pulmonary hypoplasia. It is unlikely to prevent or reverse renal damage

Fetal karyotyping should be considered before or during therapeutic interventions.

POST-MORTEM EXAMINATION OF FETUSES

- An experienced perinatal pathologist should be asked to examine all mid-trimester spontaneous abortions and those induced because of suspected congenital malformations.
- This will allow accurate counselling of the families, and audit of the screening and diagnostic tests. (see also p. 178).
- Prior fully informed written consent *must* be obtained.

FURTHER READING

Chamberlain G and Steer P (eds) 2001 Turnbull's Obstetrics (3rd edition). Churchill Livingstone, Edinburgh
James D K, Steer PJ, Weiner CP, Gonik B (eds)1999 High Risk Pregnancy— Management Options (2nd edn) Saunders, London
RCOG 1997 Report of RCOG Working Party. Ultrasound Screening for Fetal Abnormalities. RCOG, London
RCOG 2000 Routine Ultrasound Screening in Pregnancy. Protocol, Standards and Training. RCOG, London

5. Assessment of fetal growth and well-being

NORMAL FETAL GROWTH

Fetal growth and fetal size are often confused in clinical practice: babies below the 10th centile, or > 2 standard deviations below the expected mean for the gestation, are defined by the WHO as small for gestational age (SGA).

Growth restriction is a reduction of growth velocity and therefore the diagnosis can only be made after estimating size on at least 2 occasions. The estimated fetal weight will not follow the projected growth pattern i.e. the baby is not fulfilling it's growth potential.

The average weights of normal fetuses as pregnancy progresses are given in the box.

Average weight of a normal fetus	
Gestational age (weeks)	Approx. weight (g)
10	5
20	300
30	1500
40	3400

About 95% of birthweights fall within a normal distribution curve but the remaining 5% show a prolonged tail of low birthweight, which is discussed below.

FACTORS AFFECTING FETAL GROWTH AND SIZE

Physiological factors

Genetic control
- This predominates in the first half of pregnancy, but environmental factors and other constraints give rise to greater variability in the second half of pregnancy.
- About 15% of total birthweight variation is attributable to the fetal genotype.

Fetal sex
- On average males weigh 150–200 g more than females at term.
- There is no difference up to 33 weeks' gestation.

Race
The approximate mean birthweight for six ethnic groups are given in the box.

Ethnic group	Approx. mean birthweight (g)
Europeans	3200
East and South-west Asians	3100
Indonesians and Africans	3000
Indians	2900

These differences do not solely depend on race; nutritional and socioeconomic factors are likely to be involved.

Parental height and weight
- The paternal contribution is solely genetic.
- Maternal height and weight have independent effects on birthweight.
- Tall, heavy mothers will have babies up to 500 g heavier than short, light mothers.

Maternal age
Teenage mothers and those over 35 years of age tend to have smaller babies (as well as an increased incidence of congenital anomaly). Socioeconomic factors also play a role.

Birth order
Birthweight rises from first to second pregnancies by about 130 g, with a smaller rise in the third pregnancy. This may be associated with increased maternal weight.

Multiple pregnancy
Twin growth is similar to singletons up to 32 weeks but decreases thereafter. Dizygotic twins tend to be heavier than monozygotic. No weight-for-gestation standards exist for multiple pregnancy.

Socioeconomic factors
The average birthweight of babies born into social classes I and II (professional and managerial) is 150 g greater than for babies born into social classes IV and V. This may be related to maternal size, age and smoking habits rather than to nutritional status.

In general, the growing fetus is protected against the effects of maternal deprivation unless they are very severe.

Pathological markers for reduced fetal growth
- *Previous obstetric history*: Women whose first pregnancy ended in stillbirth (but not miscarriage), or in birth of a growth-restricted baby, tend to have relatively small babies in subsequent pregnancies.
- *Smoking*: Smoking in pregnancy reduces the mean birthweight by 100–200 g from 34 weeks' gestation onwards.
- *Altitude*: Birthweight falls by about 100 g for every 1000 metres of altitude.
- Excessive alcohol ingestion (see p. 123).
- Pre-eclampsia and related disorders.
- Congenital malformation of fetus.
- Fetal or maternal infections.
- Multiple pregnancy.

WEIGHT-FOR-GESTATION STANDARDS

Weight-for-gestation standards are statistical reference levels that enable babies from similar populations to be defined and compared in a uniform manner in terms of weight and gestational age.

Standard percentile values for birthweight are usually derived from cross-sectional studies and reflect fetal size but *not* fetal growth (see below).

They need to be established for each population (see Further Reading).

Clinical use of weight-for-gestation standards
Size (as assessed by weight) at birth is important because the prognosis for an infant is more dependent on birthweight than gestational age.

Most of the infants in whom problems will arise are found in the group weighing less than the 10th percentile for gestational age and sex. These infants are termed 'small-for-dates' (SFD) or 'small-for-gestational-age' (SGA).

Criticisms of weight-for-gestation standards
- Cross-sectional data obtained at birth may not reflect longitudinal fetal growth.
- The weight of babies born at a given gestational age may not be representative of the babies at the same gestational age who remain in utero.
- The charts do not identify those babies whose growth has been restricted but whose birthweight falls above the 10th percentile.
- The charts do not correctly classify those babies who are normally grown but whose weight is below the 10th percentile for gestational age and sex.

Despite these criticisms the 10th percentile cut-off for gestational age and sex for defining SGA infants is useful in clinical practice because low birth weight is associated with a higher perinatal mortality and increased risks of cardiovascular disease in later life. However, the majority are normal.

Classification of SGA fetuses:

1. Normal small
2. Abnormal small—i.e. an early viral insult or a chromosomal disorder. Symmetrical small abdominal and head circumference and normal dopplers.
3. 'Starved small' due to placental dysfunction, for example secondary to PET. Abdominal circumference below the 2nd standard deviation and abnormal dopplers.

ASSESSMENT OF FETAL STATE

ASSESSMENT OF GESTATIONAL AGE AND/OR FETAL GROWTH

- Menstrual history is an unreliable guide to gestational age in up to 45% of women.
- Measurement of the crown–rump (C–R) length by ultrasound scan in the first trimester most accurately determines the gestational age of a fetus.

Growth

- Serial clinical assessment of *fundal height* (as height in cm above symphysis pubis) provides a guide to fetal growth and is a useful part of screening for size in a low-risk antenatal population.
- The estimated fetal weight, and, therefore, size, is best calculated from the fetal abdominal and head circumferences. In clinical practice the abdominal circumference alone is often used.
- *Growth is different from size, and at least two measurements of size are required to measure growth velocity.*

FETAL WELL-BEING

There are no direct tests of fetal well being, and, therefore, the whole clinical picture needs to be interpreted rather than just the test results.

FETAL MOVEMENTS

- A daily count of perceived fetal movements from 28 weeks' gestation is a simple and inexpensive routine screening device for monitoring fetal well-being.
- Advice should be sought if fewer than 10 movements are perceived within 12 hours or if the mother feels that 'the baby is not moving'.

- Other tests of fetal welfare can then be applied.

Criticisms of fetal movement counts
- A large number of fetal movements may not be perceived.
- There are great variations in the number of fetal movements from day to day in individual women and from woman to woman.
- The sensitivity and specificity of the method is low.
- One randomised trial suggests a clear benefit, but another does not.
- Less than 1 in 1000 women might benefit from formal fetal movement counting, using late fetal death as an outcome.
- Formal counting provokes anxiety in about 25% of women. Another 50% are reassured by it.

ANTENATAL FETAL HEART RATE RECORDING

- An antenatal CTG or 'non-stress test' (NST) is still widely used in the UK as a test of fetal welfare despite lack of evidence of benefit from prospective, properly controlled trials (see Enkin in Further Reading). CTGs seem to be better at detecting acute hypoxia, secondary to an event, rather than the chronic hypoxia seen in growth restriction.
- The major hazard is over-interpretation, which results in unnecessary intervention.
- In the clinical setting, some reassurance can be obtained from a normal result. The important feature that suggests that the fetus is in good health is the presence of discrete accelerations in response to fetal movements (a 'reactive trace').
- Failure to show reactivity early in the trace is not necessarily abnormal because the fetus has 'rest–activity' cycles and the mean period of rest is about 40 minutes.
- Baseline irregularity is an important feature, but:
  - the earlier the gestation the more unreactive the normal trace is
  - the time from 28–32 weeks is a transitional period for the development of baseline irregularity.
- *Decelerations in relation to contractions accompanied by loss of baseline irregularity are a serious prognostic sign.*

ULTRASOUND INVESTIGATIONS

Ultrasound is used in a number of different ways to assess fetal well being, as described below.

Liquor volume
A number of methods are used to measure liquor volume.

- Most commonly the deepest pool is measured. It should normally be between 2 and 8 cm. Liquor volumes change with gestation but the above general limits apply throughout.

- Sometimes the deepest pool is measured in 4 quadrants and the depths averaged (the 'amniotic fluid index' or AFI). It appears to provide no added advantage over the above simpler method.

Oligohydramnios is a significantly reduced liquor volume. It may be a sign of chronic fetal hypoxia due to decreased renal perfusion and a consequent reduction in fetal urine output.

ANOMALIES
Ultrasound can identify markers for chromosomal abnormalities and occasionally the stigmata of early viral infection (e.g. cerebral calcification).

- Severe growth restriction with otherwise normal liquor volume and doppler studies raises the possibility of a chromosomal abnormality. This is even greater in the presence of polyhydramnios.

Biophysical profile (BPP) scoring
BPP scoring uses a fetal heart rate (FHR) monitor and a real-time ultrasound machine to assess five 'biophysical' variables:

- fetal breathing movements
- discrete body or limb movements
- fetal tone
- FHR
- amniotic fluid volume.

The technique and interpretation are described in Further reading.

BPP scoring does not seem to significantly improve fetal outcome. It may, however, still be of value in women at high risk of fetal problems because a normal result is reassuring (but only for up to 24 hours).

Doppler studies
Doppler ultrasound is used to assess blood flow in fetal arteries and has been shown to be useful in managing pregnancies complicated by fetal growth restriction (FGR) but not as a screening test in a low risk population.

- It does not measure flow directly, but this is inferred from analysis of the wave-like patterns ('wave forms') on the ultrasound screen to produce the *pulsatility index* (PI) and *resistance index* (RI). A value of more than 2 standard deviations above normal for these indices is indicative of significantly reduced flow.
- Alterations in blood flow can be an early indication of fetal compromise because part of the normal fetal response to inadequate nutrition is to redistribute blood flow from peripheral viscera to the brain.
  - Progressively greater vascular resistance is indicated by absent then reversed end-diastolic blood flow and indicates increasing fetal compromise.

- A reduction in the RI for the middle cerebral artery indicates an increase in blood flow to the head and, therefore, a decrease more peripherally suggesting the possibility of fetal compromise.

CORDOCENTESIS

Cordocentesis is not a normal part of the assessment of a small baby, except where an urgent karyotype may help with the management of the pregnancy.

MANAGEMENT OF THE GROWTH RESTRICTED FETUS

- The management of FGR depends on severity and gestation.
- At term the neonatal risks are minimal and, therefore, the threshold for delivery can be lower than at earlier gestations.
- Before 34 weeks steroids should be considered before delivery.
- When FGR is suspected doppler studies are more accurate and result in less unnecessary intervention than CTG alone. They can be performed between 1 and 3 times per week depending on the clinical circumstances.
- At gestations less than 28 weeks' it may be appropriate to monitor a growth restricted fetus with abnormal doppler studies using daily CTGs as they change later in the pathophysiology of FGR. This can allow some prolongation of gestation which, combined with the opportunity to give steroids, may improve outcome.

Delivery of the growth restricted fetus

- Caesarean section may be appropriate for fetuses with abnormal dopplers.
- In the presence of normal doppler patterns labour is usually well tolerated and can be managed routinely as long as there is continous CTG monitoring as the fetal reserve is less and the fetus can become acidotic more quickly than normal.

FURTHER READING

Bobrow C S, Soothill P W. Fetal growth velocity: a cautionary tale. Lancet 1999; 353: 1460

RCOG Green Top Guideline: The Investigation and management of the small-for-gestational-age fetus. www.rcog.org.uk/guidelines.

6. Medical and surgical problems in pregnancy

Not all conditions that may affect the pregnant woman can be discussed here. Inclusion depends on frequency of occurrence or, in less common conditions, seriousness of its effects. For greater detail see 'Further Reading' at the end of each section.

The diagnosis and management of many medical and surgical problems in pregnancy is complicated by several factors:

- The infrequency of their presentation.
- The lack of awareness of obstetric staff and midwives of general medical and surgical conditions.
- The lack of awareness of many physicians and surgeons and some anaesthetists of the impact of pregnancy on conditions with which they are otherwise familiar.
- Failures of communication.

CARDIOVASCULAR SYSTEM

HYPERTENSIVE AND ASSOCIATED DISORDERS OF PREGNANCY

Measurement of blood pressure
- Measure with woman sitting or lying on her side with a 15–30° tilt.
- The diastolic blood pressure (DBP) is best taken at the point of disappearance of the sound [Korotkoff phase 5 (K5)] rather than the point of muffling (K4).
- If K5 is audible at zero pressure use K4 and make a note to that effect.
- Automated sphygmomanometers tend to underestimate DBP, particularly in severe hypertension.
- In time the use of conventional sphygmomanometers will be superseded by more accurate and consistent electronic instruments.

Definition
Hypertension is a physical sign and *not* a disease. It is defined as two consecutive measurements of diastolic blood pressure (DBP) ≥90 mmHg 4 or more hours apart or one measurement ≥110 mmHg.

- A DBP of 90 mmHg corresponds to the point at which the perinatal mortality rate begins to rise in population studies, and is

approximately the mean +3 SD in mid-pregnancy, the mean +2 SD from 34 to 37 weeks, and the mean +1 SD at term.
- The use of systolic blood pressure (SBP) or the calculation of mean arterial pressure does not add to the prognostic significance and is more complicated.

Severe hypertension is a DBP ≥120 mmHg on one occasion *or* a DBP ≥110 mmHg on two consecutive occasions 4 or more hours apart. Levels at or above this are associated with an increased maternal risk (see p. 000).

Proteinuria is defined as ≥300 mg protein in a 24 h urine collection *or* a protein/creatinine ratio of >30 mg protein/mmol creatinine.

- Reagent strips are a useful screening test but false positive tests occur in 26% 'trace' reactions and up to 6% '+' reactions.
- False positive and negative errors can be minimised by using mid-stream urine samples with a pH of <8 and SG <1.030.

Clinical classification of hypertensive disorders of pregnancy
(After Davey & MacGillivray 1988—see Further reading)

Gestational hypertension and/or proteinuria
Hypertension and/or proteinuria developing during pregnancy, labour, or in the puerperium in a previously normotensive non-proteinuric woman. This includes gestational hypertension (without proteinuria) and pre-eclampsia (i.e. gestational proteinuric hypertension).

Gestational hypertension and chronic renal disease
Hypertension and/or proteinuria in pregnancy in a woman with chronic hypertension or chronic renal disease diagnosed before. But beware, pre-eclampsia can be superimposed on chronic hypertension.

Eclampsia
The occurrence of generalized convulsions during pregnancy or labour or within 7 days of delivery not caused by epilepsy or other convulsive disorder.

Pre-eclampsia (PET)
Pre-eclampsia is a multi-system disorder of endothelium peculiar to pregnancy. It is usually characterized by hypertension, renal impairment and fluid retention, and often accompanied by proteinuria and some degree of intravascular coagulation.

- It is associated with maternal mal-adaptation to pregnancy.
- Although it usually develops in later pregnancy, it occurs as a result of events around implantation.
  - It is totally dependent on the presence of trophoblast.
  - The pathology begins in the placental bed. Abnormal placentation is central to the development of pre-eclampsia.

- Pre-eclampsia is the commonest cause of FGR in non-malformed infants and of elective pre-term delivery.
- Perinatal death is increased in severe disease of early onset (10–15 fold) and when eclampsia or HELLP syndrome (Haemolysis, Elevated Liver enzymes and Low Platelets) supervene.

Predisposing factors

Primigravidity—the incidence of severe (proteinuric) pre-eclampsia in a first pregnancy is around 6%.

- It occurs in about 2% of all second pregnancies rising to 12% if severe pre-eclampsia (with FGR) was present in the first, and falling to under 1% if the first was a singleton, normotensive pregnancy.
- Pregnancy by a new partner may increase the risk to that of a first pregnancy.
- No protection is offered by an early spontaneous or induced abortion.
- *Age*—the incidence is slightly increased in very young primigravidae and more markedly in older primigravidae.

Genetic—Both maternal and fetal genes may contribute.

- The *maternal* component is either due to a dominant gene with varying penetrance or is 'multifactorial'. The risks are as shown:

Relative affected	Excess risk in woman being considered
Mother	× 4–5
Sister	× 3–4
Grandmother	× 2–3

- The *fetal* component may reflect expression of paternal genes
- The risk is increased when there is a strong family history of hypertension, other cardiovascular disorders or autoimmune disease.
- There is no significant racial preponderance

Medical—Among the predisposing factors are:

- pre-existing hypertension
- acquired or inherited thrombophilia (see p. 80)
- migraines
- diabetes mellitus

Socioeconomic—The incidence increases as socioeconomic status deteriorates. This may be associated with poor maternal nutrition. The failure of specific studies of dietary supplements to show benefit does not rule out the long-term absence of nutrients in diet as contributing to the increased risk.

- The incidence is lower in women who smoke, but the fetal outlook is worse in smokers who develop pre-eclampsia.

Obstetric—There is a strong association with:

- hydatidiform mole
- multiple pregnancy (particularly monochorionic twins)
- fetal triploidy
- fetal trisomy 13
- placental hydrops

Environmental—seasonal and climatic variations in incidence (particularly for eclampsia) remain unproven.

Postulated mechanism for development of PET
Events in early pregnancy

The mother fails either totally or partially to adapt physiologically (see p. 11 for normal adaptive mechanisms). For example:

- Trophoblast fails to invade maternal spiral arterioles.
- Maternal plasma volume fails to expand.
- The predominance of vasodilatory mediators, e.g. prostacyclin (PGI_2) and nitric oxide (NO), in the endothelium does not occur so vessels remain responsive to vasoconstrictors. There is also augmented sympathetic vasoconstrictor activity.
- The placental bed fails to become a 'low-pressure supply system'.
- The physiological inflammatory type response of normal pregnancy (see Redman et al in 'Further reading') is exaggerated.

Prodromal phase
- The placenta is perfused under high pressure.
- Circulating factors (e.g. vascular endothelial growth factor and other cytokines) are involved in a vicious cycle of endothelial damage. The vascular damage is increased yet further in a complex relationship of activated platelets, neutrophils and free radicals that produces the characteristic 'acute atherosis' and micro-thrombi formation.
- Spiral arterioles become partially or totally occluded.
- Placental perfusion to the fetus decreases and fetal growth begins to be impaired.
- Infarction of placental lobules may occur (this increases the risk of placental abruption).
- Endothelial damage begins to extend throughout the maternal vascular tree.

Clinical phase

This classically occurs in the third trimester, but it may happen earlier but seldom before 20 weeks'.

The syndrome affects each woman differently. Not all aspects are apparent in each case. Every system can be affected to a variable and sometimes severe degree.

Prediction and prevention of pre-eclampsia

Among the suggested *predictive tests* are:

- plasma fibrinectin
- serum AFP, hCG or inhibin
- urinary kallikrein/creatinine ratio
- uterine artery velocity waveforms
- angiotensin II sensitivity test

No test, singly or in combination, has been found to be sufficiently reliable.

Prevention—For analysis of clinical trials see 'Further reading'.

- Salt restriction, high protein diet, and diuretics are not effective.
- *Fatty acids*—recent trials of *fish oils* suggest some preventative effect but data on perinatal outcome are as yet inconclusive. Trials of *evening primrose oil* are still too small to provide guidance.
- *Calcium* may provide some protection against PET proportional to the degree of risk and if calcium intake is low early in pregnancy. No benefit in outcome has yet been demonstrated. It may be worth considering in women at high risk with low dietary calcium.
- *Anti-thrombotic and anti-platelet agents*
  - *Low-dose aspirin* (70–100 mg/day) suppresses production of thromboxane A_2 by platelets in vitro without significantly affecting prostacyclin.
    - The evidence about effectiveness remains unclear.
    - The results of large trials do not support routine prophylactic or therapeutic use in women judged to be at added risk of pre-eclampsia or FGR.
    - However, a review of 39 trials (see Duley *et al.* in Further reading) concludes that low-dose aspirin is associated with a 15% decrease in pre-eclampsia, a 14% fall in the risk of perinatal death and an 8% reduction in the risk of pre-term birth.
    - Despite earlier concerns, there does not seem to be any additional risk of ante- or post-partum haemorrhage.
    - Women should be allowed to make their choice on the basis of the above information.
  - Heparin/warfarin—trial evidence is inadequate. Anecdotal reports suggest no benefit and some serious side effects.
- *Anti-oxidants*—Vitamins C and E are scavengers of free oxygen radicals and, thereby, reduce the oxidative stress implicated as a factor in the vascular damage that occurs in pre-eclampsia. The one trial to date suggests that vitamins C (1000 mg/day) and E (400 IU/day) may reduce the risk. Larger studies are needed to assess the extent of any benefit and risk of fetal side effects.

Maternal clinical aspects of PET

Cardiovascular and pulmonary effects

- Hypertension is the commonest manifestation.

- Peripheral oedema occurs due to 'leaky' endothelium.
- Severe pre-eclampsia is a high cardiac output state with inappropriately high systemic vascular resistance. Left ventricular function is hyper-dynamic: cardiac failure may supervene in the most severe cases.
- Pulmonary oedema may arise due to an imbalance between a reduced colloid osmotic pressure and the pulmonary capillary wedge pressure. It can also be precipitated by intravenous fluid overload during treatment without proper monitoring.

Pulmonary causes [i.e. pulmonary oedema or acute respiratory distress syndrome (ARDS)] accounted for 11 and 8 maternal deaths in the UK in 1991–93 and 1994–96 respectively but only 1 in 1997–99.

The kidney
Glomerular endothelial cells swell, blocking the capillaries. (this 'glomerular endotheliosis' is characteristic but not pathognomonic).

Impairment of renal function may result in a rise in plasma urate (an early feature), urea and creatinine.

- Proteinuria develops: pre-eclampsia is the commonest cause of heavy proteinuria in pregnancy.
- Hypoalbuminaemia can lead to gross generalised oedema and the nephrotic syndrome. Manage in consultation with a nephrologist.

The liver

Liver involvement must be considered in all cases of severe pre-eclampsia.

- Hepato-cellular damage can occur due to fibrin deposits in the sinusoids.
- Epigastric pain (due to hepatic oedema and distension of the liver capsule), nausea and vomiting are associated with fulminating pre-eclampsia.
- In some cases, jaundice and severe liver damage can follow, often out of proportion to other signs and symptoms.
- The potentially dangerous HELLP syndrome must be considered in severe cases. See below.
- Subcapsular haemorrhages and even liver rupture may occur.

Coagulation

The physiological changes in the clotting system in pregnancy are outlined on p. 12.

- Increasingly generalised endothelial damage commonly causes slight intravascular coagulation shown by increased platelet turnover and a fall in platelet count (which can be severe in some cases).
- DIC is a rare but serious end point in some cases.
- Haemolysis can occur due to fibrinogen-associated red cell aggregation.

HELLP syndrome
- It occurs in about 20% of cases of severe pre-eclampsia with a similar risk of recurrence in subsequent pregnancies.
- It may present initially with vague flu-like symptoms that are not recognised. As a result of this and lack of medical awareness, there is often a delay in diagnosis (average 8 days).

Diagnosis depends on assessment of platelet count ($<150 \times 10^9$/l) and hepatic dysfunction determined by raised liver enzymes [particularly aspartate transaminase (AST) and/or γ-glutamyl transferase (γGT) but not alkaline phosphatase which is normally raised because it is produced by the placenta]. *Note that liver function tests are lower in normal pregnancy than the non-pregnant reference ranges.*

Management
- Involvement of a senior obstetrician with experience of the condition is mandatory in all cases.
- Help may need to be sought from a tertiary referral centre to which transfer may be indicated, but only if the maternal condition permits.
- In all cases liver, renal and coagulation status must be assessed at least daily and more frequently in more severe cases.
- Mild cases can be managed as clinical circumstances suggest. If the pregnancy is at or near term, vaginal delivery may be possible.
- In moderate cases over 34 weeks' prompt delivery by caesarean section is indicated. Careful judgement is required about best management if before 34 weeks'.
- In severe cases coagulation status and hypertension must be controlled before proceeding to deliver by caesarean section whatever the gestation.
- High dose steroids (dexamethasone 10 mg i.v. 12 hourly to delivery) may allow some safe prolongation of pregnancy but only for 1–2 days. This regimen may also allow more rapid recovery if used after delivery (see Further reading).
- Regional anaesthesia is not advised if the maternal platelet count is less than 100×10^9/l and contra-indicated if other measures of coagulation are abnormal.
- Close monitoring of moderate and severe cases is required in a high-dependency or intensive care unit for at least 48 h after delivery.

Central nervous system
- Among the signs of CNS involvement are atypical headache, visual disturbances hyper-reflexia, ankle clonus, restlessness and agitation.
- Vasoconstriction of cerebral vessels occurs (probably as a protective mechanism against severe hypertension). At a mean arterial pressure of about 130–150 mmHg this mechanism begins to fail, and small vessel walls are damaged and disrupted.

- This can lead to cerebral oedema, haemorrhages and infarcts—all associated with eclampsia.

Eclampsia
For definition see p. 59.

- It occurs in less than 1% of women with pre-eclampsia and the incidence in the UK is about 5/10 000 maternities.
- The timing of seizures is antenatal in 38%, intrapartum in 18% and postpartum in 44% of cases. Postpartum fits usually occur within 24 hours of delivery, but may occur up to 7 days later.
- Signs and symptoms of impending eclampsia usually include severe hypertension and proteinuria with epigastric pain, nausea, vomiting and signs of CNS involvement. Retinal oedema, haemorrhages and even papilloedema may occur.
- However, there are no recognisable prodromal signs or symptoms in up to 20% of cases.
- Eclampsia is still a significant contributor to maternal mortality with 8 and 5 women dying after eclamptic seizures in 1994–96 and 1997–99 respectively. The fatality rate per case is about 2% and 35% of women will have at least one major complication.

Maternal mortality and pre-eclampsia/eclampsia
The main causes of deaths (and numbers) due to 'hypertensive disorders of pregnancy' from 1985 to 1999 are given in Table 6.1.

Table 6.1   Maternal mortality in the UK, 1985–1999

	1985–87	1988–90	1991–93	1994–96	1997–99
Cerebral	11	14	5	7	7
Intracerebral Haemorrhage	11	10	5	3	7
Subarachnoid	–	2	nil	1	nil
Infarct/oedema	–	2	nil	3	nil
Pulmonary	11	10	11	8	1
ARDS*	9	9	8	6	1
Oedema	2	1	3	2	0
Hepatic	1	1	nil	3	2
Other	3	2	4	2	5
Total	27	27	20	20	16

*ARDS, adult respiratory distress syndrome

Management of gestational hypertension and pre-eclampsia
The principles are:

- Early recognition of the symptomless syndrome.
- Awareness of serious nature of the condition in its severe form without over-reacting to mild disease.
- Agreed guidelines for admission to hospital, investigation, and use of antihypertensive and anticonvulsant therapy.
- Well-timed delivery to pre-empt serious maternal or fetal complications.
- Postnatal follow up and counselling for future pregnancies.

Clinical observation and investigation
Examination (over and above routine):

- Palpation of the femoral pulses (to exclude coarctation of aorta)
- Check for hyper-reflexia and ankle clonus
- Look at optic fundi for silver wiring, arterio-venous nipping, exudates and haemorrhage

Laboratory investigation

- Proteinuria (see p. 59). If present also check urine microscopy and culture to exclude urinary infection.
- Serum urate levels increase early in pre-eclampsia. Levels >350 µmol/l are abnormal in pregnancy but gradually increasing levels are more significant.
- Serum urea and creatinine. Rising levels are significant but not so sensitive indicators of pre-eclampsia as uric acid. The upper limits of normal in pregnancy are 5 mmol/l for serum urea and 100 µmol/l for creatinine, but trends are even more important than specific levels.
- Platelet count gradually falls if DIC is occurring.
- Liver function. Liver enzymes should be checked once persistent proteinuria is present, or if platelet count is significantly reduced.
- Coagulation studies should be carried out if platelet count is reduced and in severe disease.
- Tests of fetal growth and well-being (see p. 51).
- Each of these tests should be repeated as often as is clinically necessary.

Management of mild/moderate gestational hypertension
The principles are:

- Uncomplicated hypertension is suitable for careful supervision at home by the primary health care team.
- Sedatives or tranquillisers are contra-indicated.
- Antihypertensive therapy is not required (see below).
- Admission to hospital is indicated when:
  - SBP is 160 and/or DBP 100 mmHg or greater.

- Significant proteinuria (see p. 59) is detected in a clean (i.e. mid-stream) urine sample in the absence of a urinary infection.
- The patient is symptomatic with, for example, visual disturbances, unusual headache, epigastric pain, or vomiting (URGENT!).
- There is clinical evidence of intrauterine growth retardation.
- Tests of fetal welfare have deteriorated (see p. 51).
- A previous bad obstetric history suggests that closer surveillance would be worthwhile.

Management of severe hypertension

- The maternal risks of cerebro-vascular accident and of left ventricular or renal failure begin to increase significantly when hypertension is severe.
- The choice has then to be made between delivery and antihypertensive therapy.
- Among the factors to be considered are:
  - Gestational age—it is seldom justified to commence long-term oral therapy from 34 weeks.
  - The severity of other signs and symptoms.
  - Availability of intensive neonatal care facilities.
- *Treatment neither influences the progression of underlying pre-eclampsia nor significantly improves fetal outcome.* It helps to protect the mother and enables many pregnancies to continue that otherwise would be ended because of maternal risk.

Control of acute severe hypertension

- There is no consensus on the optimum acute treatment.
- The important objective is to reduce the blood pressure to safe levels (but not too low).
- Parenteral hydralazine is used most commonly but oral nifedipine should be considered (see below). For more detailed discussion see Further reading.

Longer-term control of severe hypertension (see Further reading)

- There is still insufficient trial evidence to determine whether the benefits outweigh any disadvantages.
- If it is to be used, the suggested indications are:
  - DBP ≥100 mmHg
  - Pregnancy ≤34 weeks
  - Fetal and maternal state otherwise good
- Among the drugs used are those shown in Table 6.2.
- There is no single ideal drug. In some cases combined therapy can be useful if used with care. For specific details see BNF in Further reading.
- Angiotensin converting enzymes (ACE) inhibitors have deleterious fetal effects and are contraindicated in pregnancy. If a woman with chronic hypertension becomes pregnant on an ACE inhibitor, change to another anti-hypertensive agent.

Table 6.2   Drugs used for long-term control of severe hypertension

Drug	Effect	Comments
α-methyl dopa	Centrally acting α-adrenergic inhibitor-still the drug of first choice	May cause drowsiness initially and depression in some women
Hydralazine	Relaxes arteriolar smooth muscle fall in vascular resistance (VR)	Mainly used parenterally for acute severe hypertension. Commonly causes flushing and headache
Labetolol	Combined α- and β-adrenoceptor agonist → fall in VR	Can cause postural hypotension. Can be used intravenously in acute severe hypertension or orally for longer term treatment
Nifedipine	Calcium channel blocking agent → relaxes vascular smooth muscle	Although not licensed for use in pregnancy it is used widely. It can be given orally for acute severe H/T and as a second agent in longer term management. It can cause flushing & headache. Larger RCTs are required
Prazosin	Reduces VR by selective competitive inhibition of α$_1$ adrenergic receptors	May be useful as a second agent
Glyceryl tri-nitrate	Relaxes arterial smooth muscle	Can cause flushing, headache and postural hypotension. Not licensed for use in pregnancy.

- Diuretics have not been shown to be beneficial. Their use has been discouraged in pre-eclampsia because they further reduce circulating blood volume.

Timing of delivery
- The most common grounds for delivery are:
  - Progressive fetal compromise (i.e. when the baby is safer delivered).
  - Unacceptable risk to maternal health (e.g. uncontrollable BP, impending renal failure or heart failure, HELLP syndrome, DIC, eclampsia).
- The mode of delivery (caesarean section versus vaginal) depends on:
  - the seriousness of the situation,
  - the gestational age
  - the degree of fetal/maternal compromise

- Regional (epidural or spinal) analgesia is the method of choice for labour (as long as a coagulation defect has been excluded).
- Appropriate facilities for the care of the newborn infant must be available.
- *Avoid NSAIDs for post-operative analgesia because of the risk of renal failure when used in the presence of severe pre-eclampsia.*

Fluid balance and plasma volume expansion

- Restriction of i.v. fluids to less than 1 litre following delivery of women with severe pre-eclampsia reduces the risk of pulmonary oedema without affecting renal function.
- Diuretics are contraindicated because they aggravate hypovolaemia and can precipitate renal failure.
- Plasma volume expansion accompanied by vasodilator drugs (e.g. hydralazine) may have a role in some severe cases with the following provisos:
  - It must be used only in high-dependency units where invasive monitoring (e.g. to measure pulmonary capillary wedge pressure; PCWP) is available.
  - Only small volumes (e.g. haemaccel 200–600 ml) are necessary.
  - Blind therapy is very dangerous and can lead to pulmonary oedema and death.
  - CVP monitoring may not be adequate. Measurement of PCWP may be required (CVP does not correlate with PCWP when the former is >6 mmHg).

Management of eclampsia

- *Prevention of convulsions*—despite magnesium sulphate having been used for many years in the USA for the prevention of eclampsia, clear evidence of benefit is lacking (see Thornton 2000 in Further reading). The results of a major trial in the UK are awaited.
- *General management:*
  - Place woman in left lateral position and secure airway. Give oxygen
  - Insert urinary catheter to monitor urine output
  - Check for disorders of electrolyte balance and disseminated intravascular coagulation
- *Control of convulsions:*
  - Magnesium sulphate ($MgSO_4$) is the drug of choice for treatment of eclampsia. It reduces neuromuscular irritability and cerebral vasospasm. Intramuscular injection is painful.
  - A suggested regime is:
    - loading dose of 4 g i.v. over 5–10 minutes
    - i.v. infusion of 1 g/h for 24 h
    - treat recurrent seizures with a further i.v. bolus of 2 g over 5 min.
  - Treatment is monitored clinically by checking:
    - respiratory rate (>16/min)—treat respiratory depression with calcium gluconate 1 g i.v. over 10 minutes.

- urine output (>25 ml/h)—if less than this monitor serum levels of magnesium.
- presence of knee jerks—if deep tendon reflexes are absent withhold MgSO$_4$ until they return.
- If seizures persist despite MgSO$_4$, consider diazepam or thiopentone under anaesthetic guidance. Intubation, IPPV and muscle relaxants may be required.

Control of hypertension—see p. 68.

Delivery of the infant
- Caesarean section is the method of choice but only when the eclampsia is under control. If eclampsia supervenes when the patient is well advanced in labour vaginal delivery may be possible.

Long-term outlook
In the absence of any underlying predisposing condition, women who develop severe pre-eclampsia or eclampsia are not at increased risk of developing chronic hypertension in later life.

Patients with severe early onset pre-eclampsia should be screened for predisposing conditions (e.g. chronic hypertension and acquired or inherited thrombophilia).

Pre-existing hypertension and pregnancy
Among the possible causes are:

- Essential hypertension—the outlook is good in this condition but pre-eclampsia may supervene. Management of the hypertension is as described above.
- Coarctation of the aorta.
- Renal hypertension—see p. 105.
- Phaeochromocytoma—see p. 86.
- Autoimmune connective tissue disorders—see p. 99.

CARDIAC DISEASE

The New York Heart Association classification of cardiac functional status is summarised in Table 6.3. (for reference see James *et al* in Further reading)

The haemodynamic changes that occur during pregnancy (see p. 11) impose an increased burden on the mother's heart. This causes no problems for healthy women but may do so in women with cardiac disease.

The incidence of significant heart disease (Classes II–IV) in pregnancy is about 1%.

An increasing number of women with *congenital heart defects* (CHD) are reaching childbearing age as a result of improved medical and surgical management.

Table 6.3   Classification of cardiac functional status

Class I	No limitation of physical activity
Class II	Slight limitation—ordinary physical activity results in fatigue, palpitations, dyspnoea or angina
Class III	Marked limitation—less than ordinary physical activity results in above
Class IV	Inability to perform any physical activity without discomfort—cardiac insufficiency or angina may be present even at rest.

Maternal risks

Maternal death
In 1997–99 cardiac disease was the joint most common cause of maternal death.

The main categories of causes since 1991 have been:

Type of heart disease	%
Congenital	30
Ischaemic	15
Other (e.g. cardiomyopathy, myocarditis)	55

The conditions in which maternal death occurred most commonly are influenced by the prevalence of the condition and the nature and extent of the associated cardiac disease.

The conditions found most commonly were:

• Congenital defects:
  • Aortic valve disease
  • Any condition causing pulmonary hypertension
• Acquired disease:
  • Cardiomyopathy/myocarditis
  • Myocardial infarction
  • Dissection of aorta.

Over the past 15 years about 10% of cardiac deaths were due to endocarditis.

The risk markers for myocardial infarction in pregnancy include smoking, hypertension, diabetes mellitus and familial hyper-cholesterolaemia.

Mortality risk associated with individual conditions provides a better guide to the risk for each woman affected. Table 6.4 is derived from 'Cardiac Disease in Pregnancy' ACOG 1992 (for reference see James *et al* in Further reading).

Table 6.4

Group	Case-specific maternal mortality (%)	Conditions
1	< 1	Atrial & ventricular septal defects Pulmonary/tricuspid valve disease Tetralogy of Fallot (corrected) Mitral stenosis—woman in classes I & II Porcine valve replacement
2	5–15	Mitral stenosis with atrial fibrillation &/or woman in classes III & IV Aortic stenosis Coarctation of aorta (uncomplicated) Tetralogy of Fallot (uncorrected) Previous myocardial infarct Marfan's syndrome with normal aorta
3	25–50	Any condition associated with pulmonary hypertension Coarctation of aorta (complicated) Marfan's syndrome with aortic involvement

Fetal risks

The risks of low birth weight are increased but there is no direct increase in perinatal mortality.

If the mother has CHD there is a 5–10% risk of CHD in the fetus (but not necessarily the same defect). There is also some increased risk if another family member has CHD.

Pre-conception counselling

This is important for women with known heart disease because:

- Cardiac status can be determined.
- Treatment can be optimised.
- A specific plan can be prepared for pregnancy.
- Surgery can be advised in those women in whom pregnancy would add a severe but correctable burden (e.g. tight mitral stenosis).
- Advice can be given to those women at high risk during pregnancy (see Group 3 in Table 6.4). The fact that pregnancy may be best avoided in these conditions must be imparted.

Antenatal management

- Care should be delivered jointly headed by an obstetrician trained in maternal medicine and a cardiologist with a specific interest in this area.
- A care plan should be discussed with the woman and communicated to her GP and any referring obstetrician.

- In women who have conditions causing severe pulmonary hypertension (e.g. Eisenmenger's syndrome) it may be necessary to discuss termination of pregnancy in maternal interests. This must be done sympathetically and compassionately.

Aims and objectives of antenatal care:
In addition to the risk management aims of routine antenatal care particular attention should be paid to the following:

- Cardiac status by echocardiography when first seen and then as indicated by condition (e.g. at each visit in women in mortality risk groups 2 & 3).
- Fetal echocardiography can be offered at 20 weeks' in women with CHD to check on anatomy of fetal heart.
- Ensure adequate rest.
- Strongly advise against smoking.
- Prevent anaemia.
- Treat respiratory infection promptly.
- Be watchful for incipient pulmonary congestion and arrhythmias.
- Invite an obstetric anaesthetist to meet women in Classes II to IV prior to delivery.

Dissection of the aorta should always be considered in a pregnant woman complaining of severe chest pain. At least a chest X-ray is mandatory in such cases.

Management of labour
The following are among the suggested general guidelines. Specific cases may need higher dependency care. This should be discussed in good time with the cardiological and anaesthetic team.

- The presumption should be for vaginal delivery at term unless there are clear reasons to the contrary. Induction of labour is necessary only for obstetric reasons.
- When patient starts labour with good cardiac reserve the risk of heart failure is low.
- Good evidence on preventing endocarditis is lacking. The current consensus in the UK is that it is not necessary to cover labour with antibiotics except in women with prosthetic heart valves.
- Control any infusion of parenteral fluids very strictly.
- Provide adequate analgesia—epidural anaesthesia is safe in experienced hands as long as hypotension is avoided; it is contraindicated in Eisenmenger's syndrome and cardiomyopathies.
- Avoid aorto-caval compression.
- Shorten the second stage by use of 'lift-out' forceps or vacuum extractor (without raising legs into lithotomy position if possible).
- Avoid ergometrine in the third stage.
- Do not attempt caesarean section in the presence of heart failure.
- Have oxygen and relevant drugs immediately available.
- Avoid beta-sympathomimetic drugs in women with pre-existing heart disease.

SPECIFIC PROBLEMS

Cardiac failure
The principles of diagnosis and treatment are the same as in the non-pregnant patient.

- It can occur even in young asymptomatic women with cardiac disease at any stage of pregnancy.
- Sudden cardiac decompensation is more likely to occur shortly after delivery.

Acute pulmonary oedema
This is a medical emergency that demands immediate attention.

- Nurse in semi-recumbent position, give oxygen and keep airways clear.
- Give intravenous morphine, aminophylline, frusemide and digoxin (if not previously digitalised).
- In labour, the fetus must take second place until the situation is under control.

Tachyarrythmias
- *Atrial fibrillation* is a medical emergency requiring bed rest in hospital and digitalisation. The advice of a cardiologist must always be sought. Anticoagulation may also be indicated.
- *Atrial tachycardia* can precipitate heart failure rapidly. It often responds to carotid sinus pressure.

Cardiac valve prostheses and pregnancy (see Sadler *et al.* 2000 Further reading)

- Mechanical mitral valves:
  - Women on warfarin throughout pregnancy have a high rate of pregnancy loss.
  - Women on heparin have a high fetal survival but an almost 30% risk of thromboembolism.
- Pregnancies are more successful in women with bioprosthetic or homograft valves.

THROMBOSIS AND THROMBO-EMBOLISM

The shift towards coagulation and away from fibrinolysis during normal pregnancy is discussed on p. 13.

Venous thromboembolism (VTE)
VTE arises as a result of interaction among a variety of inherited and acquired factors. Virchow's triad of a hypercoagulable state, venous stasis and vascular damage predisposing to VTE are present in normal pregnancy resulting in an increased risk of VTE.

- The risk of VTE in a pregnant woman is about 5 times that for a non-pregnant woman of a similar age. Table 6.5 shows the

Table 6.5   (see Greer, 1999 in Further reading)

DVT (incidence/1000 pregnancies)	Antenatal	Postnatal
Women under 35 years of age	0.6	0.3
Women 35 years of age or over	1.2	0.7

estimated incidence of deep vein thrombosis (DVT) associated with pregnancy.
- DVT complicates about 2% of caesarean sections
- The risk of recurrence in a woman with a past history of thrombo-embolism occurring in pregnancy or while on 'the pill' is about 12% (majority postnatal)

Factors associated with increased risk of VTE following caesarean section
The RCOG have issued guidelines on prophylaxis against VTE in women having caesarean section (see Further reading).

Slight increase in risk:

- Elective caesarean section in an uncomplicated pregnancy with no other risk markers
- Blood groups other than O
- Action: requires only early mobilisation and hydration.

Moderate increase in risk:

- Maternal age >35 years
- Parity 4 or more
- Obesity (>80 kg)
- Gross varicose veins
- Proteinuric pre-eclampsia
- Emergency caesarean section
- Immobility before surgery (>4 days)
- Sickle-cell disease, major intercurrent illness or infection
- Action: use heparin (see below) or anti- embolism stockings.

High risk:

- 3 or more moderate risk factors
- Personal or family history of thrombosis
- Acquired or inherited 'thrombophilia' (see p. 80)
- Major surgery (e.g. caesarean hysterectomy)
- Action: Antenatal prophylaxis required when factors 1 to 3 are present. Use heparin and anti-embolism stockings.

Prevention of VTE
Since no RCTs have been done management can only be based on observational studies and expert opinion. Table 6.6 contains a recommended regimen (based on McColl et al, 1999 in Further reading).

Table 6.6   Recommended regimens for VTE

Risk of VTE	Regimen
Very high • previous VTE on anticoagulants • antithrombin deficiency (in consultation with haematologist)	From confirmation of pregnancy: • Low-molecular weight heparin (LMWH) twice daily with dose adjusted as necessary by anti-factor Xa measurements (target levels 0.35–0.7 IU/ml 3–4 hours after injection) • Graduated elastic compression stockings
High • Previous VTE not on anticoagulants • Protein C deficiency and FH of VTE • Homozygous Factor V Leiden (FVL) or prothrombin mutation • Combined thrombophilias	From about 24 weeks' (earlier if other risk markers present) or 4–6 weeks before gestation at which a previous VTE occurred: • Fixed dose LMWH • Graduated elastic compression stockings • Postpartum anticoagulation for 12 weeks
Moderate • Combinatioin of heterozygous FVL, prothrombin mutation, protein S deficiency and FH of VTE	• Graduated elastic compression stockings • Monitor for other risks of VTE • Postpartum anticoagulation for 6 weeks
Relatively low risk of VTE • Heterozygous FVL or prothrombin mutation • No personal or FH of VTE	Monitor for additional risks of VTE and intervene if indicated.

Pregnant women travelling by air: The risk of DVT may be increased ×2–3 by long-distance flights even in the non-pregnant. The current best advice (see RCOG SAC Opinion Paper in Further reading) for women who are pregnant or in the puerperium based on low-grade evidence is as follows:

• *General measures for all*: Practice isometric calf exercises, walk around cabin frequently; avoid dehydration; avoid alcohol and caffeine.
• *Compression stockings*: Recommended for all if flight >4 hours; for shorter flights only if there are additional risk factors (see above).
• *Low molecular weight heparin (LMWH)*: on day of, and day following travel for women undergoing flights >4 hours who have additional risk factors (alternative low dose aspirin for three days before and on day of travel for those unable to take LMWH).

Clinical aspects of DVT in pregnancy

- The most common clinical features are pain, local tenderness, swelling, oedema, a positive Homan's sign (pain in calf on dorsiflexion of foot), a change in leg colour and temperature and a palpable thrombosed vein.
- Most cases are less obvious and some are silent. *Clinical diagnosis is, therefore, unreliable.*
- Lower abdominal pain, mild pyrexia and leucocytosis may be present and lead to suspicion of an infective condition (e.g. UTI or appendicitis).
- DVT occurs more commonly in the ileo-femoral rather than the calf veins (72 and 9%, respectively) and over 80% are left-sided.
- Superficial thrombo-phlebitis does not carry a significant risk of thrombo-embolism unless it extends to the deep veins.

Diagnosis of DVT

Objective diagnosis is important both because of the potential consequences of failing to detect its presence and the long-term implications of a false positive diagnosis for contraception and future pregnancies. *It is, however, not easy to achieve in pregnancy.*

There is no single agreed optimal diagnostic technique. The following is a pragmatic guide based on the current conflicting evidence:

- Real time or duplex ultrasonography is the first choice investigation.
- Impedance plethysmography can be used if it is available.
- Venography is still the 'gold standard' but is invasive. It may be negative in the presence of ileo-femoral thrombosis. It is indicated if non-invasive tests are equivocal.
- MRI scanning may be indicated if there is strong suspicion of ileo-femoral thrombosis.
- If VTE is suspected clinically, treatment with unfractionated (UF) heparin or LMWH should normally be given until the diagnosis is excluded.

Hazards of DVT

The main hazards are of pulmonary embolism, chronic vascular insufficiency and their sequelae.

Pulmonary thrombo-embolism (PTE)

- The main signs and symptoms are pleuritic pain, haemoptysis, dyspnoea and varying degrees of shock.
- Consider also if there is no other obvious explanation for tachycardia, pyrexia or bronchospasm.
- There may be no prior clinical evidence of DVT.

Investigation of suspected PTE

- Chest X-ray, ECG and blood gas analysis have their place but are not definitive.

- A ventilation–perfusion isotope (VQ) lung scan should be requested (a perfusion scan alone may suffice in the first instance). The radiation dose involved is low.
- Pulmonary angiography is rarely necessary may need to be considered if clinical suspicion is high but other tests are inconclusive.
- If strong clinical suspicion persists despite tests suggesting a low probability treatment should be started. The tests can be repeated in 7 days and treatment discontinued if they are negative.

Chronic vascular insufficiency
- As many as two-thirds of women develop long-term deep-vein insufficiency in the affected leg after a DVT in pregnancy.
- The risk may be reduced by wearing graduated elastic compression stockings on the affected leg for 2 years after the acute event.

Maternal mortality from VTE
- Untreated PE has a case specific mortality of 13%.
- Maternal deaths in the UK rose from 32 (15/million maternities) in 1991–93 to 48 (22/million maternities) in 1994–96. They fell to 35 (16.5/million maternities) in 1997–99 possibly due to greater recognition of risk markers and criteria for prophylaxis (see above).

Anticoagulation in pregnancy (see Further reading)
The indications for full anticoagulation in pregnancy are:

- VTE in index pregnancy
- Metal prosthetic heart valves
- Very high-risk cases of acquired or inherited thrombophilia.

Heparin: does not cross the placenta or into breast milk so there is no added risk to the fetus. Its action is to inhibit thrombin and factors IX, X, XI and XII.

- Side effects of long-term therapy include allergic reactions, thrombocytopenia and maternal osteopenia, which is dose and duration dependent with some unpredictable individual susceptibility.

Warfarin: inhibits the synthesis of vitamin K-dependent clotting factors (II, VII, IX and X).

- It crosses the placenta readily but is not significant in breast milk.
- It is best avoided in the first trimester because of a 2–4% risk of a characteristic embryopathy (nasal hypoplasia, stippled epiphyses, eye anomalies and developmental delays).
- Control must be tight and under strict expert supervision. In general the INR should be between 2.0 and 2.5.
- Even with meticulous control there is an increased risk of fetal haemorrhage.
- Its anticoagulant effect cannot be reversed rapidly.

- Heparin therapy is preferred unless the benefits of warfarin outweigh the risks.
- The indications for warfarin in pregnancy are:
  - Some prosthetic heart valves (e.g. Starr–Edwards, Bjork–Shiley)
  - Women with antiphospholipid syndrome and previous cerebral arterial thrombosis that recurs despite heparin prophylaxis.
  - Major side-effects from heparin (e.g. marked allergic reaction, severe osteopenia or thrombocytopenia) in women at high-risk of VTE.
- Because of the increased risk of haemorrhage change to heparin at 36 weeks' gestation if possible. If labour supervenes while the patient is taking warfarin it can be counteracted in the maternal (but not the fetal) circulation with fresh frozen plasma.
- Some women wish to transfer to warfarin after delivery.
- Breast-feeding is not contraindicated.

Dextran 70 is best avoided during pregnancy due to the risk of maternal anaphylaxis.

Treatment of established VTE in pregnancy

Acute therapy
- Subcutaneous UF heparin is as effective as i.v. UF heparin for the initial management of DVT.
- LMWH has been found to be more effective in non-pregnant subjects with lower mortality and fewer haemorrhagic complications. It is also simpler; women can be treated as outpatients after the initial acute phase and the dose response curve may be more predictable. It may have a lower risk of osteopaenia than UF heparin. Further studies are needed in pregnancy.
- Check platelet count 7–9 days after commencing treatment.
- The leg should be elevated initially and graduated elastic compression stockings worn. Mobilisation while wearing the stockings should be encouraged.
- A temporary caval filter may occasionally be required with recurrent PTE or when anticoagulation is contraindicated.
- Women who remain in shock an hour after the acute event have a high risk of dying. Advice should be sought on embolectomy or thrombolytic therapy despite the risks.

Maintenance therapy
- LMWH twice daily with dose adjusted as necessary by anti-factor Xa measurements (target levels 0.35–0.7 IU/ml 3–4 hours after injection).
- Graduated elastic compression stockings.

Labour and delivery
- Spontaneous labour should be allowed if possible.
- Temporarily discontinue heparin once labour is established.

- There may be a small risk of spinal or epidural haematoma with LMWH. Thus, if spinal or epidural block is required:
  - Site it at least 12 hours after the last injection
  - Delay further dose for at least two hours
  - Remove catheter 12–24 h after last dose and delay further dose by 2 h once more.

After delivery

- LMWH can generally be recommenced 12 hours following delivery.
- Conversion to warfarin can occur if desired 1–2 days after delivery and heparin discontinued once the INR has been in the therapeutic range for 3 consecutive days.
- Breast-feeding is *not* contraindicated.
- Thromboprophylaxis should continue for at least 6 and possibly 12 weeks. The longer time is recommended by some in light of the late deaths that can occur.

THROMBOPHILIAS

Definition

A group of disorders with an increased tendency to VTE due to an inherited or acquired defect in, or deficiency of a natural anticoagulant. There is also some association with recurrent second-trimester miscarriage, unexplained fetal death and severe early onset pre-eclampsia.

Inherited thrombophilias

The main inherited thrombophilias are:

- Antithrombin deficiency types I & II
- Protein C deficiency
- Protein S deficiency
- Factor V Leiden mutation
- Prothrombin gene mutation
- Hyperhomocystinaemia.

Antithrombin deficiency

Type 1 or quantitative deficiency (antithrombin activity and antigen levels decreased) is rare but is associated with a 1 in 3 risk of VTE in pregnancy. Type II or qualitative deficiency (normal but functionally abnormal levels) occurs in 1–2/1000 individuals. The risk of VTE in pregnancy is about 1 in 40.

Protein C and protein S deficiency

Protein C deficiency occurs in about 2/1000 of the population. The associated risk of VTE in pregnancy is about 1 in 110. The prevalence of *protein S* deficiency is not known.

Factor V Leiden mutation

This is due to a single amino acid substitution (glutamine for arginine) that renders factor Va resistant to proteolysis by activated protein C (APC).

- It is found in about 5% of individuals of European origin but is very rare in native populations outside Europe.
- Heterozygosity is associated with a 5–10 fold lifetime increase in a risk of VTE.
- This rises to 80–100 fold in the uncommon homozygous individuals.
- Other precipitating factors are usually required (e.g. pregnancy, surgery or use of the combined o.c. pill) for VTE to occur.
- Pregnancy in a heterozygous woman is associated with a risk of VTE of about 1 in 400 risk (relative risk about 4). The risk is greater post-partum.
- The APC sensitivity ratio cannot be used for screening in pregnancy when APC resistance may be present (see p. 13). The test is also affected by oral anticoagulants, heparin, antiphospholipid antibodies and other rare gene defects in factor V. In these circumstances a modified APC test is advised.

Prothrombin gene mutation (G20210A)

- It occurs in 1–3% of the population.
- Plasma prothrombin levels are raised.
- There is an associated 2–4-fold increase in risk of VTE (relative risk about 15) that rises further when, as occasionally happens, it co-exists with factor V Leiden mutation.
- There is no screening test. Detection depends on PCR techniques.

Hyperhomocystinaemia

The enzyme methylenetetrahyrofolate reductase (MTHFR) is important for homocysteine metabolism. Individuals who are homozygous for a gene mutation in MTHFR and who are folate deficient have elevated fasting levels of homocysteine. This may cause oxidative endothelial damage and, as a result, lead to an increased risk of both arterial and venous thromboembolism.

- No increased risk in VTE has yet been demonstrated in pregnancy in the absence of folate deficiency.

Acquired thrombophilia

Antiphospholipid syndrome (APS)

This is the presence of circulating antiphospholipid antibodies (aPL) and possibly lupus anticoagulant (LA) combined with one or more characteristic clinical features. The most important of these are:

- Vascular thrombosis (both arterial & venous)
- Thrombocytopenia
- Endocarditis
- Three or more 1st trimester miscarriages
- One or more fetal losses in 2nd or 3rd trimester
- One or more births before 34 weeks' because of severe PET or placental insufficiency

APS may be secondary to SLE (see p. 99) or primary (i.e. without any other evidence of autoimmune disease).

Management of APS
The aims are to prevent maternal thrombosis and optimise fetal outcome.

- *Pre-pregnancy:*
  - Full discussion with woman to allow informed choice
  - Commence low-dose aspirin when pregnancy test positive
  - Early presentation to allow assessment, planning of antenatal care timing of start of heparin therapy or change to heparin from warfarin if applicable.
- *Women with previous thrombosis*—see p. 76
- *Women with characteristic pregnancy problems:*
  - Treat with aspirin and LMWH. Current best evidence suggests that this should continue to 34 weeks.
  - High dose corticosteroids confer no benefit and increase maternal risk.
  - Intravenous immunoglobulin may have a role but only in those women who develop pregnancy complications despite pregnancy complications.

Screening for thrombophilia
- Routine screening is not justified.
- Screening should be offered *before pregnancy* to women with a personal or family history of VTE and possibly to those with recurrent fetal loss.
- More widespread screening (e.g. in women with pre-eclampsia, placental abruption or FGR) cannot yet be justified on available evidence.

Screening tests should include:

- Full blood count
- Antithrombin and protein C activities
- Total and free protein S antigens
- (PCR for MTHFR gene mutation is not routinely included)
- Coagulation screen
- Lupus inhibitor and anti-cardiolipin antibodies
- Factor V and prothrombin gene status.

INHERITED BLEEDING DISORDERS IN PREGNANCY

- *Von Willebrand's disease (vWD)* is the commonest with a prevalence of 1–3%.
  - Type I vWD forms 75% and is inherited as an autosomal dominant trait. The production of normally functioning von Willebrand factor (vWf) is reduced resulting in a secondary defect in factor VIII.

- Type II vWD (about 25% of cases) is predominantly also an autosomal dominant trait and is associated with a qualitative defect in vWF.
- Type III vWD is rare but bleeding problems are severe. It is autosomal recessive.
- *Haemophilias A (Factor VIII deficiency) and B (Factor IX deficiency)* are X-linked disorders. Clotting factor levels in a carrier are usually around 50% of normal (because only one X chromosome is affected) but she may have very low VIII or IX levels due to random deletion of one of each pair of X chromosomes (lyonisation). This may put her at risk of severe bleeding. *Factor XI deficiency* occurs rarely.
- An *acquired postpartum haemophilia* has been described in which antibodies develop to factor VIII. It may result in very severe bleeding and has a high morbidity and mortality.

Management of inherited bleeding disorders:
The main aspects are:

- Close collaboration with a local haemophilia centre.
- Assessment of women in families with these disorders before pregnancy to identify affected or carrier status.
- Prenatal diagnosis—mainly in carriers of haemophilia or severe forms of vWD (clotting status must be known beforehand and prophylaxis arranged if needs be).
- Establishment of clear management guidelines for uncommon but potentially serious complications.
- Check levels of clotting factors at booking and in third trimester as it may not be possible for the tests to be done in an emergency.
- Labour and delivery:
  - Affected fetuses are potentially at risk from haemorrhage and scalp clips. Prolonged second stage and instrumental delivery (save perhaps for low-cavity forceps) are best avoided.
  - Regional anaesthesia can be offered *if coagulation status is normal*.
  - Assess coagulation status of infant on cord blood.
- *Bleeding complications:*
  - The main risks are following abortion or post partum. This is because the pregnancy induced rise in clotting factors falls rapidly after delivery.
  - Minimise maternal genital tract and perineal trauma at delivery.
  - Prophylaxis is by desmopressin or clotting factor concentrates when appropriate.

CENTRAL NERVOUS SYSTEM

EPILEPSY

Pre-pregnancy counselling is important for women with epilepsy in order to:

- Check their anticonvulsant therapy for need, safety and dosage.
  - Adjust the drugs as necessary- the current advice is that sodium valproate is best avoided in pregnancy unless there is no safer and effective alternative (see below).
  - Some women may be temporarily able to stop at least some of their medication before conception and recommence it at about 16 weeks.
- Allay their many fears about pregnancy and nursing a small baby.
- Give advice about commencing folic acid.

Pregnancy does not provoke epilepsy in mothers but the frequency of seizures may increase because anticonvulsants are cleared more quickly and, perhaps, compliance is less during pregnancy.

There were 19 and 9 maternal deaths associated with epilepsy in 1994–96 and 1997–99, respectively. The reason for the fall is not clear.

Sudden unexpected death can occur but is uncommon when the epilepsy is well controlled.

- This risk should be part of the information given to the pregnant woman with epilepsy who is considering stopping anticonvulsants because of perceived risks to the fetus.
- Women with epilepsy who discover themselves to be unexpectedly pregnant should NOT stop taking their medication.

The risk of an epileptic mother having an epileptic baby is about 1 in 40.

Teratogenicity of anticonvulsants
The incidence of congenital malformations is increased two to three-fold in infants of women on anticonvulsants.

The period of greatest risk is at organogenesis (i.e. around the first 56 days of pregnancy).

No one drug is free of risk, but phenytoin (alone or in combination) and now sodium valproate seem to be implicated most frequently. Among the *severe abnormalities* are:

- Spina bifida—sodium valproate is associated with fetal spina bifida in about 1% of 'at risk' pregnancies.
- Cleft lip and/or palate (increased 10-fold).
- Congenital heart defect (increased 4-fold).
- Malformations of bladder and sexual organs.
- Malformations of ribs, unseparated fingers or toes.
- Retarded growth, delayed development and, occasionally, mental retardation.

Among the other problems are:

- Possible characteristic facial appearance: wide-spaced eyes, low posterior hair line, short neck, prominent brow and trigoncephaly. These may be associated with later impaired intellectual development.
- Small fingers and toes.

Management
- Folic acid from before conception throughout pregnancy.
- Adjust anticonvulsant dose preferably with a single drug to control seizures using serum levels as a guide.
- Offer detailed fetal anomaly scan at 20 weeks'.
- Vitamin K can be offered to mothers during last 4 weeks of pregnancy and should be given to all neonates to reduce risk of haemorrhage.
- Breast-feeding is *not* contraindicated.

Status epilepticus is best treated with intravenous diazepam. The airway must be kept patent and oxygen administered.

For further information see the British Epilepsy Association website.

MULTIPLE SCLEROSIS

The rate of relapse falls during pregnancy especially in the third trimester. It increases during the first 3 months post-partum before returning to the pre-pregnancy rate.

MYASTHENIA GRAVIS

This is a rare auto-immune condition with a peak incidence between 20 and 30 years of age frequently associated with a thymoma or thymic lymphoid hyperplasia.

- It produces rapid fatigue and weakness of voluntary muscles.
- Pregnancy does not worsen the disease but exacerbations can occur (most frequently in the puerperium) in up to 30% of women.
- The antibody can cross the placenta and cause a transient (or rarely permanent) effect on fetal voluntary muscles.
- Among the drugs that can exacerbate it are sedatives, tranquillisers, analgesics and narcotics.

Treatment is with anticholinesterase drugs such as neostigmine (with atropine) or pyridostigmine. Corticosteroids or ACTH may also be effective.

- Labour may be shorter than usual but the effort of the second stage can be tiring. Elective forceps delivery is usually indicated.
- General anaesthesia requiring muscle relaxation can result in prolonged paralysis of voluntary muscles.

ENDOCRINE SYSTEM

ADRENAL CORTEX

Addison's disease (primary hypoadrenalism) complicates pregnancy rarely.

- If diagnosed and treated before pregnancy, corticosteroid therapy must continue.
- Additional supplementation will be necessary at times of stress (e.g. labour) or if any infection occurs.

Cushing's syndrome is a rare but serious condition in pregnancy.

- Fetal loss is common and there is a significant risk to the mother's life.
- The main causes are pituitary adenoma, and adrenocortical adenoma or carcinoma.
- The presentation is as in the non-pregnant.

ADRENAL MEDULLA

Phaeochromocytoma complicates pregnancy rarely, but the consequences for the mothers are serious if it goes undetected. Only about half the cases are diagnosed antenatally.

- Women may present with sustained or paroxysmal hypertension. The other classical symptoms of headache, palpitations and excess sweating may not occur in pregnancy.
- It can cause sudden collapse in pregnancy, labour or the puerperium.
- It should be excluded:
  - when severe or intermittent hypertension occurs (particularly in early pregnancy)
  - in the presence of above 'classical' symptoms
  - in women with a family history of phaeochromocytoma or associated syndromes (e.g. neurofibromatosis or multiple endocrine neoplasia).

Diagnosis: estimation of catecholamines in a properly collected 24-hour urine sample. Ultrasound may detect a suprarenal mass. CT scan or MRI are useful for further localisation.

Treatment: The first priority is alpha-adrenergic blockade using phenoxybenzamine.

Surgical removal of the tumour can be considered with elective caesarean section. Specialist anaesthesia is required, and initial postoperative management must be in an intensive care unit.

DIABETES MELLITUS (DM)

Definition

Fasting venous plasma glucose concentration ≥7.8 mmol/l and ≥11.0 mmol/l 2 hours after a 75 g oral glucose load; *or* one of these plus symptoms and signs (polydipsia, polyuria, weight loss).

Impaired glucose tolerance (IGT) is said to be present if the fasting level is <8.0 mmol/l but rises to 8.0–10.9 mmol/l 2 hours after 75 g oral glucose load.

Risks associated with pre-existing insulin dependent diabetes mellitus (IDDM)

All risks are increased by poor control of diabetes (especially if keto-acidosis develops) and by inadequate obstetric supervision.

Maternal
- Retinopathy, nephropathy and neuropathy may be worsened.
- Obstetric complications (e.g. polyhydramnios, pre-term labour, pre-eclampsia).
- Infections—particularly urinary and monilial.

Fetal
- Congenital malformations in general (and cranio-spinal and cardiac defects in particular) are increased 3–4 fold. This is related to hyperglycaemia during organogenesis. Sacral agenesis is a rare anomaly specifically associated with IDDM.
- Macrosomia (i.e. birthweight <4000 g) occurs in up to 30% of women with an abnormal GTT.
  - It is associated with an increased risk of difficult delivery
  - Antenatal prediction of macrosomia leads to a marked increase in delivery by caesarean section without a significant reduction in the incidence of shoulder dystocia (see p. 159) or birth injury.
- FGR may occur if maternal diabetes is complicated by micro-vascular disease.
- Perinatal mortality (PNM) is still increased (about 5-fold) despite the St Vincent declaration of 1989 aiming for near normal pregnancy outcomes among women with IDDM.
  - Sudden unexpected fetal death (SUFD) is increased risk during the last 4–6 weeks of pregnancy
- Neonatal problems—birth trauma, hyaline membrane disease, hypoglycaemia, hypomagnesaemia, hypocalcaemia, jaundice.

Management of IDDM in pregnancy

Pre-pregnancy counselling allows:

- General advice—e.g. about tight diabetic control (particularly around conception and in the early weeks of pregnancy) and folate supplements (4–5 mg/day)
- Planning for pregnancy (including early booking for antenatal care)
- Review of diet
- Examination of optic fundi
- Establishment of good blood glucose control.

Antenatal care for women with IDDM should be jointly between obstetrician and diabetes specialist. The following is a guide to optimal diabetic control:

- High-fibre diet with correct calorific intake and CHO content
- Blood glucose profiles two or three times/week at home using filter-paper strips or a reflectance meter

- Tests are carried out before and 2 hours after each meal and last thing at night
  - Pre- and post-prandial levels of <5.0 and <7.0 mmol/l respectively are ideal
- Regular urinalysis (mainly to check on CHO loss)
- Regular glycosylated haemoglobin HbA$_1$c estimations (to provide retrospective information on the validity of home glucose monitoring)
- *Insulin treatment*—combined soluble and intermediate-acting insulins morning and evening or intermittent soluble insulin with each meal (three times a day) and an intermediate acting insulin in the evening. Human or highly purified porcine insulins reduce the risk of developing antibodies (which can cross the placenta).
  - The woman's family should be instructed on the use of *glucagons* for hypoglycaemic attacks.

Maternal health:

- Monitor weight, optic fundi, blood pressure, and renal function

Fetal welfare:

- Carry out baseline scans to confirm gestational age and a detailed anomaly scan at 20 weeks' (especially for cranio-spinal and cardiac defects).
- Continue with serial scans for reduced and, particularly, excess fetal growth.
- Assess fetal well-being (see p. 51) regularly from 28 weeks.
- If macrosomia arises check ultrasound scans for fetal cardiac enlargement.

Admission to hospital is indicated if:

- Good glucose control cannot be achieved as an outpatient
- Severe H/T or pre-eclampsia develop
- Weight gain is excessive
- Renal function deteriorates
- Fetal well-being causes concern.

Labour and delivery
When diabetes is well controlled and *pregnancy is uncomplicated* induction of labour between 38 and 40 weeks should be advised.

- During labour close control of blood glucose is achieved by a continuous infusion of soluble insulin (usually 50 units in 50 ml normal saline), and a separate infusion of 5% dextrose with KCl (10 mmol in 500 ml) added. The dextrose and KCl infusion should run at a constant rate (100 ml/h).
- Regular blood glucose monitoring should be undertaken and the insulin infusion titrated to keep levels between 5 and 7 mmol/l.
- If a syntocinon infusion is necessary this should be made up using normal saline.

- Continuous electronic fetal monitoring is advised.

If labour is induced an induction-delivery interval of < 24 hours should be aimed for.

If *elective caesarean section* is planned, careful control is necessary before, during and afterwards until the woman can eat and drink normally.

If *pre-term labour* supervenes, β-sympathomimetics and steroids are best avoided but, if absolutely necessary, can be covered by appropriate insulin infusions.

Postnatal care
- Insulin sensitivity increases immediately after delivery of the placenta. The required dose of insulin therefore fails quickly and careful monitoring is necessary.
- Hypoglycaemia is common in the neonate and must be treated promptly.
- Breast-feeding is to be encouraged.

Gestational diabetes
The clinical validity of the concept of gestational diabetes based on the oral glucose tolerance test (GTT) for the index pregnancy is questionable.

The current evidence (see Enkin *et al* in Further reading) suggests that:

- The GTT is not reproducible at least 50–70% of the time.
- The small increase in PNM is associated with the reason for testing rather than the result.
- Treatment of women with an abnormal GTT has *not* been shown to improve fetal outcome.
- The GTT is of limited value in identifying women at risk of fetal macrosomia and the majority of macrosomic infants will be born to women with a normal GTT.

Thus available evidence does *not* provide evidence of any benefit from either selective or routine screening for IGT/DM in the index pregnancy.

THYROID GLAND

Hyperthyroidism

This complicates 2/1000 pregnancies but it has usually been diagnosed and treated before pregnancy.

- The main cause is Graves' disease, but toxic multinodular or solitary nodular goitre may occur.
- Solitary nodules require careful evaluation because of the risk of malignancy. Fine-needle aspiration is used for diagnosis.

Management in pregnancy
- Carbimazole or propylthiouracil cross the placenta and can, therefore, affect the fetal thyroid. However, the balance of risk is in favour of use.
- Repeat thyroid function tests 3-monthly.
- Beta-blockers may be required to control serious peripheral effects of thyrotoxicosis.
- No special management is necessary for labour or delivery.
- Breastfeeding is not necessarily contraindicated.
- Babies should be screened for hypothyroidism.

Hypothyroidism
Treated hypothyroidism due to auto-immune disease or following partial thyroidectomy occurs in about 9/1000 pregnancies.

Myxoedema rarely presents in pregnancy because sufferers tend to be infertile.

Management in pregnancy
- Continue thyroid replacement therapy
- Check TFTs 3-monthly
- Breast-feeding is not contraindicated.
- If mother has previously had:
  - thyrotoxicosis check for neonatal thyrotoxicosis
  - auto-immune thyroiditis check baby for hypothyroidism.

Children born to mothers with mild or *sub-clinical hypothyroidism* may score lower in IQ tests than children of healthy mothers. Screening of all pregnant women (by measuring thyroid-stimulating hormone; TSH) early in pregnancy has been proposed. In addition to the logistic problems of this policy there is, as yet, no evidence that screening followed by treatment of those with mild hypothyroidism will provide real benefit (see Pop *et al* in Further reading).

Postpartum thyroiditis
This is a poorly recognised condition that may occur in 5–9% of pregnancies.

- It presents with fatigue, palpitations or other features of mild hyperthyroidism 2 to 4 months postpartum, and is often confused with 'postpartum blues'.
- Up to 25% of affected women will have a first-degree relative with a history of thyroid disease. Such women should be screened for thyroid antibodies at booking.

Diagnosis: T_3 and T_4 levels are raised. Radioactive iodine uptake is low. Thyroid antimicrosomal antibodies are present.

Treatment: It is usually a self-limiting condition, but hypothyroidism may persist in a small minority. In the thyrotoxic phase β-blocking agents may be used. In the hypothyroid phase thyroxine can be given for 4 to 6 months.

GASTRO-INTESTINAL SYSTEM

Gastro-oesophageal reflux, hiatus hernia and peptic ulceration

The lower oesophageal sphincter relaxes under the influence of pregnancy hormones. Reflux of acid gastric contents leads to *heartburn*. This can also be due to a 'sliding' *hiatus hernia*.

Management
- Frequent small meals; advise patient to avoid lying flat; simple antacids.
- If no relief is obtained 'floating' antacids, or metoclopramide, can be tried.

Peptic ulceration
- Use non-absorbable antacids or H_2 receptor blockers
- Consider anti-*Helicobacter pylori* therapy in women with proven duodenal ulcer where the organism has been identified and surgery may otherwise be thought necessary.
- Avoid steroids.

LIVER DISEASE

JAUNDICE DUE TO PREGNANCY

Intrahepatic cholestasis (ICP—20% of cases) (see Milkiewicz *et al* in Further reading)

The incidence in Europe is 0.1–1.5% of pregnancies rising to up to 16% in some S. American countries.

Aetiology
It is multifactorial in origin involving genetic, environmental and hormonal factors. Metabolites of both oestradiol and particularly progesterone have important roles. The underlying problem may be a genetic minor malfunction of biliary canalicular transporters that become overloaded in face of the high levels of sex hormones in pregnancy. It is possible that fetal inheritance of the mutation may make it more susceptible to the complications noted below.

Clinical features
The patient has pruritus (most pronounced in the palms and soles) usually in the second half of pregnancy that is often difficult to control. Jaundice occurs only in the most severe and prolonged cases.

- It is associated with an increased risk of:
  - pre-term labour (in up to 60% of cases)
  - fetal distress (in up to 33% of cases)
  - perinatal death (in about 2% of cases).

- Pruritus usually subsides within a few days of delivery.
- There is a 60–80% chance of recurrence in subsequent pregnancies.
- It may also occur in association with oestrogen-containing oral contraceptives.
- It does not lead to chronic liver disease.

Management

- Measure bilirubin (raised in 25% of cases), transaminases (raised in 60% of cases) and bile salts (raised in most patients).
- Exclude other causes if liver function is abnormal (particularly if this persists after delivery).
- If non-specific anti-pruritic remedies are not effective urso-deoxycholic acid will usually reduce itching and abnormalities in liver function tests. (*Note:* it is not currently licensed for use in pregnancy but no adverse effects have emerged when it has been used.)
- Parenteral vitamin K is required if jaundice causes prolongation of the prothrombin time leading to an increased risk of post-partum haemorrhage.
- Monitoring of fetal welfare (see p. 54) is advised but its value has not been demonstrated.
- The balance of risks and the poor predictive value of tests of fetal welfare suggest that elective induction of labour may be indicated from 37 weeks'.
- Vitamin K supplements should be given to the baby.

JAUNDICE COMPLICATING PRE-ECLAMPSIA—see p. 63.

ACUTE FATTY LIVER IN PREGNANCY

This is a rare but serious disorder induced by pregnancy the underlying cause of which is not known.

- It usually occurs in the 3rd trimester and can cause liver failure with high rates of maternal and perinatal death.
- Diagnosis is by exclusion and depends mainly on clinical criteria. Liver biopsy is too risky to contemplate in the acute phase.
- The clinical features include severe vomiting, extreme fatigue, upper abdominal pain and jaundice leading to drowsiness and confusion.

Management

- The principles of management are recognition of the condition, maternal resuscitation and fetal monitoring.
- Care should be in a high-dependency or intensive care unit. Multidisciplinary teamwork is required.
- Urgent delivery is indicated once maternal condition allows.
- If possible vaginal delivery should be aimed for because it is less risky for the mother. Whatever the route meticulous haemostasis is vital.
- Convalescence is prolonged and postnatal depression is common.

INTERCURRENT JAUNDICE IN PREGNANCY

Viral hepatitis (40% of cases)—see p. 112.

Cholelithiasis (6% of cases)
Modern ultrasound or transhepatic cholangiography may be useful in confirming the diagnosis. Cholecystectomy (including by laparoscopy) can be carried out in pregnancy if necessary, preferably not earlier or later than the second trimester.

PRE-EXISTING LIVER DISEASE

Pregnancy is uncommon in the presence of cirrhosis due, for example, to active chronic hepatitis, or primary biliary cirrhosis.

The prognosis is good for mother and baby in familial non-haemolytic jaundice (e.g. Gilbert's and the Dubin–Johnson syndromes). Pregnancy may increase jaundice in the latter.

INFLAMMATORY BOWEL DISEASE

ULCERATIVE COLITIS

This does not affect pregnancy adversely.

Pregnancy does not increase the chance of relapse of quiescent colitis, but if the colitis arises *de novo* in pregnancy or the puerperium it carries a poor prognosis.

- Treatment can continue during pregnancy with rectal and systemic steroids and/or sulphasalazine.
- In the presence of an ileostomy most pregnancies proceed to normal vaginal delivery.

CROHN'S DISEASE

- There may be a small adverse effect on fetal outcome due to the disease.
- The condition itself is usually unaffected by pregnancy.
- Deterioration is most likely in the puerperium.
- It should be managed in the same manner as in the non-pregnant.

HAEMATOLOGICAL SYSTEM

ANAEMIA

The haemoglobin (Hb) concentration fails during pregnancy (but not normally below 10.4 g/dl) because the physiological increase in plasma volume outstrips that of the red cell mass.

- The average requirement for iron is about 4 mg/day increasing as the pregnancy progresses. Although the normal diet contains up to 25 mg/day of iron only about 10% of this is absorbed. Iron stores, therefore, fall during pregnancy. Hb levels do not fall for several weeks after the stores are exhausted.
- Routine supplementation with iron and folate is not required in well-nourished communities.

Iron deficiency anaemia
The blood film is hypochromic and microcytic. MCH is decreased; serum ferritin levels are low (<15 µg/l) and iron-binding capacity is increased.

- This is a major health problem in developing countries.

Treatment
Increase dietary sources of iron (e.g. meat, fish, eggs and spinach) and supplement with oral iron and folate (because there is often an underlying folate deficiency).

- If gastrointestinal intolerance to iron occurs change to a chelated or delayed release preparation.
- Parenteral iron is rarely necessary.
- Blood transfusion may be necessary for severe symptomatic anaemia.

Megaloblastic anaemia
In women of reproductive age this is almost always due to folate deficiency

The blood film is normochromic and macrocytic.

Treatment
Increase dietary sources of folate (as for iron) and prescribe 5–15 mg folic acid orally daily.

HAEMOGLOBINOPATHIES

These inherited defects are a major cause of morbidity and mortality worldwide and particularly among those from E. Mediterranean, Middle-East, parts of India, SE Asia, Africa and the West Indies.

For genetics and prenatal diagnosis see p. 40.

Sickle-cell disease
The commonest (in descending order) are Hb-SS, SC and SThal.

They are associated with an increased risk of miscarriage, FGR, pre-eclampsia, pre-term delivery and both perinatal and maternal death.

Antenatal screening
Routine Hb electrophoresis is indicated in communities with a high prevalence of these conditions. Also check the partners of affected women to assess the risk of the fetus being affected.

Sickling crises

Hb-A and its abnormal variants function similarly when well-oxygenated but the latter polymerise when deoxygenated. The red cells become sickle-shaped and occlude vessels causing widespread vascular damage, severe pain and haemolytic anaemia.

Crises occur most commonly in the 3rd trimester and around delivery. Women with Hb-SC may be at particular risk during late pregnancy.

Treatment—prompt intervention is required including hydration, oxygen, treatment of any infection and, if necessary, exchange transfusion.

Prevention—the only successful preventive treatment is blood transfusion (3–4 units) at 6-week intervals. The potential benefit is counterbalanced by the risks of the transfusions (e.g. adverse reactions, transmission of hepatitis or HIV and the production of atypical antibodies). Further trials are required of routine transfusion from 26–28 weeks but it may be justified in affected women with multiple pregnancies.

Sickle-cell trait (Hb-A/S)

This is usually benign, but sickling cases occur under extreme hypoxia, dehydration or acidosis.

THALASSAEMIAS

β-thalassaemia major (homozygous)—pregnancy is very uncommon.

β-thalassaemia minor (heterozygous)—screening is by detection of poorly haemoglobinised cells (i.e. a low MCV and MCH in the booking full-blood count. The diagnosis is confirmed by finding raised HbA_2 with or without raised HbF.

α-thalassaemia major is incompatible with survival. The fetus usually develops hydrops with an increased risk of severe pre-eclampsia.

α-thalassaemia minor:

- α^+-thalassaemia—one of the two α-genes deleted
- α^0-thalassaemia—both genes deleted

Carrier women, particularly those with α^0-thalassaemia, tend to become anaemic in pregnancy. They can be detected at their booking visit by finding typically abnormal red cell indices (MCV and MCH reduced; MCHC normal or slightly reduced).

Diagnosis is only by globin chain synthesis studies or DNA analysis of nucleated cells.

HBH disease is an intermediate form of α-thalassaemia with only one functional α-gene and an unstable haemoglobin formed from the β-chain. Patients have a chronic haemolytic anaemia and circulating HbH that is found by Hb electrophoresis.

Treatment
- Iron and folate supplements can be given safely in α^+ and α^0 thalassaemia.
- Folate only is given in HBH disease.
- Parenteral iron is contraindicated because of the risk of iron overload.
- Transfusion may be required for anaemia at term.

RHESUS ISO-IMMUNISATION

The Rh factor
Each Rh gene is made up of three components from three allelomorphic pairs—C or c, D or d, E or e. Each parent passes on either the first or second half of his/her full genotype, e.g. CDe/cde parents hand on their CDe or cde.

- All Rh-negative people have 'd' in each half of the genotype. Where 'D' occurs in both halves of the genotype a parent is homozygous and passes on only the Rh-D-positive gene.
- Clinically significant rhesus iso-immunisation is usually against the D antigen but antibodies to C or E (and more rarely to other blood groups such as Kell, Kidd and Duffy) may also cause problems.

Sensitisation
- It may occur antenatally in 1–2% of previously unsensitised Rh-D negative women in the absence of any overt complications.
- It usually occurs at parturition due to feto-maternal haemorrhage (particularly at caesarean section).
- Other sensitising events include abortion (threatened, spontaneous or induced after 12 weeks'), invasive prenatal diagnosis, antepartum haemorrhage, external cephalic version, closed abdominal injury, intrauterine death.

Prevention
The continued occurrence of Rh iso-immunisation is due to failure to give any or enough anti-D when indicated.

Anti-D immunoglobulin 500 i.u. (100 µg) can eliminate up to 4.0 ml of Rh-D-positive blood from the maternal circulation.

- It should be given in this dose to:
  - Rh-D negative primigravidae and other previously unsensitised women at 28 and 34 weeks. This would reduce the incidence of Rh sensitisation by at least a factor of 8.
  - all Rh-D-negative women preferably within 60, but no later than 72, hours of delivering an Rh-D-positive infant (or if Rh status is unknown) from 20 weeks' gestation or after a severe placental abruption.
- If a Kleihauer test demonstrates a feto-maternal transfusion (FMT) of >4.0 ml additional anti-D must be given at a dose of 125 i.u. per additional ml.

- 250 i.u. (50 µg) should be given to Rh-D-negative women as soon as possible after a potentially sensitising event. Any FMT >2.0 ml requires additional anti-D.

Detection and prediction of severity
- Check for Rh antibodies in unsensitised women at booking, 28, 32 and 36 weeks.
- Obstetric history:
  - It tends to become more severe in successive pregnancies.
  - If at least one child has died from rhesus haemolytic disease the chance of this pregnancy ending successfully is less than 50%.

Husband's genotype:
About 75% of the fathers of affected children are homozygous $(R_1 R_1)$.

Maternal antibody levels:
- Once antibodies are detected they must be measured at least monthly thereafter.
- Serum antibody protein levels are of greater predictive value than antibody titres.
- A rapid increase suggests that acute haemolysis will be occurring in the fetus and amniotic fluid analysis is necessary.

Amniotic fluid analysis:
- Maternal IgG crosses the placenta and will cause a fetal haemolytic anaemia.
- Amniotic fluid bilirubin concentrations correlate well with the severity of the haemolysis.
- Spectrophotometry at an optical density (OD) of 450 nm shows a peak directly proportional to the quantity of bilirubin.
- If a previous pregnancy has been complicated by Rh-iso-immunisation, the first amniocentesis should be 10 weeks before the earliest previous intrauterine transfusion, intrauterine death or delivery of fatally or severely affected infant, but not before 20 weeks, gestation.
- The second should be 3 to 4 weeks later. The necessity for, and interval between, subsequent amniocenteses are determined by bilirubin levels.

Fetal blood sampling (under ultrasound guidance) to check fetal haematocrit is indicated in patients at risk of severe early disease or if amniotic fluid analysis in later second and third trimesters suggests that the baby is severely affected.

Intrauterine transfusion
If the fetus is severely affected between 24 and 31 weeks' gestation direct intravascular fetal blood transfusion (IVT) can be carried out under ultrasound guidance; transfusions can be repeated fortnightly.

It is particularly useful if hydrops is present, but should be carried out only in specialised centres.

Intraperitoneal transfusion can be used in conjunction with IVT in the absence of hydrops.

Testing the baby at birth

Cord blood is taken routinely from the babies of all Rh-D-negative mothers for Hb and film, Coombs' test and bilirubin levels.

THROMBOCYTOPENIA

Platelet mass and turnover increase in pregnancy. The count may fall slightly in normal pregnancy.

Thrombocytopenia is defined as a platelet count below $100 \times 10^9 \, l^{-1}$ but major clinical concern arises at counts at or below $50 \times 10^9 \, l^{-1}$.

The main causes of maternal thrombocytopenia in pregnancy are 'benign' gestational, auto-immune, pre-eclampsia related (see p. 63), DIC or the rare haemolytic uraemic syndrome and thrombotic thrombocytopenic purpura (see Further reading).

'Benign' gestational thrombocytopenia

This causes mild to moderate thrombocytopenia in about 7% of pregnancies. It seems to have no adverse effects on the mother or fetus. The diagnosis is more likely if the platelet count is known to have been normal before pregnancy and other causes have been excluded as far as possible.

Auto-immune (or idiopathic) thrombocytopenia (ITP)

This affects about 1/1000 pregnancies. IgG antiplatelet auto-antibodies bind to platelet-specific antigens and cause them to be sequestered in the spleen.

Maternal risks have been overstated. The major hazard is postpartum haemorrhage with an incidence of over 30% if platelet count is below $100 \times 10^9 \, l^{-1}$.

Fetal risk

The principal fetal risk is *intracranial haemorrhage* (ICH) but this too has been overstated. IgG antiplatelet antibodies cross the placenta, but maternal platelet count is a poor predictor of fetal/neonatal thrombocytopaenia. A normal platelet count in a woman who has had a splenectomy does not mean that the fetus will be unaffected.

There is no evidence that elective caesarean section reduces the risk, but it is indicated in the pre-term infant and for breech presentation.

Investigation of mother with ITP

- If platelet count $\geq 100 \times 10^9 \, l^{-1}$ check it at booking, 28, and 34 weeks, and at onset of labour.
- If count $< 50 \times 10^9 \, l^{-1}$, or if there is haemorrhage, exclude other causes.

Investigation of fetus
- Antenatal ultrasound can help to exclude intracranial haemorrhage in utero.
- Fetal scalp sampling in labour is not helpful.
- Cordocentesis will give an accurate picture of the fetal state but its morbidity does not justify its use save in exceptional circumstances.

Treatment
- Corticosteroids if maternal platelet count $<50 \times 10^9 \, l^{-1}$.
- Immunoglobulin infusion is best restricted to steroid resistant cases.
- Platelet transfusions give only short-lived benefit. They can be used to cover delivery if platelet count is $<30 \times 10^9 \, l^{-1}$.
- Any woman who has had a splenectomy should take daily oral penicillin for life to protect against pneumococcal infections.

Feto-maternal allo-immune thrombocytopenia (FMAITP)
The major risk is intracranial haemorrhage that occurs in 10–30% of affected pregnancies (5–10% before birth).

The majority of cases in a caucasian population are due to antibodies against the platelet antigens HPA-1a (75%) or HPA-5b (20%).

- Maternal platelets are normal but the fetus is at significant risk of intracranial haemorrhage.
- 50% of cases occur in the first pregnancy and it recurs in almost all subsequent pregnancies in which the fetus is antigen positive.
- There is still no routine antenatal screening test and usually no clues exist until the delivery of an affected baby.

Management
Ideal management is still not clear. If FMAITP has been confirmed in a previous pregnancy:

- Refer to a specialist centre (preferably before the next pregnancy).
- Check for maternal anti-platelet antibodies and maternal and paternal HPA status.
- Fetal HPA status can be ascertained by PCR on cell culture from *amniocentesis*.

The fetal platelet count can also be determined by *cordocentesis* and serial fetal platelet transfusions can be given if required.

Elective caesarean section is indicated if the fetal platelet count is $<50 \times 10^9 \, l^{-1}$.

IMMUNE SYSTEM

SYSTEMIC LUPUS ERYTHEMATOSUS (SLE)

This is a multisystem disease of unknown aetiology that tends to occur in women of reproductive age.

- The diagnosis rests on the presence of criteria suggested by the American Rheumatism Association (see Tan *et al*, in Further reading).
- The most helpful serological tests are anti-nuclear factor and anti-DNA antibodies.
- Pregnancy has no specific effects on SLE except for an increased risk of exacerbation during the puerperium.
- Women with SLE in pregnancy have an increased risk of:
  - First-trimester pregnancy loss
  - Lupus nephritis
  - Pre-eclampsia
  - Transient neonatal SLE—permanent congenital heart block (CHB) may occur in association with anti-Ro antibodies.
- A seemingly healthy woman delivering a baby with CHB should be observed for the development of SLE.

Management during pregnancy
- Close antenatal supervision is necessary with particular attention to serial measurements of blood pressure, renal function and fetal growth.
- The mainstay of treatment is maternal corticosteroid therapy but azathioprine may be needed in some circumstances.
- Consider low-dose aspirin.
- The timing of delivery depends on the severity of the condition, and deteriorating renal function may be an indication for early delivery.
- If the fetus has congenital heart block then caesarean section is warranted.

Lupus anticoagulant (LA) see p. 81, also known as lupus inhibitor. Other immune conditions are considered under system headings.

MUSCULO-SKELETAL SYSTEM

LOW BACK PAIN

This is one of the commonest pregnancy symptoms with over 30% of women reporting significant disability from it. It is due to the mechanical effects of pregnancy and hormonally mediated relaxation of pelvic joints.

Symptomatic relief may be obtained by reducing physical activity, rest and heat to the back. Simple analgesics should be used for pain relief. Surgery is contra-indicated.

PELVIC ARTHROPATHY

Pelvic girdle relaxation occurs physiologically in pregnancy. Separation of the pubic symphysis may be associated with pain (that can be severe) in the pubic area and groin as well as the hips and lower back. In severe cases there may be a waddling gait or limp. The symphysis pubis is tender.

The degree of symphyseal separation may not correlate with severity of symptoms.

Management includes analgesics as required, minimising exacerbating factors and rest. Pelvic support and, in severe cases, use of a walker or elbow crutches may be required. The risk of DVT must be considered if the woman is immobile (see p. 76).

Leg separation should be kept to a minimum in labour.

Spontaneous recovery is usual. Surgical fixation of the joint is rarely indicated.

NEOPLASTIC DISEASE

Pregnancy does not usually adversely affect the course of malignant disease.

CERVICAL INTRA-EPITHELIAL NEOPLASIA (CIN)

- Offer a cervical smear at the booking antenatal clinic if the woman has never had one before or not within the past 5 years.
- If the smear is abnormal carry out colposcopy (colposcopically-directed biopsies can be taken safely in pregnancy).
- CIN should be serially observed for the remainder of pregnancy and dealt with definitively at the end of the puerperium.

MICRO-INVASIVE CARCINOMA OF THE CERVIX

- Counsel regarding delaying treatment until fetal viability is reached then deliver and treat definitively (see p. 296)

INVASIVE CARCINOMA OF THE CERVIX

This poses several clinical problems in pregnancy:

- If discovered under 22 weeks' gestation advise termination followed by definitive treatment (see p. 297).
- Between 22 and 26 weeks it may be justifiable to counsel awaiting fetal viability. Then deliver in consultation with a neonatal paediatrician.
- Current evidence suggests that the mode of delivery does not affect prognosis.
- It was the cause of 1 indirect maternal death in 1997–99.

OVARIAN CANCER

Ovarian tumours of all varieties are said to complicate 1 in 1000 pregnancies, although only 1 in 20 are malignant. The frequency of tumour types is as in the non-pregnant woman (see p. 308).

Ultrasound is useful for detection of ovarian swellings.

- Treat as in the non-pregnant woman (see p. 314).
- The prognosis seems to be better for ovarian cancer in pregnancy with a 5-year survival rate of up to 75% compared with an overall 25%. This reflects the nature of the tumours in this age group.

BREAST CANCER

The prognosis for women who are pregnant at the time of diagnosis is no different from the non-pregnant when matched for disease stage.

- In the first half of pregnancy, treatment should be as for the non-pregnant woman.
  - Tamoxifen is probably best avoided in pregnancy.
  - Termination of pregnancy is not routinely necessary. The issue must be dealt with very compassionately. Current evidence suggests:
    - TOP does not improve prognosis.
    - Children of women treated for breast cancer do not appear to have an increased incidence of birth defects or childhood cancer.
- In the second half of pregnancy, delivery is advised if the fetus is viable; treatment can then begin. It may be justifiable to delay treatment for a short time to await fetal viability in some cases.

There now appears to be no contraindication to breast-feeding if it is possible following treatment.

If fertility is preserved, further pregnancies can be embarked on if desired after a post-treatment interval of at least 2 years.

LYMPHOMAS

Hodgkin's disease

This affects about 1 in 6000 pregnant women.

- Treatment should not be withheld during pregnancy except, perhaps, for early stage disease.
- In the first half of pregnancy, radiotherapy can be carried out with shielding of the uterus and ovaries.
- In women with advanced disease combination chemotherapy is usually used.
- Each case needs individual management plans.

Non-Hodgkin's lymphoma (NHL) is rarely associated with pregnancy.

Malignant melanoma
- Pregnancy appears to have no significant influence on survival.
- Termination of pregnancy is not indicated.
- Management of a melanoma found in pregnancy is as for the non-pregnant woman.
- Transplacental spread to the fetus can occur.
- Pregnancy is probably best avoided for 3 years following excision because most recurrences occur within that time.

PSYCHIATRIC CONDITIONS

POST-PARTUM 'BLUES'

This is not an illness but rather a transient mild disturbance characterised by:

- weeping
- irritability
- variation in mood
- feelings of helplessness
- sensitivity to criticism
- poor sleep
- It occurs in at least 50% of postpartum women, usually develops around the third day, and may last for a few hours or days.
- Treatment is by psychological support and reassurance.

DEPRESSIVE ILLNESS

Characterised by tiredness, lethargy, irritability and anxiety which may be more prominent than depression. It may affect at least 10% of women.

- Often brought on by psycho-social stress, and there may be a previous psychiatric history.
- Peak incidence is 3 months postpartum though depression during pregnancy is more common than previously thought.
- Maternal death from suicide occurred in 10 women from 1997–99.
- Treatment is by psychological and practical support and antidepressant drugs as necessary. Lithium should be used only when no other treatment is effective.
- A programme of postnatal care designed for the individual needs of each mother rather than the current emphasis on routine examinations has been shown to reduce depression at 4 months' postpartum (see MacArthur *et al* 2002 in Further reading').

PUERPERAL PSYCHOSIS

The incidence is about 2 per 1000 live births.

It presents either as an affective disorder with depression or hypomania, or schizophrenia with delusions and hallucinations.

- It often begins within 4 days of delivery.

- A psychiatrist must be consulted because there is risk of suicide and harm to or neglect of the baby. In 1997–99 it was associated with 9 maternal deaths.
- There is an increased risk of psychotic illness in the future, including during further pregnancies.
- Monoamine oxidase inhibitors are best avoided in pregnancy, but withdrawal must be gradual if treatment is changed.

RESPIRATORY DISEASES

BRONCHIAL ASTHMA

- Pregnancy has no consistent effect on asthma, and cases should be managed medically in the normal manner using sympathomimetic bronchodilators (e.g. salbutamol or orciprenaline) or disodium cromoglycate.
- If steroids are used, or have been recently, cover labour (for anaesthesia) with hydrocortisone (inhaled steroids do not need parenteral cover during labour).
- Status asthmaticus is treated by steroids in high doses, bronchodilators and artificial ventilation, if necessary.
- In 1997–99, there were 5 maternal deaths from asthma.

PULMONARY TUBERCULOSIS

- If the diagnosis is made during pregnancy treat with isoniazid and PAS or ethambutol.
- Breast-feeding is contraindicated if the patient has sputum-positive TB.
- The infant requires BCG vaccination and should be separated from the mother only if she has open TB and until Mantoux conversion.

CYSTIC FIBROSIS

Pregnancy occurs in women with all degrees of severity. Contraceptive advice and counselling about the risk of passing on the CF gene are, therefore, important. For pre-natal counselling see p. 39.

- Outcome for the baby is generally good but variable for the mother in proportion to her pulmonary function. There were 2 maternal deaths among women with cystic fibrosis in 1997–99.
- Combined care should be undertaken by respiratory physician and obstetrician trained in maternal medicine.
- Pregnancy should be advised against in women with *cor pulmonale*, pulmonary hypertension or when forced expiratory volume is <50% than expected.

URINARY SYSTEM

URINARY TRACT INFECTIONS

Asymptomatic bacteriuria is the presence of >100 000 organisms/ml in cultured urine in the absence of any symptoms.

- It occurs in about 5% of pregnancies
- *Escherichia coli (E. coli)* is the infecting organism in 90% of cases
- It progresses to acute pyelonephritis in 25–40% of pregnant women.
- Routine culture of a mid-stream urine (MSU) should be performed at booking because:
  - Detection and treatment prevents at least two-thirds of the cases of acute pyelonephritis.
  - Maternal anaemia and FGR may be more common in untreated cases.
  - Recurrent bacteriuria is common.

Acute pyelonephritis usually presents as a febrile illness with loin pain and vomiting.

- It needs to be differentiated from other causes of an acute abdomen.
- It is associated with pre-term labour and, sometimes, fetal death.
- Blood cultures should be taken in severe cases. *E. coli* is the commonest infecting organism.
- Treatment with appropriate antibiotic should begin while urine culture and sensitivity results are awaited. It should continue in full therapeutic doses for 3 to 6 weeks.
- Thereafter, urine culture should be performed from each antenatal visit.
- If it recurs consider maintenance antibacterial therapy for the remainder of pregnancy and for 2 weeks postpartum.

CHRONIC RENAL DISEASE

- Among the renal diseases affecting pregnancy are:
  - Chronic pyelonephritis—good prognosis if renal function adequate and normotensive
  - Chronic glomerulonephritis—women more liable to develop superadded pre-eclampsia
  - Polycystic kidneys—prognosis depends on renal function and level of BP
  - Lupus nephropathy—see p. 100.
  - Diabetic nephropathy—see p. 87.
- Pregnancy does not usually adversely affect most renal diseases with the possible exception of membrano-proliferative glomerulonephritis and lupus nephropathy.

- Both fertility and the outcome of pregnancy are proportional to the severity of renal impairment rather than specific diseases.
- Pregnancy is not advisable in women whose plasma creatinine levels are ≥200 µmol/l and whose DBP is ≥90 mmHg.

Regular antenatal assessment of the following should be carried out:

- Maternal blood pressure, renal function and urine cultures
- Fetal growth and well-being (see p. 54)

RENAL AND URETERIC CALCULI

- Pregnancy does not predispose to stone formation.
- Pain is the commonest presenting symptom.
- There may be a co-existent urinary infection.
- If this diagnosis is suspected, intravenous urography is indicated if at least two of the following are present:
  - Microscopic haematuria
  - Recurrent symptoms referable to urinary tract
  - Sterile urine culture when symptoms suggest pyelonephritis.
- Management is initially conservative, with hydration, antibiotics and analgesia. Surgery is rarely necessary.

RENAL ALLOGRAFTS AND PREGNANCY

- Chronic haemodialysis is associated with infertility, and successful pregnancy is uncommon in women receiving this treatment.
- Renal transplantation restores fertility in proportion to reproductive age and allograft function.
- Pre-pregnancy counselling using the following guidelines:
  - At least 18 months since transplant
  - Renal function stable, with no proteinuria and plasma creatinine ≤200 µmol/l
  - Normotensive (or nearly so)
  - No evidence of graft rejection
  - Immunosuppressive therapy at maintenance levels.
- All pregnancy care must be shared between obstetrician and nephrologist.
- The following general guide applies:
  - In addition to routine, maternal assessment should include screening for anaemia, any infection, and superadded pre-eclampsia.
  - Graft rejection is no more or less common.
  - Immunosuppressive therapy should be maintained.
  - Vaginal delivery should be aimed for. Caesarean section is indicated for obstetric reasons only.
  - Steroid doses need to be increased to cover delivery.
- Fetal outcome is surprisingly good, although pre-term delivery (elective and spontaneous) and FGR are more common.
  - Congenital malformations are no more common.

- Neonates may be more prone to viral or other infections.
- Data are still lacking as to whether breast-feeding is to be encouraged or not.

FURTHER READING

British National Formulary published by British Medical Association and Royal Pharmaceutical Society of Great Britain—consult latest edition

Chamberlain G and Steer P (eds) 2001 Turnbull's Obstetrics, 3rd edn. Churchill Livingstone, Edinburgh

Davey DA MacGillivray I 1988 The classification and definition of the hypertensive disorders of pregnancy. American Journal of Obstetrics & Gynecology 158: 892–8

Davison JM 1999 Chronic renal disease in pregnancy. The Obstetrician & Gynaecologist 1: 29–32

De Swiet M, Shennan A 1996 Blood pressure measurement in pregnancy. British Journal of Obstetrics and Gynaecology 103: 862

Duley L, Henderson-Smart D, Knight M, King J 2001 Antiplatelet drugs for prevention of pre-eclampsia and its consequences: systematic review. British Medical Journal 322: 329–33

Econimedes DL, Kadir RA, Lee CA 1999 Inherited bleeding disorders in obstetrics & gynaecology. British Journal of Obstetrics and Gynaecology 106: 5–13

Edenborough F P, Mackenzie WE, Stableforth DE 2000 The outcome of 72 pregnancies in 55 women with cystic fibrosis in the UK 1977–1996. British Journal of Obstetrics and Gynaecology 107: 254–261

Enkin M, Keirse MJNC, Neilson J, et al 2000 A guide to effective care in pregnancy and childbirth 3rd ed Oxford University Press, Oxford

Geary M 1997 The HELLP syndrome. British Journal of Obstetrics and Gynaecology 104: 887–891

Greer IA 1999 Thrombosis in pregnancy: maternal and fetal issues. Lancet 353: 1258–1265

Hadley A, Soothill P (eds) 2002 Alloimmune disorders of pregnancy. Cambridge University Press, Cambridge

James DK, Steer PJ, Weiner CP, Gonik B (eds) 1999 High Risk Pregnancy—Management Options, 2nd edn. Saunders, London

Knox TA, Olans LB (1996) Liver Disease in Pregnancy. New England Journal of Medicine 335: 569–575

Lakasing L, Nelson-Piercy C 1999 Anticoagulation in pregnancy. Contemporary Reviews in Obstetrics & Gynaecology 11: 239–242

Langford K, Nelson-Piercy C 1999 Antophospholipid syndrome in pregnancy. Contemporary Reviews in Obstetrics & Gynaecology 11: 93–98

Letsky EA, Greaves M 1996 Guidelines for the investigation and management of thrombocytopaenia and neonatal allo-immune thrombocytopaenia. British Journal of Haematology 95: 21–26

MacArthur C, Winter HR, Bick DE et al 2002 Effects of redesigned community postnatal care on womens' health 4 months after birth: a cluster RCT. Lancet; 359: 378–85

McColl MD, Walker ID, Greer IA 1999 The role of inherited thrombophilia in venous thromboembolism associated with pregnancy. British Journal of Obstetrics and Gynaecology 106: 756–66

Milkiewicz P, Elias E, Williamson C, Weaver J 2002 Obstetric cholestasis British Medical Journal 324: 123–4

Nelson-Piercy C, Moore-Gillon J 1996 Asthma in pregnancy. British Journal of Hospital Medicine 55: 115–7

Pop VJ, van Baar AL, Vuksma T 1999 Should all pregnant women be screened for hypothyroidism? Lancet 354: 1224–5

Redman CW, Sacks GP, Sargent IL 1999 Preeclampsia: an excessive maternal inflammatory response to pregnancy. American Journal of Obstetrics and Gynecology 180: 499–506

Reports on Confidential Enquiries into Maternal Deaths in the United Kingdom 1994–6 and 1997–9. HMSO, London

RCOG 1995 Report of the RCOG Working Party on Prophylaxis Against Thromboembolism in Gynaecology and Obstetrics. RCOG, London

RCOG 1997 Pregnancy after Breast Cancer: Guideline No 12. RCOG, London

RCOG 2001 Thromboembolic Disease in Pregnancy and the Puerperium: Acute Management. Guideline 28. RCOG, London

RCOG 1999 Use of Anti-D Immunoglobulin for Rh Prophylaxis: Guideline No 22. RCOG, London

RCOG 2001 Scientific Advisory Committee Opinion Paper

Sadler L, McCowan L, White H, et al 2000 Pregnancy outcomes and cardiac complications in women with mechanical, bioprosthetic and homograft valves. British Journal of Obstetrics and Gynaecology 107: 245–53

Smith P, Anthony J, Johanson R 2000 Nifedipine in pregnancy. British Journal of Obstetrics and Gynaecology 107: 299–307

Tan E M, et al 1982 The 1982 revised criteria for the classification of systemic lupus erythematosus. Arthritis and Rheumatism 25: 1271–7

Thornton JG 2000 Prophylactic anticonvulsants for pre-eclampsia? British Journal of Obstetrics and Gynaecology 107: 839–40

Walsh SW (ed)1998 Endocrinology of Pre-Eclampsia. Seminars in Reproductive Endocrinology 16: 1–105

Yassin AS, Eyong E, Turner P 2000 Orthopaedic complications of pregnancy. The Obstetrician & Gynaecologist 2: 41–44

7. Maternal and fetal infections

RUBELLA
Naturally acquired infection confers life-long immunity

Prevention by vaccination
- The policy of routine vaccination of girls in their early teens has made a major contribution to prevention of rubella infection in pregnancy.
- Antenatal testing for rubella antibody should be routine even when noted to be positive in a previous pregnancy.
- Non-immune women should be offered vaccination within 7 days of delivery.
- The vaccine is a live-attenuated virus and, although no cases of fetal rubella infection have been noted after vaccination, it should be avoided for 3 months before and during pregnancy.
- Accidental vaccination during pregnancy is not an indication for termination.

Clinical features
- The incubation period is 14–18 days. Affected women are infectious for the last week of incubation and the first week after the rash appears. Only laboratory tests can confirm that a rash is due to rubella.
- The virus damages mitosis which retards cell division. Major malformations are likely if infection occurs during the critical stage of organogenesis.
- The frequency of congenital infection after maternal rubella with a rash is:
  - >80% in the first trimester
  - 50% at 13–14 weeks
  - 25% at the end of the second trimester.
- Among the congenital defects associated (singly or in combination) with maternal rubella are:
  - Congenital heart disease
  - Eye lesions—cataract, chorio-retinitis, microphthalmia, glaucoma
  - Deafness

- An 'expanded syndrome' involving the liver, spleen, brain and skeleton which may lead to abortion, stillbirth, FGR, microcephaly, or mental retardation.
- Rubella-associated defects are present in almost all infants infected before 11 weeks (mainly cardiac lesions and deafness), and in 35% of those infected at 13–16 weeks (mainly deafness). Infection after 16 weeks is not usually associated with defects.

Management after maternal exposure
- Test the mother for rubella-specific IgM.
- If there is no antibody or only low titres repeat the tests 25 to 28 days after exposure:
  - No rise is reassuring.
  - A rise in titre of four-fold or more confirms recent infection.
- If infection is confirmed advice will depend on the gestation:
  - In early pregnancy chorionic villus sampling (CVS; see p. 47) can be used to locate the rubella virus in the placenta/fetus by *in situ* hybridisation.
  - In later pregnancy, fetal blood sample can be considered. Monitor fetal growth and welfare.

CYTOMEGALOVIRUS (CMV)

- CMV is the commonest primary viral infection of pregnant women. It is usually subclinical (95%).
- It may account for up to 10% of mental retardation in children up to 6 years of age.
- The information box lists some other consequences of CMV.

CMV: other consequences	
Generalised effects	Abortion, stillbirth, FGR, failure to thrive
Neurological effects	Microcephaly, cerebral palsy, optic, atrophy, deafness
Other effects	Thrombocytopenic purpura, jaundice, pneumonia

- However, of congenitally infected infants, less than 10% have serious handicaps, and only a minority of these could be detected before 28 weeks.
- Congenital infection follows primary (75%) or reinfection (25%) of the mother.
- In light of this, and since no treatment is available, routine screening of pregnant women to detect evidence of primary infection is not clinically useful.
- The virus is excreted in breast milk.
- Only CMV-negative blood should be used for transfusion in sero-negative pregnant women and all newborn infants.

VARICELLA ZOSTER (CHICKENPOX)

- Over 80% of children have had chickenpox by 10 years of age and >85% of adults who cannot remember having it are immune on testing.
- The incidence of primary infections during pregnancy is 1–3/1000 pregnancies.
- The effects on the mother range from the typical rash to life threatening viral pneumonitis, hepatitis, encephalitis (rarely).
- About 2% of fetuses are affected if maternal infection occurs in the first 20 weeks of pregnancy. The *fetal varicella syndrome* may include:
  - scarring (with dermatomal distribution)
  - eye defects;microphthalmia,chorioretinitis
  - hypoplasia of bone and muscle of a limb (usually on same side as scarring)
  - neurological abnormalities (mental retardation, microcephaly, dysfunction of bowel & bladder sphincters).
- Zoster immune globulin should be given to affected women in early pregnancy and to the infants of women affected in late pregnancy.

HUMAN PARVOVIRUS B19

- This causes 'erythema infectiosum' (Fifth disease or 'slapped cheek syndrome') possibly preceded by a non-specific febrile illness.
- The incidence is <1% of pregnancies.
- Most women with B19 infection in pregnancy have a normal infant but it may inhibit fetal erythropoiesis. This can cause severe fetal anaemia, ascites and hydrops, which can be corrected by intrauterine transfusion.

SEXUALLY TRANSMITTED DISEASES (STDs)

HUMAN PAPILLOMA VIRUS (HPV-WART VIRUS)

- This is the commonest STD
- Warts tend to grow in pregnancy—they can be treated by trichloracetic acid

HERPES SIMPLEX VIRUS (HSV)

- HSV type 2 causes 70% of herpetic genital-tract infections. Small vulval or vaginal vesicles may become painful ulcers. Diagnosis is by culture in special viral culture medium. Aciclovir cream reduces the duration of signs and symptoms.
- The fetus has no intrinsic immunity to the virus and no passive immunity during a primary maternal infection. Transmission of

herpes infection from mother to the fetus/baby is high (40%) after vaginal delivery in primary maternal infection but low (<2% in the UK) if infection is recurrent.
- The following policy is therefore suggested.

Primary infection with active genital lesions
- Delivery by caesarean section if labour occurs and if membranes intact, or within 4 hours of membrane rupture. Take viral swabs from baby (treat with aciclovir if positive or if membranes ruptured).
- If more than 4 hours since membrane rupture allow vaginal delivery because caesarean section will not reduce risk of neonatal infection.
- Take viral swabs from baby and treat him/her with aciclovir.

Secondary infection with active genital lesions
- Although the perceived risk of neonatal infection is much less, its extent is not fully known. The above policy may be adopted in the absence of good evidence to the contrary.
- Prophylactic aciclovir given near term may reduce the rate of recurrent HSV lesions at delivery, although evidence is limited and aciclovir is not licensed for use in pregnancy.
- In the Netherlands, women with recurrent genital herpes at delivery have been allowed vaginal birth since 1987. This has not resulted in an increase of neonatal herpes.
- Asymptomatic viral shedding is neither predictable or preventable. A diagnosis of neonatal herpes should be considered if the infant becomes ill unexpectedly in the first weeks of life even in the absence of risk factors for HSV infection.

HEPATITIS B VIRUS (HBV)

- Most adults recover fully and become immune after HBV infection. 10% become carriers.
- All pregnant women should be routinely screened for the HBV surface antigen (HBsAg) at booking (or when they present if previously unscreened).
- The fetus is at risk if the mother:
  - has recently had acute HBV infection (which may have been asymptomatic)
  - carries the surface antigen (HBsAg$^+$), are positive for the core antigen (eAg$^+$) but have not developed antibodies to it (eAb$^-$) or are eAg$^-$/eAb$^-$.
- Carriers who have antibodies to the e antigen of the virus (eAb+) are not infectious but should not be blood donors.
- Risks of transmissions to the fetus are given in the box.

Maternal immune status	Risk of transmission to fetus
eAg$^+$	90%
eAg$^-$/eAb$^-$	40%
eAb$^+$	10%

- Infants of HBsAg-positive mothers should be given Hep.B gammaglobulin (HBIG) within 12 hours of birth and an initial dose of HBV vaccine within 7 days. Give further doses of vaccine at 1 and 6 months. Test for HBsAg at 12–15 months.
- Advice about breast-feeding is controversial.

HEPATITIS C VIRUS (HCV)

- This is the major cause of non-A, non-B post-transfusion hepatitis and a frequent cause of sporadic hepatitis in the USA and Western Europe.
- The risk of sexual transmission is much lower than for HBV but the inoculation risk (IR) categories are as shown below (p. 115).
- Up to 80% of those infected become chronic carriers, with many progressing slowly to chronic active hepatitis and cirrhosis.
- The acute phase is often asymptomatic.
- Vertical transmission during pregnancy is much less likely than with HBV (with the possible exception of HIV$^+$ women).
- Routine screening for HCV in pregnancy is currently unwarranted.
- Pregnant women at high risk of HCV infection should have antibody testing and their infants observed for the development of hepatitis.
- HCV infection does not seem to increase the risk of pregnancy complications nor does pregnancy have any effect on HCV hepatitis.
- Although severe HCV infections have been successfully treated with interferon α, this should not be used in pregnancy because of the risk of maternal side-effects and unknown effects on the fetus.
- Avoid fetal blood sample/scalp electrode.

HUMAN IMMUNODEFICIENCY VIRUS (HIV) INFECTION

See Further reading for fuller discussion.
- Each year in the UK, around 300 children are born to women who are infected with HIV.
- Over 20 million people are infected with HIV worldwide.
- HIV infections are most commonly acquired in Europe through i.v. drug abuse. Heterosexually acquired HIV is not common in the UK but is increasing, particularly among women with a partner in a 'high risk' group (see below).

- In some areas in sub-Saharan Africa 10–30% of pregnant women are HIV infected and the incidence is increasing rapidly in SE Asia.
- The risk of mother-to-child transmission ranges from about 15–30% with lowest rates in Europe and highest in Africa.
- Transmission depends on many factors, including viral load and biological/genetic variation of HIV; presence of neutralising antibody; presence of chorio-amnionitis or other STDs; mode of delivery and breast-feeding.
- Initial reports suggested that pregnancy may increase the progression to symptomatic infection by accelerating the depletion of helper T lymphocytes and the resulting immunodeficiency. However, this has not been supported by more recent studies.
- Multidisciplinary care involving the obstetrician, HIV physician, GP and midwife is key to management.

Antenatal HIV testing
- UK data for 1997 indicated that over 70% of pregnant women with HIV infection were undiagnosed at the time of delivery.
- Voluntary antenatal screening (with informed consent) particularly of 'high-risk' women (see below) provides the opportunity to reduce risk of transmission and offer prophylactic treatment. The adverse consequences (e.g. anxiety, stigma and possible discrimination) need to be considered.
- The Department of Health has set national targets for HIV screening in the UK. By December 2002 all health authorities should have achieved an increase in uptake of antenatal testing to 90%.
- About 50% of women found to be HIV infected during pregnancy are likely to progress to acquired immune deficiency syndrome (AIDS) or the AIDS Related Complex (ARC) in 2–6 years.
- Special precautions should still be taken in handling blood and other body fluids from women at 'high risk' who refuse HIV testing (see below).

Vertical transmission
- HIV infection can occur *in utero*, during labour or delivery and from breast-feeding:
  - Intrauterine infection is defined by detection of HIV in blood from the infant (by culture or PCR) within 48 hours of birth.
  - Intrapartum infection is presumed when test results are negative in the first week of life but become positive between days 7–90 in an infant who is not breast fed.
- These definitions need to be kept under review.
- Probably about 70% of transmission occurs in late pregnancy and labour.

Reduction of vertical transmission
- Treatment of other STDs.
- Avoidance of illicit drug use.
- Anti-retroviral therapy (e.g. Zidovudine) for the mother during pregnancy/delivery and for the infant after birth.

- Combination therapy comprising zidovudine plus a second nucleoside reverse transcriptase inhibitor, and a non-nucleoside reverse transcriptase inhibitor or protease inhibitor are increasingly being recommended.
- Reduction in peri-partum exposure, e.g:
  - Delivery by caesarean section for HIV-positive women. The European Collaborative Study (see Further reading) suggested a 50% reduction in transmission with this policy.
  - Avoidance of intrapartum invasive procedures (e.g. fetal scalp electrode or blood sampling).
- Avoid breast-feeding wherever possible—in developing countries the risk of *not* breast-feeding may be the greater.
- The above measures may reduce vertical transmission to as low as 2%.
- Passive immunotherapy for baby and/or mother is being evaluated.
- Active immunisation is undergoing preliminary studies in the USA.

INOCULATION RISK (IR) WOMEN

- The information box gives those women with an increased likelihood of carrying hepatitis B virus, HIV or other agents spread by inoculation.

Inoculation risk women

- Known or suspected AIDS or ARC
- HIV antibody-positive

- HBsAg-positive/anti HBe-negative
- History of acute hepatitis in past 6 weeks[1]
- Chronic active hepatitis or cirrhosis[1]

- Childhood spent in developing world[2]
- Visit to Central Africa in past 5 years[2]
- Treated using blood products[2]

- Sexual partners of HIV-risk men[2]

- Intravenous drug abusers

[1]Can be excluded if found to be HBsAg-negative but eAg+ and eAb+
[2]Can be excluded if HIV-negative and more than 1 year since last exposure

- Babies of HIV-positive mothers are also at risk.
- All blood or other body fluids being sent to laboratories from IR women must be clearly identified. All personnel dealing with IR women should be immunised against HBV.

RISK TO MEDICAL & NURSING PERSONNEL

- The risk of HIV seroconversion after a single needlestick or sharps injury is <0.5%.

- Without vaccination, the risk of acquiring hepatitis B from an HBeAg⁺ patient after a single exposure by needle stick or sharps injury may be as high as 30%.
- All personnel at risk must be vaccinated against HBV (and seroconversion confirmed).

CARE OF IR WOMEN IN LABOUR AND POSTNATALLY

- Make sure there is a well defined policy for caring for all inoculation-risk (IR) patients including those who are HIV-positive.
- It is advised that those looking after IR women in labour should:
  - Wear adequate eye protection, protective clothing and double gloves, particularly for operative delivery
  - Avoid needle stick injuries
  - Handle body fluids with care and dispose of soiled garments as per above policy
  - Sterilise instruments by autoclave
  - Try to avoid use of fetal scalp clip and sampling to minimise risk of transmission to neonate
  - Warn paediatricians of forthcoming delivery
  - Avoid mouth-operated suction devices.

TREPONEMAL INFECTIONS

- Syphilis, yaws and pinta are all caused by treponemes which are indistinguishable morphologically and serologically.
- Clinically apparent syphilis is rare in pregnancy in the UK, but failure to diagnose it can have severe long-term effects on mother and child. Routine antenatal screening is, therefore, still indicated and cost effective.
- Syphilis is still rife in developing countries.

Screening for syphilis

- Blood is taken at booking for VDRL (Venereal Disease Reference Laboratory) or RPR (Reiter protein reagin) and TPHA (*Treponema pallidum* haemagglutination) tests.
- More specific testing is necessary if screening tests are positive, there is a history of contact or there is clinical evidence of syphilis.
- FTA[abs] (fluorescent treponemal antibody-absorbed) is the most sensitive test for syphilis.

Biological false-positive reactions (BFPR) are much commoner than true infections and may occur spontaneously in pregnancy, after blood transfusion or recent vaccination as well as many other conditions (e.g. SLE). FTA[abs] is negative in BFPR detected by other tests.

Treatment of syphilis

- Use penicillin unless the patient is allergic. (If allergy is mild use cephaloridine: if severe, use erythromycin.)
- It may be best to re-treat women in subsequent pregnancies.

Congenital syphilis

- Syphilis can have serious effects on every organ and system in the developing fetus and early maternal syphilis carries a high rate of fetal infection.
- Adequate treatment of the mother before 16 weeks of pregnancy will prevent infection in virtually all cases. Treatment after this time will still be effective in most cases.

OTHER INFECTIONS

GROUP B STREPTOCOCCAL (GBS) INFECTION

- In the UK, 15–20% of women carry GBS in the vagina at delivery.
- 40–70% of infants of mothers colonised antenatally with GBS are themselves colonised, but <1% develop evidence of infection affected by it.
- Nevertheless, GBS infections are one of the commonest infective causes of neonatal morbidity and mortality in the developed world with an incidence of 1–4 in 1000 births.
- Among the particular risk factors for the fetus are:
  - pre-term delivery
  - premature rupture of membranes before 37 weeks'
  - rupture of membranes for >18 hours at any gestational age
  - multiple births
  - maternal pyrexia in labour
  - a previous affected child.
- The mortality rate for perinatal infection can be as high as 80% despite early recognition and prompt treatment.
- Routine screening for maternal colonisation and treatment if GBS positive is controversial. The American Association of Pediatrics (AAP) has recommended routine screening at 26–28 weeks' with intrapartum antibiotic therapy for colonised women who have any of the above risk factors. However, review of the evidence so far (see Further reading) suggests that:
  - GBS is only temporarily eradicated by short term antibiotic therapy during pregancy
  - if treatment is based on a positive culture at 28 weeks up to 50% will be negative at delivery: and up to 15% of culture-negative women at 28 weeks will be culture-positive by delivery. Thus, some women would be overtreated while others would be undertreated.
- The current conclusion, which must be kept under review, is that there is insufficient firm evidence to support routine screening for GBS during pregnancy and antibiotic treatment for women found to be positive.
- However, the presence of GBS in the vagina after premature rupture of the membranes may be an indication for delivery and treatment of the infant.

BAPM recommendations for GBS

- Give intrapartum antibiotic prophylaxis specifically for GBS to the following women:
  - GBS known to be present in the vagina at any time during pregnancy
  - GBS known to be present in the urine at any time during pregnancy
  - GBS infection in a previous baby
- Give broad spectrum antibiotics when clinically indicated and ensure the regime includes adequate GBS cover in the following situations:
  - Chorioamnionitis diagnosed or suspected clinically
  - Pre-term prolonged rupture of membranes
- Consider giving inrapartum antibiotic prophylaxis in the following situations:
  - Labour is pre-term
  - Prolonged rupture of membranes in labour
  - Fever in labour

- Recommendations of the British Association of Perinatal Medicine (BAPM) are given in the information box.

GROUP A STREPTOCOCCAL (GAS) INFECTION

GAS septicaemia caused 5 maternal deaths in the UK from 1997–99. All patients died of respiratory or multi-organ failure within 24 hours of becoming ill.

These cases illustrate the virulence of GAS even in the modern antibiotic era.

BACTERIAL VAGINOSIS (BV)

- This is due to replacement of the normal vaginal flora predominately with anaerobes as is described on p. 324.
- Its presence has been associated with a ×2 increase in intra-amniotic infection and preterm birth.
- Treatment for *symptomatic* BV during pregnancy can be with intravaginal clindamycin cream or metronidazole gel.
- The effect of treatment on asymptomatic women with BV has not yet been fully evaluated. Published trials to date have not shown a significant reduction in pre-term labour.

TOXOPLASMOSIS

- Toxoplasmosis is a systemic infection caused by the protozoon *Toxoplasma gondii*. It is either asymptomatic or confused with 'flu' or other pregnancy symptoms.
- The best estimate of the incidence in pregnant women in the UK is about 2/1000.

- When acquired in pregnancy it can cause fetal infection with potentially severe sequelae, such as cerebral calcification, hydrocephalus and chorio-retinitis. The risks vary according to gestational age at infection:
  - During the first trimester, transmission to the fetus occurs in about 10% of infections. Fetal death or severe sequelae are likely.
  - During the second trimester, transmission is frequent with a high risk of congenital infection.
  - During the third trimester, transmission is very frequent but the risk of problems at birth is low. However, as many as 80% of children may develop chorio-retinitis in later years.
- The best policy is prevention by avoiding undercooked meat, unpasteurised milk, and contact with cat litter; washing all garden produce well and hands after gardening.

Testing and treating the mother
- Routine screening is not of proven benefit in the UK in light of current knowledge (see Further reading). This needs to be kept under review.
- Serological testing should be carried out on suspicion, looking for specific IgM antibody. If positive, repeat for confirmation and to check for rising antibody titres.
- If current infection is confirmed treatment of the mother with spiramycin for the remainder of pregnancy will reduce transplacental infection by 60%.

Testing and treating the fetus
- If current infection is confirmed in the mother consider the following:
  - Carry out amniocentesis and cordocentesis. Infection is confirmed if these samples contain specific IgM antibodies.
  - Check for ventricular dilatation by ultrasound at 20–22 weeks.
  - If the fetus is infected and ventricular dilatation is present counsel couple regarding termination.
  - If fetus is infected but seems normal, or parents do not wish to consider termination, treat with pyrimethamine, sulphadiazine and folinic acid for 3 weeks, alternating with spiramycin for 3 weeks for remainder of pregnancy.
  - Continue ultrasound monitoring of ventricles.
- After birth:
  - Send samples of placenta, amniotic fluid, cord and maternal blood for serology.
  - Carry out detailed clinical examination including cranial X-ray and ultrasound and ophthalmoscopy.
  - If toxoplasmosis suspected treat as above for a year.
- A further pregnancy can be embarked on once the anti-Toxoplasma IgM has disappeared. This can take from 6 months to 2 years

LISTERIOSIS

- Caused by *Listeria monocytogenes*, which is widely distributed.
- The rate of listeriosis is about 1 in 10 000 births in the UK.
- The source is usually dairy products, vegetables, meat and meat products (e.g. paté), poultry or shellfish. Pasteurisation may not eradicate the organism. It thrives at 4°C (see Further reading).
- It should be considered in all cases of 'flu'-like pyrexial illness in pregnancy, mid trimester miscarriage or pre-term delivery (particularly if the amniotic fluid is meconium stained).
- If suspected, take vaginal swabs for Gram-staining and culture, and blood cultures.
- After birth, the placenta should be examined for the organism.
- A live-born infant may develop a generalised infection, including meningitis and pneumonia.
- The organism is sensitive to a wide range of antibiotics, including ampicillin.

TUBERCULOSIS

- Among those for whom screening for TB infection should be considered in pregnancy are:
  - women in close contact with a known or suspected case
  - those recently arrived from an endemic area (e.g. Africa or Asia)
  - women who are HIV⁺ and/or i.v. drug abusers
- Diagnosis is confirmed by PPD skin testing; chest X-ray and 3 sputum samples

Treatment

- Active disease—use isoniazid (INH) with rifampicin, or ethambutol (or both) and continue until course is completed.
- If PPD⁺ but no other evidence of active disease, consider INH prophylaxis.
- If INH is prescribed, monitor liver function and give pyridoxine supplements to reduce risk of CNS toxicity.
- The baby should receive BCG vaccination. Breast-feeding is *not* contraindicated.

MALARIA

- Malaria must be considered in non-endemic areas among immigrants or tourists returning from endemic areas suffering from unexplained pyrexia.
- Parasites are seen on thick and thin blood smears.
- Treat with chloroquine if possible.
- Advise pregnant women to avoid travel to endemic areas especially those with drug-resistant strains. If such travel is unavoidable prophylaxis is strongly advised.

FURTHER READING

British Association for Perinatal medicine—www.bapm-london.org

Burrow GN, Ferris TF 1999 Medical Complications During Pregnancy (5th edn); Saunders, Philadelphia

Creasy RK, Resnik R 1998 Maternal Fetal Medicine, 4th edn. Saunders, Philadelphia

Drug and Therapeutics Bulletin 1999 HIV in pregnancy and early childhood. 37 (9): 65–67

James DK, Steer PJ, Weiner CP, Gonik B (eds) 1999 High Risk Pregnancy-Management Options, 2nd edn. Saunders, London

Nicoll A, Peckham C 1999 Reducing vertical transmission of HIV in the UK. British Medical Journal 319: 1211–1222

Ohlsson A, Myhr TL 1994 Intrapartum prophylaxis of perinatal GBS infections: a critical review of RCTs. American Journal of Obstetrics and Gynecology 170: 910–17

Reducing Mother to Child Transmissions of HIV Infection in the United Kingdom. Executive summary and recommendations. 1998. RCPCH London

RCOG 1992 Prenatal screening for Toxoplasmosis in the UK. Report of a Multidisciplinary Working Party. RCOG, London

RCOG 2001 Why Mothers Die? Report on Confidential Enquiries into Maternal Deaths in the United Kingdom 1997–9. RCOG, London

RCOG Guideline No.13 2001 Chickenpox in Pregnancy. RCOG, London

Smith J, Cowan FM, Munday P 1998 The management of herpes simplex virus infection in pregnancy. British Journal of Obstetrics and Gynaecology 105:255–268

Standing Medical Advisory Committee 1992 The diagnosis and treatment of suspected Listeriosis in pregnancy—Report of a Working Group

The European Mode of Delivery Collaboration. 1999 Elective caesarean-section versus vaginal delivery in the prevention of vertical HIV-1 transmission: a randomised clinical trial. Lancet 353: 1035–1039

Towers CV 1995 GBS: the US controversy. Lancet 346: 197–99

8. Drugs and pregnancy

DRUGS USED FOR THERAPY

The following are among the factors to consider when prescribing any drug during pregnancy and lactation:

- Most drugs, except those with a molecular weight >1000, cross the placenta and are excreted in breast milk.
- The timing of exposure to a 'teratogen' is an important factor in determining the nature and extent of adverse effects:
  - 'Pre-embryonic phase' (days 0–14 after conception)—tends to be an 'all or nothing effect' i.e. damage to all or most cells leads to death: if only a small number of undifferentiated cells are involved normal development is likely.
  - Embryonic phase (weeks 3–8)—this is most crucial period for organogenesis and is, therefore, the time of greatest theoretical risk of congenital malformation. Very few drugs, however, have been conclusively shown to be teratogenic.
  - Fetal phase (week 9 to birth)—fetal growth and development can be impaired by drugs taken during this phase. Drugs which cross the placenta may have direct actions on the fetus (e.g. warfarin may cause intra-cerebral and retroplacental haemorrhage). Some drugs given close to term or during labour may affect the neonate (e.g. diazepam or pethidine).
- Even non-prescription drugs, such as cough medicines (containing iodides), can be harmful; ointments applied to the nipple may be harmful if ingested by the infant.
- Drugs taken by the male partner and excreted in sperm must also be considered, e.g. finasteride for prostatic hypertrophy may be teratogenic to a male fetus; griseofulvin may damage sperm.

PRINCIPLES FOR PRESCRIBING DURING PREGNANCY AND LACTATION

- Drugs should be prescribed for a pregnant woman only when the indications are clear and specific, and the expected benefit to the mother is greater than the risk to the fetus.
- If at all possible, avoid all drugs in the first trimester (even non-prescription drugs).

- Prescribe drugs that have been well tried in pregnancy in preference to newer preparations.
- Drugs may be prescribed to a pregnant woman for fetal therapy (e.g. digoxin or flecainide for fetal arrythmias).
- Use the smallest effective dose for the shortest therapeutic time.

GUIDE TO PRESCRIBING DURING PREGNANCY AND LACTATION

- This can be found in the most current editions of the British National Formulary. See also other suggested Further reading.
- A National Teratology Information Service has been established to provide information on all aspects of drug use in pregnancy (Tel: 0191 232 1525).

DRUGS OF ABUSE

MATERNAL CIGARETTE SMOKING

This is associated with an increased risk of low birthweight, microcephaly and facial clefts.

It is probably the commonest preventable risk marker for late fetal death.

There is a long-term relation between smoking in pregnancy and the intellectual development of the offspring. These effects are due to:

- a direct feto-placental effect of nicotine and its metabolites.
- reduced fetal oxygenation.

ALCOHOL AND PREGNANCY

Excessive chronic alcohol ingestion is usually defined as >80 g/day (equivalent to at least eight large glasses of wine).

- It is associated with a group of fetal problems—the fetal alcohol syndrome. The incidence in North America is 1–2 in 1000 births. It is less common in the UK despite a high level of alcohol abuse in society.
- The principal features of the fetal alcohol syndrome are mental retardation, growth restriction and facial anomalies. Other congenital anomalies are also said to be more common.
- The effects of moderate alcohol ingestion (up to 40 g/day) are much more difficult to assess because an accurate drink history is difficult to obtain, and its effects are compounded by other variables such as smoking, social class, age and parity.
- There may be some women in whom the fetus is particularly susceptible to damage from even moderate alcohol ingestion.

MARIJUANA SMOKING

This is associated with a reduction in birthweight. This could be due to:

- the direct effect of cannabis
- reduced fetal oxygenation
- increase in maternal heart rate and blood pressure
- there may also be a synergistic action with cocaine.

HEROIN ABUSE

This is associated with an increased risk of pre-term delivery and low birthweight. A significant number of newborns have signs of withdrawal—up to 85% if mothers injected heroin, and over 30% for those who smoked it.

COCAINE OR 'CRACK' ABUSE

This causes marked vasoconstrictive effects on uteroplacental and fetal vessels.

- This can cause miscarriage, placental abruption, growth restriction, premature delivery, fetal distress and congenital malformations.
- It may affect the neurobehavioural development of the infant and is associated with an increased incidence of sudden infant death.

MATERNAL DEATH AND SUBSTANCE ABUSE

There were 7 deaths from drug abuse (mainly overdoses) and 4 in women who abused alcohol in 1997–99.

FURTHER READING

Briggs GG, Freeman RK, Yaffe SJ 1998 Drugs in Pregnancy and Lactation, 5th Edn. Williams and Wilkins, Maryland

British National Formulary 2001 Number 42 *et seq*. BMA and Pharmaceutical Society of Great Britain, London

Pre-conception, Pregnancy and Prescribing 1996 Drug and Therapeutic Bulletin 4: 25–27

Rubin P 2000 Prescribing in Pregnancy, 3rd Edn. BMJ, London

9. Other pregnancy problems

Definition
Bleeding from the genital tract from 24 completed weeks of pregnancy to the birth of the baby, including the first and second stages of labour.

Sources
- Separation of a placenta lying partly or wholly within the lower uterine segment—*placenta praevia.*
- Separation of a normally situated placenta—*abruptio placentae.*
- Fetal/Cord Bleeding—*vasa praevia.*
- Lesions of the cervix or vagina.
- Unknown.

Incidence
2–5% of pregnancies progressing beyond 24 weeks' gestation.

PLACENTA PRAEVIA

Definition
The placenta lies partially or wholly within the lower uterine segment. The simplest clinical classification is *minor degree* (placenta encroaches on lower segment but does not cover internal os) and *major degree* (placenta covers internal os).

Maternal risks
Among them are:

- *Postpartum haemorrhage*—the risk is increased because of the less efficient contractility of the lower uterine segment.
- *Abnormally adherent placenta (placenta accreta; see p. 170)*—may occur in about 15% of women with placenta praevia. If the woman has been delivered by caesarean section in a previous pregnancy the relative risk of adherent placenta is increased >2000. In some cases the trophoblast will have invaded through the entire thickness of the myometrium (*placenta percreta*).

- *Anaesthetic and surgical complications*—more likely if caesarean section is carried out by inexperienced medical personnel as an emergency in face of major haemorrhage.
- *Recurrence*—4–8% of women who have had placenta praevia in one pregnancy will have it again in the next.
- *Maternal death*—in 1997–99 there were 3 direct deaths due to placenta praevia in the UK.

Fetal risks
Among them are:

- Pre-term delivery.
- Fetal growth restriction (FGR)—particularly if multiple episodes of bleeding occur.
- Both placenta praevia and abruption are associated with a two-fold increase in the incidence of congenital malformations.
- Fetal haemorrhage—particularly in the presence of *vasa praevia*. This maybe partly explain the increased incidence of cerebral palsy.

Clinical features
- Vaginal bleeding—slight, moderate or heavy, most commonly occurring between 32 and 37 weeks' gestation.
- The bleeding is usually painless (in the absence of labour).
- It may have been preceded by several slight 'warning haemorrhages'.
- The abdomen is usually soft and non-tender to palpation, and the fetal heart can be heard.
- The presenting part is high, or the lie is oblique or transverse; breech presentation is common. (A persistently high presenting part or variable lie should raise the suspicion of *placenta praevia* even in the absence of vaginal bleeding.)

Management
- From home: organise immediate admission. *Do not perform a vaginal examination* because it may provoke profuse bleeding. Stop oral intake—mother may need an anaesthetic.
- In hospital: manage expectantly if haemorrhage is not severe and pregnancy has not reached 36–37 weeks:
  - localise placenta by ultrasound (see below)
  - a gentle speculum examination can be carried out when bleeding has ceased for at least 24 hours
  - keep 2 units of blood cross-matched as clinical judgement dictates
  - check for feto-maternal transfusion in Rh-D-negative women and give anti-D immunoglobulin as necessary
  - monitor fetal welfare (see p. 54)
  - the current recommendation from the RCOG is for inpatient care for third trimester. Outpatient care has not been properly assessed and should be offered only in the context of clinical trials.

Indications for intervention
- Heavy bleeding or continuous oozing is compromising maternal or fetal health.
- Moderate or heavy bleeding occurs when the pregnancy has reached 37 completed weeks or more.
- Expectant management has allowed the pregnancy to reach 38 weeks.

Mode of intervention
- If the diagnosis of a major degree of placenta praevia is certain and maternal and/or fetal health are in jeopardy, or if there is a malpresentation, carry out caesarean section.
- Where the placenta is more than 2 cm away from the internal os it may be appropriate to allow a vaginal delivery.

Localisation of the placenta
- Ultrasound is the method of choice—transvaginal scanning appears to be both safe and effective where there is difficulty visualising the placenta with abdominal scanning.
  - MRI may be appropriate, particularly where accreta is suspected.
- If a low-lying placenta is detected early in pregnancy the scans should be repeated later in pregnancy (at about 32 weeks) because the placenta may seem to 'migrate' away from the lower segment as it forms in late pregnancy.
  - Only 1 in 10 placentae thought to be low-lying early in pregnancy persists as clinically relevant placenta praevia towards term.
- A low-lying placenta discovered during an ultrasound examination for another reason and in the absence of bleeding can be managed as follows:
  - before 28 weeks—repeat the scan in 1 month
  - after 28 weeks—discuss the findings with the patient and advise her to avoid coitus. If she lives a long distance from the hospital, or if there are other adverse circumstances, it may be advisable to admit her to hospital. Repeat the scan each month.

ABRUPTIO PLACENTAE

Definition
- Haemorrhage arising from a normally situated placenta.
- *Revealed haemorrhage*—the blood tracks between the membrane and the uterine wall and escapes at the introitus.
- *Concealed haemorrhage*—a large haematoma forms between the placenta and the uterus. No external bleeding occurs.
- *Mixed haemorrhage*—combines features of the above. This is the most common.

Associated factors
- High parity and poor nutrition
- Pre-eclampsia—due to associated placental bed pathology

- Sudden reduction in uterine volume, e.g. when a patient with hydramnios loses a large volume of liquor
- External cephalic version (occasionally)
- Direct trauma (rarely)
- Smoking
- Drugs of abuse especially cocaine
- Previous abruption.

Maternal risks
- *Disseminated intravascular coagulation* (DIC) after release of thromboplastins —see page 172
- *Hypovolaemic shock*—blood loss is often underestimated, particularly if 'concealed'
- *Postpartum haemorrhage* (see p. 168)—associated with DIC or bleeding into myometrium, which interferes with uterine contraction ('Couvelaire uterus')
- *Renal failure*—acute tubular necrosis may result from hypovolaemia and intravascular coagulation within the kidney
- *Maternal death*—there were three direct deaths from placental abruption in the UK between 1997 and 1999
- *Recurrence*—may be as high as 17% after one and 25% after two previous placental abruptions.

Fetal risks
- *FGR*— mainly due to association with pre-eclampsia (see p. 59)
- *Perinatal death*—APH (probably mostly due to abruption) accounts for over 10% of all stillbirths (see p. 175)
- *Perinatal morbidity*—including 'birth asphyxia'.

Clinical features of severe placental abruption
- Intense, constant abdominal pain with or without vaginal bleeding
- A degree of shock out of proportion to extent of blood loss
- Tender, hard uterus perhaps large for dates and increasing in size
- Fetal parts may be difficult to feel
- 'Fetal distress' or absent fetal heart.

Later features
- DIC
- Oliguria (or anuria in really severe cases).

Differential diagnosis
Among them are:

- placenta praevia
- uterine rupture
- degeneration of a fibroid
- rectus sheath haematoma
- acute hydramnios
- acute surgical conditions.

Management
- Single episode of slight bleeding, mother and fetus in good condition:

- before 36 weeks' gestation—manage conservatively (as for placenta praevia) and monitor fetal welfare regularly (see p. 54)
- induce labour (if indicated) at 38 to 40 weeks.
- Severe abruption:
  - begin resuscitation at home before transfer to hospital
  - admit by ambulance with a trained paramedic crew (accompanied by midwife or GP if possible)
  - correct shock and hypovolaemia with intravenous fluids. Monitor central venous pressure and urine volume.
  - expedite delivery by amniotomy and judicious oxytocin
  - monitor FHR continuously—a trace suggestive of an acidotic (hypoxic) fetus indicates the need for delivery by caesarean section
  - a case can be made for caesarean section in some situations in which the fetus is already dead, such as when the cervix is tightly shut and amniotomy is impossible; e.g. there is, as yet, no DIC but if the uterus were not to be emptied quickly the risk of its developing would be high
  - *beware of postpartum haemorrhage.* Hysterectomy may be necessary in some rare circumstances. It must neither be carried out too soon nor too late! The judgement of a senior obstetrician is mandatory.

OTHER CAUSES OF ANTEPARTUM HAEMORRHAGE

LOCAL CAUSES

For example, vaginitis, cervical polyp or cervical ectropion. It may rarely be due to carcinoma of cervix. A gentle speculum examination will help to detect these.

UNKNOWN CAUSE

- Do not ignore antepartum haemorrhage even if its cause cannot be determined. There is a high incidence of pre-term delivery in this group.
- Fetal welfare should be monitored for the remainder of pregnancy with the patient in or out of hospital as clinical circumstances dictate.

POLYHYDRAMNIOS

Definition
An excessive volume of amniotic fluid. It can be chronic or acute; the latter can mimic abruptio placentae. It is associated with major fetal anomalies and the risks of uterine overdistension.

Associated features

- Increase in placental mass, e.g. in multiple pregnancies and maternal diabetes mellitus.
- Reduced fetal swallowing, e.g. anencephaly and spina bifida.
- Reduced fetal gut area, e.g. oesophageal, duodenal and jejunal atresia.
- Hydrops fetalis.

Consequences

These are related to uterine overdistension:

- Maternal discomfort
- Unstable lie of the fetus
- Increased incidence of pre-term labour
- If the membranes rupture prematurely there is an increased risk of:
  - prolapsed cord
  - malpresentation of fetus
  - placental abruption.

Management

- Check glucose tolerance in all except minor cases.
- Ultrasound scan for fetal anomalies.
- Mild cases can be treated conservatively.
- Amniocentesis should be considered in severe cases but it often produces only brief respite and may induce pre-term labour (up to 50%).
- Test the infant for oesophageal atresia at birth.

FETAL HYDROPS

Definition

The accumulation of fluid in some or all of the serous cavities in the fetus accompanied by generalised oedema of the skin. The placenta may also be oedematous. Fetal ascites can be an early manifestation.

Causes

Although in 15–30% of cases a cause is not identifiable, among the best recognised causes are:

- Rhesus (anti-D) iso-immunisation—at one time the commonest, now rare (see p. 96).
- Occasionally—other blood group antigens such as K (Kell), Fya (Duffy) or C and E (Rhesus).

This group of cases is 'immune hydrops'.

The remainder are 'non-immune' hydrops, due for example to:

- cardiovascular lesions—e.g. many cardiac anomalies, congenital heart block, tachydysrhythmias

- chromosomal disorders—e.g. trisomies (particularly trisomy 21), Turner syndrome, triploidy
- congenital malformations—e.g. several recognised syndromes, diaphragmatic herniae, bladder neck obstruction
- haematological—e.g. β-thalassaemia, glucose-6-phosphate dehydrogenase (G-6-PD) deficiency
- twin–twin transfusion syndrome
- infections—e.g. parvovirus B19, CMV, toxoplasmosis, rubella, syphilis
- placental and umbilical cord lesions—chorioangioma, feto-maternal transfusion, umbilical vein thrombosis
- maternal conditions—severe diabetes or anaemia, hypoproteinaemia.

Incidence
- 'Immune' fetal hydrops affects 2–3% of women with anti-D or other antibodies.
- The ratio of 'non-immune' to 'immune' causes is about 9:1.
- The incidence of 'non-immune' hydrops is about 1/1000 pregnancies.

Investigation
- Antenatal detection is possible in most cases. Cases should be referred to a Fetal Medicine Specialist.
- Ultrasound is the most important for initial detection and subsequent assessment.
- Maternal blood—blood group and antibodies; and to exclude G-6-PD deficiency, β-thalassaemia, infection. Check Kleihauer test.
- Fetal heart monitoring and echocardiography may be helpful.
- Amniocentesis—karyotype; amniotic fluid AFP, CMV culture, and specific metabolic tests as indicated.
- Cordocentesis (see p. 49)—fetal blood for IgM, karyotype, DNA analysis and metabolic tests as indicated.

Management
Depends on the cause and severity of the condition.

- Those presenting before 24 weeks tend to have a worse prognosis than those presenting later.
- Currently the only cases amenable to fetal therapy (see p. 50) are those 20–30% of cases due to high output failure (e.g. anaemia, tachydysrhythmias, hydrothorax, twin–twin transfusion syndrome).

MALPRESENTATIONS

HIGH HEAD AT TERM

Though not strictly a malpresentation it may develop into one during labour.

It is common in multiparous patients, and in one third of all primigravidae the head remains unengaged at term.

Among the potential causes to be considered particularly in primigravidae are:

- greater than average angle of inclination of the brim, e.g. in black women
- a deflexed head
- head too large to enter pelvis easily—hydrocephalus; large baby
- pelvis too small
- something in the way—placenta praevia, fibroid, the head of an undiagnosed twin
- too much room for movement, e.g. hydramnios.

A trial of labour is indicated in the absence of significant causes.

VARIABLE LIE TOWARDS TERM

There is an increased risk of cord prolapse.

If the fetal lie is persistently variable from 37 weeks' gestation admission is advised lest labour begins and/or the membranes rupture with the fetal lie other than longitudinal.

- Exclude causes such as wrong dates, placenta praevia, multiple pregnancy, and pelvic tumour.
- If the lie stabilises to longitudinal, the mother can be allowed home.
- If the variable lie persists to 41 weeks consider elective caesarean section. However, many women are unwilling to wait that long so each case must be considered individually.

BREECH PRESENTATION (see p. 154)

FACE AND BROW PRESENTATION (see p. 158)

MULTIPLE PREGNANCY

Multiple pregnancy rates have increased to 14.4 per 1000 maternities, particularly due to assisted conception techniques.

- The incidence of monozygous twinning is constant at 3.5/1000 births.
- Dizygous twinning rates vary widely because they are influenced by maternal age, parity, ethnicity and assisted conception. There is also a familial tendency.
- The incidence of triplets is about $1:80^2$ and of quadruplets about $1:80^3$.
- Perinatal mortality rates are 37/1000 for twins, 52/1000 for triplets and 231/1000 for quadruplets.

- Cerebral palsy increases 8-fold with twins and 47-fold with triplets. This is particularly but not solely associated with monozygosity.

Clinical management
- Regular antenatal clinic attendance is advised because all the hazards of pregnancy are increased:
  - Major congenital malformations are twice as common as in singleton pregnancies.
  - FGR complicates about 30% of twin pregnancies.
  - Iron and folic acid supplements are advised.
  - 10% of all pre-term labours are associated with multiple pregnancy—twins are 8 times more likely to be born <32 weeks gestation.
  - Prophylactic oral tocolytic drugs do *not* reduce the risk of pre-term labour.
- Routine admission for rest has not been shown to prolong pregnancy.
- Admit if any complications supervene (e.g. pre-eclampsia) or the cervix is effacing too soon.
- Carry out serial checks of fetal growth and welfare (see p. 54).
- Intrauterine death of one twin can occur and the risk of harm to, or death of, the surviving twin is increased thereafter (particularly in monozygous twins).

The *determination of chorionicity* is important because:

- Monochorionic (MC) twins require much greater surveillance— perinatal mortality in monochorionic twins is 5 times that for dichorionic twins.
- It also allows the risks and possible interventions to be discussed with the parents, e.g. invasive testing and pregnancy reduction for higher multiples.

Ultrasound scan before 14 weeks' will allow chorionicity to be determined in almost all cases on the basis that:

- Dichorionic twins have a thicker intertwin membrane, particularly at the chorionic plate—lambda sign.
- Monochorionic twins have a thinner intertwin membrane—'T' sign.

From 14 to 20 weeks' it can be determined in about 80% of cases but it is not sufficiently reliable after 20 weeks'.

SPECIFIC PROBLEMS WITH MONOZYGOUS TWINS

- Vascular anastomoses complicate 15% of MC twins and can cause *twin–twin transfusion syndrome* resulting in problems outlined in the box.
  - Without intervention the risk of pre-term delivery is high and fetal outlook is poor.
  - Diagnosis and management depend on detailed ultrasonography and expertise most likely to be found in a recognised Fetal Medicine Unit.

Receiving twin	Donor twin
• polycythaemia	• anaemia
• acute, severe polyhydramnios (usually in the second trimester)	• severe oligo- or anhydramnios—the fetus seems to be fixed to uterine side wall—a 'stuck twin'
• fetal hydrops	• FGR

- Therapeutic amniocentesis is likely to be necessary. For more detailed management see 'High Risk Pregnancy' in Further reading.
- In *monochorionic, monoamniotic twins* (about 1% of MZ twins) the placental circulations anastomose completely and the umbilical cords may become intertwined. This can lead to *cord entanglement*, occlusion and fetal death. The risk seems to be greater before 30 weeks so elective pre-term delivery may not be indicated.

Conjoined twins comprise 1% of monozygotic twins. The extent of the conjunction is variable.

Twin reversed arterial perfusion (TRAP) sequence is a rare complication (about 1/35 000 births). It results from arterial anastomosis allowing competition between the two circulations early in pregnancy. This results in absent or rudimentary development of the head, heart and limbs in one twin—the 'acardiac twin'. The extra load on the 'pump' twin may cause heart failure with hydrops and polyhydramnios. Pre-term delivery is likely (see Further reading).

POST-TERM PREGNANCY

A pregnancy is post-term when it extends beyond 293 days (42 weeks) from the first day of the last menstrual period (LMP).

- The risk of perinatal death is low (2.4/1000 for normally formed babies) in post-term pregnancy.
- There is no reliable evidence to suggest that routine fetal surveillance (see p. 54) will detect those at particular risk (see Enkin in Further reading).
- Meta-analysis of trials of elective induction of labour for post-term pregnancy (see Enkin) suggests that:
  - such a policy is 'not associated with any major disadvantage'
  - may reduce the already small risk of perinatal death
  - does not affect vaginal operative delivery rates while slightly reducing the risk of delivery by caesarean section.
- The mother should be allowed to make an informed choice about induction of labour.

FURTHER READING

Cox C, Grady K 1999. Managing Obstetric Emergencies. Bios, London
Denbow M and Duncan K 2000 Multiple Pregnancy. Current Obstetrics &
    Gynaecology 11, 211–217
Enkin M, Keirse M, Neilson J, et al 2000 A Guide to Effective Care in
    Pregnancy and Childbirth. Oxford University Press, Oxford
James DK, Steer P, Weiner CP, Gonik B (eds) 1999 High Risk Pregnancy—
    Management Options. Saunders. Edinburgh
RCOG Green Top Guideline. Placenta Praevia – Diagnosis & Management.
    2000. London
RCOG 2001 Why Mothers Die CEMD 1997–99 RCOG Press, London
The Cochrane Collaboration 2001. www.cochrane.org

10. Labour and intrapartum problems

NORMAL LABOUR

Normal labour is characterised by:

- Regular uterine contractions
- Dilatation of the cervix
- Descent of the presenting part.

It encompasses the time from the onset of regular contractions to spontaneous vaginal delivery of the infant (within 24 hours).

UTERINE CONTRACTIONS

- Contractions begin in two 'pace-makers' near the uterotubal junctions.
- Only one is operative in each contraction that spreads like a wave over the whole uterus.
- Relaxation begins simultaneously in all areas of the uterus.

Labour is characterised by:

- Strong and sustained action of the muscle of the uterine fundus which increases as labour progresses
- Less strong contractions of the mid-zone
- Relative inactivity of the lower segment

Normal uterine contractions are characterised by:

- A frequency of one every 2 to 3 minutes with at least 1 minute between contractions
- A duration of 40 to 70 seconds
- An intensity (measured by intrauterine catheter) of around 50 mmHg with a resting tonus of <10 mmHg.

CERVICAL DILATATION

- This occurs from above downwards accompanied by effacement (thinning).
- It is caused by co-ordinated contraction and retraction of the upper segment.

• The forewaters may act as a hydrostatic wedge, and dilatation is facilitated by close apposition of the cervix and presenting part.

FIRST STAGE OF LABOUR

Latent and active phases—see Table 10.1 and Fig. 10.1.
The latent phase starts from the onset of regular uterine contractions and ends when the cervix is 2–3 cm dilated and fully effaced. It occurs because the thinning of the lower segment and cervix take a lot of uterine work before rapid dilatation can begin. In the active phase the cervix dilates at 1–3 cm per hour in primigravidae and up to 6 cm per hour in multigravidae.

Control of uterine activity in labour
Prostaglandins are, and oxytocin may be, important for the maintenance of progressive labour.

The autonomic nervous system has little or no motor function.

Progress in labour is best assessed using a *partogram* on which can be recorded:

Table 10.1   Length of first stage of labour

| | Mean length in hours (± 1 SD) | |
	Primigravidae	Multigravidae
Latent phase	9 ± 6	5 ± 4
Active phase	5 ± 3.5	2 ± 1.5

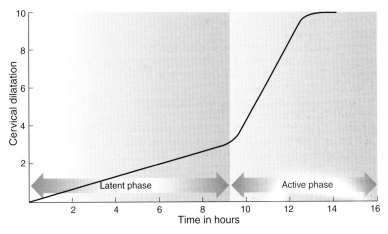

Fig 10.1   Cervical dilatation time curve

- Cervical dilatation—marked in centimetres at zero time (the time of admission to labour ward) and at every subsequent examination.
- Descent of the head (in fifths palpable above the pelvic brim).
- Contractions—frequency, duration and strength assessed for 10 minutes each half-hour.
- Fetal heart rate (see p. 150).
- Condition of the liquor and time and manner of membrane rupture.
- Moulding of the fetal skull.
- Dosage of oxytocin, if used.
- Maternal status (BP, pulse, temperature, urinalysis) and medication (including epidural block, if used).

MANAGEMENT OF NORMAL LABOUR

Each obstetric unit should set down (and review regularly) agreed guidelines for the management of labour to include a clear statement about the diagnosis of the onset of labour.

Routine perineal shaving and an enema on admission are outmoded practices.

Maternal informed choice is to be encouraged. (This includes recognition of responsibility for that choice.)

Posture
- Mobility should be encouraged during the latent phase.
- In the active phase (in the absence of complications) allow the mother to adopt the position she finds most comfortable.
- Maternal posture should at all times be as upright because:
  - the supine position tends to impair placental perfusion
  - the need for augmentation (see below) and analgesia is reduced

Normal progress
- In primigravidae delivery should be expected within 8 hours of the diagnosis of labour and achieved within 12 hours.
  Delay in primigravid labour may be due to:
  - Inefficient uterine action
  - Occipito-posterior position of the fetal head
  - True cephalo-pelvic disproportion (rarely)
- Labour is much more rapid in multiparous women, and inefficient uterine action is rare. *If delay is occurring its cause should be sought and corrected if possible.*
  Obstruction must be considered as a possible cause for prolonged labour in a multiparous woman.

Augmentation of labour in primigravidae
- This practice is widespread but remains controversial. Its aim is to achieve safe delivery within 8 hours of admission to the labour ward.

- It is usually considered if the rate of cervical dilatation is less than 1 cm per hour in the active phase of labour.
- The membranes are ruptured and oxytocin infusion is set up 1 hour later if labour does not accelerate.
- Among the contraindications are:
  - obstetric anomalies, e.g. breech presentation or multiple pregnancy.
  - fetal compromise.
- It is relatively contraindicated in multigravidae because the risk of uterine rupture is increased.
- Review of trials to date (see Enkin et al in Further reading) suggests that:
  - no beneficial effects have been demonstrated
  - women find ambulation more acceptable
  - further trials are necessary.

Oral intake in labour
- The major risk to be avoided is aspiration of gastric contents. This only occurs in the context of general anaesthesia.
- In general, therefore, low-fat, low-residue food and drink can be given to a mother during labour.
- There is no evidence that the routine use of antacids or H_2 receptor antagonists is beneficial.
- The significance of *ketonuria* is exaggerated:
  - intravenous infusions of dextrose solutions (particularly dextrose 10% are contra-indicated because of their deleterious effect on mother and baby (fetal hyponatraemia).
  - if dehydration needs to be corrected, normal saline should be infused but the volume should not exceed 3 litres/24 hours.

SECOND STAGE OF LABOUR

- It begins with full dilatation of the cervix and ends with delivery of the baby.
- Its average length in primigravidae is 40 minutes, and in multiparae is 20 minutes.
- It has two phases:
  - the *propulsive phase* from full dilatation until the presenting part has descended to the pelvic floor.
  - the *expulsive phase* which ends with delivery of the baby and is recognised by the mother's irresistible desire to bear down and/or distension of the perineum.
- A woman should not usually be encouraged to bear down until she has entered the expulsive phase.
- A prolonged propulsive phase in primigravidae due to inefficient uterine action (and not cephalo-pelvic disproportion) can be treated judiciously with oxytocin.

INDUCTION OF LABOUR

- Induction of labour can be justified when:
  - the intrauterine risks to the fetus outweigh those from delivery
  - the risk to the mother's health from the continuation of pregnancy outweighs the risk to the fetus from delivery.
- If the added risk of labour is unacceptable, delivery must be by caesarean section.
- Otherwise, labour can be induced and the maternal and fetal state monitored throughout.
- Fetal well-being should be confirmed immediately prior to induction of labour.
- A policy of offering routine induction of labour after 41 weeks reduces perinatal mortality without increasing the caesarean section rate.
- An ultrasound scan to confirm gestation should be offered before 20 weeks gestation as this reduces the need for induction for perceived post term pregnancy.
- Women who have pregnancies complicated by diabetes should be offered induction of labour prior to their estimated date for delivery (see p. 88).
- Women with pre-labour rupture of the membranes at term should be offered a choice of immediate induction of labour or expectant management. Expectant management at term should not exceed 96 hours following membrane rupture.
- 'Social' indications rarely constitute an adequate reason for induction but each situation must be considered on its merits. If offered, the cervix should be favourable.

CONTRAINDICATIONS

Absolute
- The fetal lie is not longitudinal.
- Caesarean section has been carried out in a previous pregnancy for a recurrent reason (e.g. pelvic contraction).
- Two previous caesarean sections have been performed.
- Placenta praevia.
- A tumour occupies the pelvis that will obstruct labour.

Relative
- The cervix has previously been repaired. Previous cone biopsy merits caution.
- Highly multiparous woman.

Other factors to be borne in mind
- An unfavourable cervix
- Uncertain gestational age.

HAZARDS

- *Iatrogenic prematurity*—early pregnancy dating by ultrasound reduces this risk.
- *Infection*—there is little appreciable risk in practice but amnionitis can always be detected within 36 hours of amniotomy.
- *Neonatal jaundice*—there is a small risk if the total dose of oxytocin exceeds 20 units.
- *Failed induction*—defined as failure to deliver vaginally a patient in whom safe vaginal delivery was expected. The incidence is about 2% of all inductions.

CERVICAL RIPENESS

This is assessed by a modified Bishop's score that gives marks of 0 to 3 for five cervical features—see Table 10.2.

- If the cervix is 'ripe' (score >5) induction of labour is likely to be successful
- With a score of <5 induction is more likely to fail, the latent phase will tend to be longer, and a higher total dose of medication is likely to be necessary to reach optimal uterine activity.

METHODS OF INDUCTION

- *Membrane sweeping*—should be offered to women prior to formal induction. It is associated with discomfort during the procedure and light bleeding.
- *Prostaglandins*—should be used in preference to oxytocin in both nulliparous and multiparous women with intact membranes regardless of their cervical favourability. Intravaginal PGE_2 should be used in preference to intracervical preparations, as vaginal administration is as effective but less invasive.

Table 10.2 Modified Bishop's score

	Score			
	0	1	2	3
Cervical dilatation (cm)	<1	1–2	2–4	>4
Cervical length (cm)	>4	2–4	1–2	<1
Station (cm above ischial spines)	–3	–2	–1/0	+1/+2
Consistency	Firm	Average	Soft	–
Position	Posterior	Mid/Anterior	–	–

- *Artificial rupture of membranes*—following ruptured membranes, prostaglandins and oxytocin are equally effective.

Fetal well-being should be established once contractions are established or reported.

In women with intact membranes amniotomy should be performed where feasible prior to commencement of oxytocin infusion.

Oxytocin should not be started for 6 hours following the administration of prostaglandins.

Oxytocin should be delivered through a syringe driver or an infusion pump with a non-return valve. A recommended regimen is:

- Starting dose of 1–2 milliunits/min.
- Increased at intervals of 30 minutes or more.
- Minimum dose should be used, titrated against uterine contractions aiming for a maximum of 3–4 contractions every 10 minutes.
- Adequate contractions may be established at 12 milliunits/min although doses up to 32 milliunits/min are sometimes needed.
- As labour becomes established the dose of oxytocin may need to be reduced to avoid hyper-stimulation, particularly in multigravidae.

Water intoxication has occasionally followed the infusion of large volumes of fluid containing dilute oxytocin. Confusion and convulsions can proceed to coma and even death. *This is totally avoidable*.

For more discussion see Further reading.

Fetal heart rate monitoring is necessary if induction is being carried out for fetal reasons and during oxytocin infusion.

PAIN IN LABOUR

Pain is a normal part of labour and delivery although emotional, cultural and other influences alter individual responses.

CAUSES OF PAIN IN LABOUR:

- Dilatation of the cervix
- Accumulation of pain-producing substances due to ischaemia during uterine contractions
- Pressure on other organs (e.g. bladder and rectum) or the lumbo-sacral plexus; spasm in skeletal muscles
- Distension of vagina and perineum.

Sensory pathways are T10 to L1 for both uterine body and cervix. T11 and 12 are stimulated during the latent phase when pain is not severe, T10–L1 are stimulated during the active phase. Referred pain is experienced in the dermatomes of the above segments.

FACTORS AFFECTING PAIN IN CHILDBIRTH
Physical factors

- Intensity and duration of contractions
- Speed of dilatation of cervix
- Vaginal and perineal distension
- Others, e.g. age, parity, size of infant, condition of patient.

Physiological factors
- Pain blocking, e.g. customs, culture, preparation, distractive activity
- Pain aggravating, e.g. customs, culture, fear, apprehension, anxiety, ignorance, misinformation
- Antenatal preparation of the mother and father is very important.

ANALGESIA

Antenatal education is a vital part of preparing women for the pain of labour.

METHODS FOR PAIN RELIEF
Psychological methods
- Counteract the 'fear-tension' sequence.
- Pain-relieving drugs can be used to supplement the mother's own efforts.
- With proper preparation and support, up to 30–40% of women can go through labour without requiring analgesic drugs.

Inhalational agents
- Nitrous oxide (50%) and oxygen (50%)—'Entonox' apparatus
- Inhalational agents are often used too late and too hesitantly
- They can be highly effective and appear safe for mother and baby.

Transcutaneous electrical nerve stimulation (TENS)
- This aims to reduce pain by stimulating large myelinated nerve fibres to reduce input from small myelinated and non-myelinated fibres linked to peripheral pain receptors.
- Low-intensity continuous stimulation is applied to the dermatomes associated with the pain.
- It can provide good to moderate pain relief but success depends on time spent teaching and supporting the mother before and during use.

Narcotic drugs
- e.g. intramuscular pethidine

Note: combination with a phenothiazine (e.g. promazine or promethazine) provides no additional benefit, may produce maternal and fetal tachycardia and can rarely cause an oculogyric crisis. It should, therefore, not be used.

Advantages
- Ease of administration
- Reasonably rapid analgesia
- Low incidence of serious side-effects
- Antagonists available.

Disadvantages
- Inadequate analgesia in up to 40% of patients
- Nausea and vomiting common
- Psychic disturbances common (e.g. confusion, inability to cooperate)
- Delayed gastric emptying
- Neonatal respiratory depression.

Contraindications
- Previous idiosyncratic reactions
- Current mono-amine oxidase inhibitors.

Epidural analgesia
Despite its widespread use, little is known about the short or long term effects of epidural block on mother or baby.

Lumbar analgesia will provide total or adequate analgesia in over 90% of patients.

Indications
Epidural analgesia can be helpful for:

- prolonged labour
- maternal distress
- multiple pregnancy
- instrumental delivery
- hypertension in labour
- breech presentation.

Contraindications
- Lack of experienced personnel
- Infection at the injection site
- Coagulation defects or bleeding diathesis
- Anticoagulant therapy
- Shock & hypovolaemia
- Bony abnormalities of the spinal column
- Idiosyncratic reactions to local anaesthetic agents.

Pre-existing neurological disease is not necessarily a contraindication as long as it is understood that coincidental relapses can occur unrelated to the epidural block.

Immediate maternal problems

- *Dural tap*—dural puncture by needle or catheter; it may lead to 'spinal' headache (see below).
- *Total spinal block*—loss of all sensory and motor function; can include unconsciousness, severe hypotension and apnoea; it results from subarachnoid injection of epidural dose of local anaesthetic agent.
- *Hypotension*—can be avoided by nursing the patient on her side and by the intravenous infusion of Hartmann's solution before the block is established (also used for treatment of hypotension).
- *Motor paralysis*—reduces maternal expulsive effort, tends to prevent rotation of the fetal head and makes instrumental delivery more likely. Motor block may be reduced by modification of anaesthetic agents used (see below).
- Prolongation of *second stage* of labour.
- *Toxic reactions* to local anaesthetic agents.

Delayed maternal hazards

- Severe *spinal headache* due to spinal tap.
  - Ensure adequate hydration and analgesia.
  - Infuse 1 litre of normal saline through the epidural catheter over 24 hours.
  - If no improvement within 48 hours consider a 'blood patch' (i.e. injection of up to 20 ml autologous blood into epidural space).
- *Urinary retention ?*—more usually due to method and circumstances of delivery.
- *Sepsis*—extremely unlikely if bacterial filter is used.
- Temporary diminished sensation of dermatomes affected.
- *Local backache* is an occasional temporary problem. Chronic long-term backache is not.

Fetal effects

There are no direct adverse effects on the fetus. Temporary changes in the fetal heart rate, sometimes related to hypotension, are not uncommon.

Guidelines for use

- The regional block may be continuous during labour or as a single injection for operative delivery.
- Bupivacaine (0.5, 0.375 or 0.25%) is the preferred anaesthetic—a test dose should be injected initially. Lower concentrations of Bupivicaine (0.1–0.25%) combined with an opiate (e.g. fentanyl) reduce the motor block and may allow a 'walking epidural'.
- Anaesthetic agents are often given by continuous infusion.
- Constant monitoring of maternal and fetal condition is mandatory.
- Top-up dose must be individually chosen when the patient begins to experience discomfort.

Epidural analgesia and previous caesarean section

Epidural block is permissible in any woman who is being allowed to labour having previously been delivered by caesarean section. FHR should be monitored throughout. Significant FHR abnormalities may be a sign of scar dehiscence (and see p. 171).

PRE-TERM LABOUR AND DELIVERY

Definition
Regular, painful uterine contractions accompanied by effacement and dilatation of the cervix after 20 and before 37 completed weeks of pregnancy. It accounts for 5–10% of all deliveries but 85% of neonatal deaths.

FACTORS ASSOCIATED WITH PRE-TERM DELIVERY

- Spontaneous labour—cause unknown: 40%
- Spontaneous labour due to maternal or fetal conditions other than multiple pregnancy: 25%
- Multiple pregnancy: 10%
- Elective delivery: 25%

CAUSES OF SPONTANEOUS PRE-TERM LABOUR

These are given in the information box (roughly in order of importance).

Spontaneous pre-term labour: causes	
• Multiple pregnancy	• Congenital uterine anomaly
• Antepartum haemorrhage	• Diabetes
• Intrauterine growth restriction	• Polyhydramnios
• Cervical incompetence	• Pyelonephritis
• Amnionitis	• Other infections

PREDICTION OF RISK

- No scoring system yet devised has proven itself superior to clinical judgement.
- The strongest association is with previous pre-term delivery. Among the measures suggested for prediction of high risk and possible prevention and for which no evidence of benefit exists are:
  - routine cervical examination
  - home monitoring of uterine activity
  - prophylactic beta-sympathomimetics
  - routine screening for bacterial vaginosis
  - prophylactic antibiotics
- It has, however, been suggested that the risk tends to increase the shorter the cervix measured by vaginal ultrasound from 20–28 weeks. See information box over:

Length of cervix (at or below centile)	Length of cervix (mm)	Relative risk of preterm delivery
75th	40	2
10th	26	6
5th	22	9.5
1st	13	14

MANAGEMENT

Management varies according to five main factors:

- *The state of the membranes*—it is generally inadvisable to inhibit pre-term labour when the membranes are ruptured.
- *Dilatation of the cervix*—labour is likely to progress if the cervix is >4 cm dilated
- *Gestational age*—the earlier the gestation, the more strenuous attempts to inhibit labour must be. Labour should be allowed to progress if the estimated fetal weight is >2000 g or gestation is >34 weeks.
- *The cause of pre-term labour*—delivery is indicated if fetal welfare is prejudiced.
  - Carry out an infection screen on the mother and consider amniocentesis for bacteriological culture if suspicion of chorio-amnionitis.
  - Assess fetal well-being (see p. 54).
- *The availability of neonatal intensive care facilities*—if all cots are full or facilities are inadequate consider transfer of the patient (in good time) to a unit with better facilities.

Glucocorticoid therapy and the prevention of respiratory distress syndrome

- Corticosteroids given to the mother between 24 and 34 weeks can induce pulmonary surfactant in the lungs of the immature fetus and reduce the severity of respiratory depression syndrome.
- One regimen is dexamethasone or betamethasone 12 mg i.m. on 2 successive days. Where the risk of pre-term labour is very high (e.g. triplet pregnancy) this may be repeated two-weekly to 34 weeks.

INHIBITION OF PRE-TERM LABOUR

In up to 50% of patients contractions will stop spontaneously and the pregnancy will continue to term without any treatment whatsoever.

The clinical problem is to discern correctly those in whom drug therapy is indicated.

β-sympathomimetic drugs

- These drugs (e.g. salbutamol or ritodrine hydrochloride) suppress uterine activity.
- Prolongation of pregnancy is, however, not necessarily beneficial to the fetus.
- The only true indication for their use is to delay delivery for long enough to allow:
  - glucocorticoids to stimulate fetal lung surfactant (see above)
  - transfer of the mother to a centre with adequate facilities for preterm delivery.

Potential side-effects

- Maternal tachycardia
- Hypotension
- Palpitations, headache, visual disturbances, skin flushing, nausea and vomiting
- Fetal tachycardia
- Hyperkalaemia
- Hyperglycaemia
- Rarely right heart failure may develop (usually when glucocorticoids have also been given).

Contra-indications:

- Antepartum haemorrhage
- Severe pre-eclampsia
- Maternal anti-hypertensive therapy (risk of myocardial infarction)
- Maternal cardiac disease or thyrotoxicosis
- Any other situation in which the prolongation of pregnancy could be hazardous
- Extreme caution must be exercised if the woman has diabetes, or is being treated with corticosteroids.

Other tocolytics

- Atosiban—oxytocin receptor antagonist. Licensed for the inhibition of uncomplicated pre-term labour between 24 and 33 weeks of gestation. Reported to have fewer side effects than β-sympathomimetics but more expensive.
- Indomethacin and nifedipine have also been used, but their use is unlicensed.

METHOD OF DELIVERY IN PRE-TERM LABOUR

- If the fetus is viable it must be delivered by the route least likely to cause trauma or hypoxia.
- Aim to have an experienced neonatal paediatrician present for delivery.
- In general, aim for vaginal delivery if the presentation is cephalic.
- Caesarean sections at very early gestation <26 weeks, and with infants under 1000 g, can be hazardous for the mother, and are not necessarily safer for the baby.
- The indications for caesarean section are stronger but not absolute in multiple pregnancy and breech presentation.

- Ventouse delivery should be avoided below 34 weeks.
- Pre-term labour is unpredictable and the woman may become fully dilated quickly and silently.

PRE-LABOUR RUPTURE OF THE MEMBRANES (PROM)

This is defined as rupture of the membranes before the onset of labour without reference to gestational age.

- It can be managed conservatively before 34 to 36 weeks' gestation unless intrauterine infection is present or likely to develop. In the absence of infection prophylactic erythromycin should be given for 10 days.
- A high vaginal swab should be taken on admission. If it grows any significant organisms (particularly beta-haemolytic streptococci), delivery should be expedited and the neonatal paediatricians alerted.
- Any intrauterine infection must be treated vigorously and expeditiously (see 'Further reading').
- In term pregnancies 86% of women with PROM go into labour within 24 hours and deliver satisfactorily. The rate of spontaneous labour after this is about 5% per day. In the absence of any evidence of infection or cord presentation/prolapse, the onset of labour can be awaited for 24 hours. Expectant management of women with pre-labour rupture of the membranes at term should not exceed 96 hours following membrane rupture.

INTRAPARTUM FETAL MONITORING

Prior to any form of fetal monitoring, the maternal pulse should be palpated simultaneously with fetal heart rate auscultation in order to differentiate between maternal and fetal heart rates.

The aim of monitoring is to detect fetal hypoxia. The *effects of hypoxia* depend on the fetal glycogen reserves. A growth-restricted fetus will, therefore, be affected earlier and more severely than a well-nourished fetus.

- Anaerobic glycolysis results in an accumulation of lactate. This causes a fetal metabolic acidosis.
- The fetal pCO_2 rises, causing a respiratory acidosis.
- The blood pH falls.
- Fetal heart rate (FHR) patterns change (see below) the most serious being late decelerations associated with a fetal tachycardia.

Fetal distress
The traditional diagnosis of 'fetal distress' depended predominantly on the crude observation of heart changes.

'Fetal distress' is an imprecise and rather unhelpful term. Half of all babies delivered by forceps or caesarean section because of 'fetal distress' are not hypoxic; and half of the most hypoxic babies do not exhibit classical signs of 'fetal distress'.

METHODS OF INTRAPARTUM MONITORING

Intermittent auscultation of FHR using a fetal stethoscope
- In the active stage of labour this should occur after a contraction for a minimum of 60 seconds, and at least:
  - Every 15 minutes in the first stage.
  - Every 5 minutes in the second stage.
- It is applicable to low-risk patients with no significant obstetric abnormalities.
- More intensive monitoring should be used if any risk factors are present (see below).

Continuous monitoring of FHR and uterine activity (cardiotocography; CTG)
- The FHR is obtained by an external Doppler ultrasound monitor or an electrode attached to fetal scalp.
- The monitor measures the interval between paired beats, converts it into 'beats per minute' (bpm) and registers it.
- Uterine activity can be assessed by an external strain gauge transducer or measured by intrauterine catheter.
- This is a screening technique that facilitates the detection of fetal hypoxic stress. It is not diagnostic.
- Even when the most ominous pattern is present (see below) only 50% of the babies have a low Apgar score (see p. 188) at birth.
- The use of continuous FHR recordings must therefore be backed up by measurement of fetal scalp pH (see below).

Guide to indications for continuous FHR monitoring in labour

Antepartum risk factors
- Previous caesarean section
- High multiparity
- Suspected FGR
- Hypertension/pre-eclampsia
- History of APH in this pregnancy
- Poor obstetric history
- Diabetes
- Multiple pregnancy
- Rhesus iso-immunisation
- Oligohydramnios
- Reduced fetal movements
- Abnormal antenatal FHR tracing.

Intrapartum risk factors
- FHR >160 or <110 bpm
- Meconium-stained liquor
- Prolonged labour
- Epidural anaesthesia
- Augmented or induced labour
- Pre-term labour
- Breech presentation
- Prolonged rupture of membranes.

Interpretation
The whole clinical situation must be considered particularly gestational age, stage and progress of labour.

Normal pattern
- Rate between 110 and 160 bpm observed over a 5 or 10-minute period to determine the baseline.
- Baseline irregularity/variability of ≥5 bpm.
- No significant reduction in rate during contractions.

Loss of baseline irregularity (<5 bpm)
- This is the feature most commonly associated with fetal hypoxia
- Maternal drug administration can also reduce it
- Regard as:
  - *suspicious* if it lasts for up to 40 minutes
  - *pathological* if it lasts for >90 minutes

Management: check fetal pH.

Baseline bradycardia (FHR <110 bpm)
Regard as significant if it is:

- accompanied by loss of baseline irregularity and/or decelerations (i.e. complicated bradycardia)
- and/or is <100 bpm.

Management: turn the patient on her side, give oxygen and check fetal pH.

Baseline tachycardia (FHR >160 bpm)
Management: measure fetal pH if tachycardia persists or it is accompanied by decelerations and/or loss of baseline irregularity.

Accelerations
Transient increases in FHR of 15 bpm or more and lasting 15 seconds or more. This is normal and reassuring.

Decelerations
Transient episodes of slowing of FHR below the baseline level of more than 15 bpm and lasting 15 seconds or more.

Early decelerations:

- Uniform, repetitive, periodic slowing of FHR with onset early in the contraction and return to baseline at the end of the contraction.
- It may be due to head compression, cord compression or early hypoxia.

Management: check fetal pH if the pattern deteriorates or persists.

Late decelerations:

- Uniform, repetitive, slowing of FHR with onset mid to end of the contraction and nadir more than 20 seconds after the peak of the contraction and ending after the contraction.
- The greater the lag time the more serious the significance.
- The worst picture is of shallow late decelerations, loss of baseline irregularity and tachycardia.

Management: a fetal pH measurement is mandatory.

Variable decelerations:

- Variable, repetitive, periodic slowing of FHR with rapid onset and recovery. Time relationships with contraction cycles are variable and they may occur in isolation.
- Sometimes they resemble other types of deceleration patterns in timing and shape.
- If they appear consistently, fetal hypoxia is likely.

Management: check fetal pH if the pattern persists after turning the patient on her side (or if other adverse features are present).

FHR in the second stage of labour
- The fetal heart patterns are complex and may be difficult to interpret in the second stage of labour.
- The CTG trace should be interpreted in conjunction with the pattern in the first stage of labour.
- Brief profound early decelerations are not uncommon but persistent late decelerations or prolonged bradycardia must not be ignored.

Fetal ECG
- Uses the same scalp clip as for the FHR
- It depends on analysis of the ST waveform
- The following adverse features have been suggested:
  - T/QRS ratio >0.25
  - a negative T wave
  - ST depression with T elevation
- Its main benefit is to provide reassurance in the presence of an abnormal CTG and, perhaps, reduce the rate of unnecessary caesarean sections.

Fetal blood sampling (FBS)
- FHR and scalp pH measurement are complementary.
- The former without the latter increases the caesarean section rate unnecessarily because of false positive diagnoses.
- The indications for FBS are outlined above.
  - A fetal scalp pH of 7.0 or less is strongly associated with a poor outcome (particularly if the Apgar score is 3 or under at 5 minutes)
  - A pH of 7.20 or less suggests the need to deliver
  - A base deficit of >12 mmol/l is also abnormal

Significance of meconium staining of the liquor
- Meconium is present in the liquor of about 15% of all deliveries at term and up to 40% post-term.
- It's significance as a diagnostic sign of 'fetal distress' has been over-emphasised although gross staining is more likely to be significant.

- Aspiration by the baby of the liquor heavily stained with meconium causes a severe and sometimes fatal pneumonitis.

Conclusion

The sensitivity and specificity of all methods for intrapartum monitoring of the fetus are still poor. New initiatives are still badly needed. For further discussion see NICE guidelines and Enkin *et al* in Further reading.

THE NORMAL PELVIS

AVERAGE DIAMETERS

PELVIC SHAPE—IN THE NORMAL PELVIS

- The brim is round, and the sacral promontory is not prominent.
- The angle of inclination is about 55° to the horizontal.
- The cavity is shallow with straight, non-converging walls.
- The sacrum is smoothly curved.
- In the outlet the sacro-sciatic notches are wide and shallow.
- The sacrum does not project forwards.
- The ischial spines are not prominent.
- The pubic arch is wide and domed.
- The sub-pubic angle is about 90°.
- The inter-tuberous diameter is wide

PELVIMETRY

- Clinical assessment of pelvic size and shape is only likely to be of benefit if the pelvis is severely contracted.

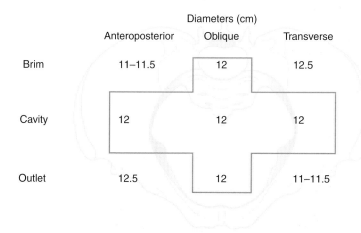

	Diameters (cm)		
	Anteroposterior	Oblique	Transverse
Brim	11–11.5	12	12.5
Cavity	12	12	12
Outlet	12.5	12	11–11.5

Fig 10.2 Normal Pelvis

- X-ray pelvimetry has been superseded in many places by CT scanning. This reduces the radiation dosage and is likely to be more accurate.
- However, the criteria for normality have not yet been set.
- Pelvimetry is of no clinical value if the presentation is cephalic.
- There is also no reliable evidence of benefit for the traditional indications of primigravid breech presentation or after caesarean section for suspected disproportion. Pelvimetry after previous caesarean section has been shown to increase caesarean section rates in subsequent pregnancies.

CEPHALO-PELVIC DISPROPORTION (CPD)

Definition: The failure of the head to pass through the pelvis safely because the pelvis is too small and/or the head too large

- CPD is more likely if maternal height is 1.5 metres or under.
- The diagnosis is made in labour if the fetal head fails to descend and the cervix to dilate. With increasing oedema of the scalp, *caput* forms and excessive moulding of the skull bones occurs.

MANAGEMENT

- Elective section is rarely necessary in primigravidae unless there are other indications e.g. a malpresentation or the true conjugate is <7.5 cm.
- Otherwise an attempt at vaginal delivery is justifiable. This is then regarded as a *trial of labour.*
  - A trial of labour should be allowed to continue for as long as progress is occurring in labour with regular forceful contractions.
  - If the woman has not delivered within 12 hours of the onset of regular contractions the situation must be reviewed critically.
  - *Such a trial of labour has no place in multigravid women or in the presence of a breech presentation.*

ABNORMALITIES OF LIE, PRESENTATION AND POSITION

BREECH PRESENTATION

Incidence
3–4% of all labours. Up to one-third are undiagnosed.

Definitions
- Frank breech (65%)—both legs extended at the knee.
- Complete breech (10%)—both legs flexed at hip and knee.
- Footling breech (25%)—one or both feet tucked underneath the buttocks; more common in multiparous women due to laxity of abdomen.

Causes
- Extended legs preventing spontaneous version
- Those conditions preventing the presenting part entering the pelvic cavity
- Uterine anomaly
- Chance.

Associations
- Fetal anomaly
- Pre-term delivery
- Multiple pregnancy.

Antenatal management
- Spontaneous version is likely up to 34 weeks but may occur later.
- External cephalic version (ECV) is safe for mother and baby in carefully selected patients and reduces the need for elective caesarean section. It should be actively offered and discussed.
- ECV is not advised before 36 weeks'. Tocolytic agents may increase success rates. Do not use in women with heart disease, diabetes or thyroid disease.
- ECV at term will reduce non-cephalic births by up to 60%. Over 95% remain cephalic.

Hazards of ECV. See the information box.

Hazards of ECV	
• Pre-term labour	• Cord accident
• Placental abruption	• Uterine rupture (if previous section)

Contraindications to ECV. See the information box.

Contraindications to ECV	
Absolute	*Relative*
• Multiple pregnancy	• Previous caesarean section
• APH	• FGR
• Ruptured membranes	• Hypertension
• Oligohydramnios	• Rhesus iso-immunisation
• Significant fetal anomaly	• High multiparity
• Caesarean section indicated for other reasons	• Anterior placenta
• Placenta praevia	• Obesity

Prerequisites for ECV
- Gestation at least 36 weeks'

- Recent ultrasound to confirm presentation, normal fetus and adequate liquor volume
- Reactive FHR
- Informed consent of mother
- Facilities for rapid progression to caesarean section, if necessary
- Rh-D-negative women must be given anti-D immunoglobulin (50 μg or more as Kleihauer test dictates).

Management of delivery
Current evidence suggests that:

- Vaginal breech delivery is safe for 97% of babies in whom there are no other risk markers (see below).
- However, the overall risk of perinatal death for the term singleton breech delivered by planned caesarean section is reduced by 75% [Relative risk (RR) 0.23; Confidence interval (CI) 0.07–0.8].

Thus, women should be offered an elective caesarean section if ECV is declined or unsuccessful.

Although there is insufficient evidence to support routine caesarean section for the delivery of the pre-term breech and the first or second breech twin, most obstetricians would now recommend caesarean section for the pre-term breech or if twin one is breech.

Some mothers will still opt for an attempt at a vaginal breech delivery and should be further assessed (see below).

Pre-delivery assessment
- There is no evidence that routine pelvimetry is beneficial. It has not been shown to improve outcome. If thought to be necessary use CT pelvimetry (see p. 154).
- Carry out ultrasound assessment of BPD, fetal mass, fetal attitude and flexion/extension of fetal head.
- Major fetal anomalies should have been excluded.

Vaginal delivery
- An attempt at vaginal delivery can be considered with:
  - Term pregnancy and fetal weight estimated at 2500–3800 g
  - Frank or complete breech
  - Presumed or demonstrated normal pelvic dimensions
  - No other complications of pregnancy (e.g. pre-eclampsia)
  - Normal fetal assessment
- Epidural anaesthesia can be useful during a breech labour but is not essential.
- Augmentation of labour with oxytocin should only be used with extreme caution and close monitoring. It is contraindicated if there is any evidence of disproportion.
- The baby should be born by the patient's own efforts with little assistance from the obstetrician (assisted breech delivery).

- Any more active intervention involving breech extraction is contraindicated because the perinatal consequences are so severe.

Caesarean section

Among the definite indications are any medical or obstetric complications that are likely to be associated with mechanical difficulties at delivery or a compromised fetus:

- Any abnormality of bony pelvis
- Fetal weight estimated at >3.8 kg
- Hyperextension of fetal head
- Previous difficult labour

- FGR
- Bad obstetric history

- Diabetes

- Severe pre-eclampsia

- Failure to progress in first stage
- Failure of descent of breech in second stage
- Any condition which would apply whatever the presentation, e.g. fetal hypoxia.

OCCIPITO-POSTERIOR POSITION

Incidence: approximately 20% in *early* labour.

If the baby's head is partially extended it does not fit into the lower uterine pole well, with the following consequences in labour:

- The membranes rupture early and the cervix is not well apposed to the cervix.
- The sinciput reaches the pelvic floor first and, therefore, rotates to the front, i.e. the occiput is posterior.
- The larger occipito-frontal diameter (10 cm) of the head presents, making its passage through the pelvis more difficult.
- The first stage of labour is prolonged.
- The moment of the forces pushes the head posteriorly causing backache and inducing bearing-down efforts before full dilatation.
- The second stage of labour may be prolonged.

The occiput may:

- Rotate anteriorly and deliver relatively easily (75%)
- Persist posteriorly (POP) and delivery spontaneously if the pelvis is capacious (i.e. face to pubes) or require assisted delivery (5%)
- Begin to rotate anteriorly but undergo deep transverse arrest at the level of the ischial spines. Instrumental delivery will be required (20%).

Predisposing factors
- Slight reduction in pelvic inlet
- Large baby

Diagnosis
Antenatally—this is inaccurate:

- the maternal abdomen may be flattened or fetal parts palpable easily on both sides of the midline.
- the head is unengaged and feels larger than usual.

Intrapartum—by vaginal examination:

- both fontanelles can be felt more easily.
- moulding and caput may make recognition difficult and palpation of an ear may be necessary for correct positioning.

Management
- Provide adequate analgesia: an epidural anaesthetic is ideal.
- Prevent 'maternal distress', ketosis and dehydration.
- Observe progress in labour carefully.
- Monitor fetal welfare.
- Syntocinon may be used *with care* only in primigravidae to encourage spontaneous rotation to occipito-anterior.

Relative cephalo-pelvic disproportion may occur and there is an increased risk of instrumental delivery and caesarean section.

The criteria for assisted delivery are discussed on p. 164.

BROW PRESENTATION

Incidence: approximately 1/1000

A brow presentation discovered antenatally may be due to:

- chance—and may correct itself spontaneously
- a swelling in the neck causing extension of the head, e.g. goitre, cystic hygroma
- spasm of the sterno-mastoid muscles.

Suspect a brow presentation in a multiparous woman with delay in the first stage of labour despite good contractions when she has delivered vaginally easily before.

Diagnosis
- Supra-orbital ridges and anterior fontanelle palpable p.v.
- Confirm by ultrasound.

Management
- In early labour a brow presentation may flex to become a vertex or extend further to a face presentation. Both are potentially deliverable vaginally.
- If the brow presentation persists into, or is discovered in, established labour delivery should be by caesarean section.

FACE PRESENTATION

Incidence: approximately 1/500. (75% mento-anterior).

A face presentation has the same causes as a brow presentation but causing full extension of the head on the neck.

In labour, anterior rotation of the chin is essential: a mento-posterior position cannot deliver vaginally.

Diagnosis
Palpation of supra-orbital ridges and the alveolar margins (confusion may arise between a face and the breech).

Management
An attempt at vaginal delivery should be allowed unless:

• Something is obstructing the entry into the pelvis.
• The pelvis is too small.
• The chin is posterior.

TRANSVERSE AND OBLIQUE LIE

Incidence: approximately 1/300

Among the causes are:

• High multiparity
• Pre-term labour
• Multiple pregnancy
• Uterine anomaly
• Hydramnios
• Obstructing tumour or placenta praevia
• Severe pelvic contraction.

Antenatal management
See p. 132.

Intrapartum management (singleton pregnancy)
In a neglected shoulder presentation an arm may well be prolapsed and the baby already dead. In these circumstances vaginal decapitation may be possible but only by an experienced operator. This is very seldom performed in the UK.

Otherwise caesarean section with decapitation *in utero* is less hazardous for the mother.

SHOULDER DYSTOCIA

Incidence: about 0.2–1%.

This is one of the most frightening obstetric emergencies

It occurs when the fetal shoulders fail to negotiate the pelvic inlet

Prompt (but not forcible) action is required to prevent fetal morbidity or mortality (see Stirrat and Taylor in 'Further reading')

Antenatal risk factors
• Mother's birthweight >90th centile
• Maternal obesity or massive weight gain

- Diabetes mellitus—can be *despite* seemingly good blood sugar control
- Prolonged pregnancy (beyond 42 completed weeks)
- Previous shoulder dystocia (10% risk of recurrence) or large baby
- Recognised macrosomia this pregnancy.

Intrapartum risk factors
First stage:

- 'dysfunctional labour'
- secondary arrest after 8 cms.

Second stage:

- midcavity arrest
- need for midcavity instrumental delivery in multiparous woman.

Prediction
- Consideration of above risk factors predicts fewer than 20% of cases!
  - Where practiced it has not reduced fetal asphyxia or trauma.
  - When interpreted too rigidly many women will have unnecessary interventions.
- Clinical prediction of excessive birthweight is unreliable.
- Ultrasound estimates are inaccurate at upper centiles.

Risks to the baby
- Neurological injury—occurs in 1–2/1000 births. It can involve:
  - cervical cord
  - brachial plexus—Erb's palsy (C5,6,7): Klumpke's palsy (C7,8,T1)
  - phrenic nerve.
- Hypoxic ischaemic encephalopathy (HIE)—0.5–1/1000 births
- Fractures: clavicle (2–3/1000); humerus (0.2–0.3/1000).

Management
- Recognition and recording of possible risk factors (keep good records!)
- Clear plan of action in guidelines
- Rapid reaction—the midwife has a vital role
- Immediate response:
  - call for help—summon experienced obstetrician, anaesthetist and paediatrician
  - place woman in 'McRoberts position', i.e. hip joints fully abducted, rotated outwards and flexed with thighs touching maternal abdomen. This encourages release of the anterior shoulder.
  - make good-sized episiotomy.
- *Next steps:*
  - Apply suprapubic pressure to try to encourage the anterior shoulder to flex and rotate transversely.

- Attempt to deliver posterior shoulder if unable to deliver anterior (adequate analgesia needed for this and manoeuvres below).
- Try to dislodge and rotate fetal shoulders vaginally (Wood's screw manoeuvre).
- Cephalic replacement following tocolysis and delivery by caesarean section (Zavanelli manoeuvre) has been described but only as a 'desperate solution'.
- Symphysiotomy may allow delivery as a last resort, but is seldom used in the UK.

MULTIPLE PREGNANCY AND LABOUR

TWINS

- Pre-term labour is common.
- Placenta praevia may be present.
- Prolapse of the cord must be watched for.
- Malpresentations are more likely—the presentations in order of frequency being:
  - Vertex: vertex
  - Vertex: breech
  - Breech: vertex
  - Breech: breech
  - Vertex: transverse
  - Breech: transverse.

POSSIBLE INDICATIONS FOR ELECTIVE CAESAREAN SECTION

- First twin presenting as a breech
- Triplets and higher multiples
- Proteinuric pre-eclampsia
- Any indication which would also apply in singleton pregnancies, e.g. FGR, APH.

MANAGEMENT OF LABOUR AND DELIVERY

- An intravenous line should be set up; a paediatrician and an anaesthetist should be present for delivery lest rapid general anaesthesia becomes necessary.
- An epidural is often useful, particularly to assist in delivery of the second twin.
- After vaginal delivery of the first twin, check the lie is longitudinal. External cephalic version is usually possible. If necessary, presentation can be checked by portable ultrasound in the delivery room. The second sac should be ruptured once uterine activity begins.
- If contractions do not begin within 15 minutes, commence an oxytocin infusion.
- If the cord of the second twin prolapses, proceed to ventouse extraction (if the presentation is cephalic) or breech extraction (if the presentation is breech).

- Anaesthesia for the latter should be epidural if already established, or general.
- *The interval between delivery of the first and second twins should be no more than 20 minutes.*
- *Beware of postpartum haemorrhage.* The third stage should be actively managed and a syntocinon infusion given if the uterus is poorly contracted.
- After delivery check placentae and membranes for zygosity. Histological confirmation is necessary.

OPERATIVE OBSTETRICS

EPISIOTOMY

The need for an episiotomy is a matter for experienced clinical judgement. 'Routine' episiotomy is no longer practiced.

Indications
Among these will be:

- When a major perineal tear appears inevitable
- In cases of fetal distress late in the second stage
- Most forceps deliveries (except low cavity forceps)
- Pre-term delivery
- Breech delivery
- Failure to advance because of perineal rigidity.

Technique
An episiotomy must be:

- Performed at the correct time—incise too early and unnecessary blood loss will result.
- Carried out with adequate local or regional anaesthesia. Failure to use anaesthesia is to be deprecated.
- Made with sharp scissors in the correct place. The medio-lateral episiotomy is more common in the UK. Midline incisions increase the risk of third degree tears. The episiotomy must always start in the midline.
- Repaired properly within as short a time of delivery as possible.

Side-effects
- *Pain.* This can be severe and is the main reason for avoiding episiotomy. It can be reduced by prompt, careful and expert repair.
- *Bleeding.* The average blood loss is about 100 ml and much larger losses are all too common.
- *Breakdown.* Inversely related to the expertise of the person repairing the episiotomy.
  - potential causes are delay in suturing, inappropriate suture materials and bad technique.

- primary repair with antibiotic cover should be carried out where possible.
- *Dyspareunia*. This can be so severe that it becomes a factor in marital breakdown.

THIRD- AND FOURTH-DEGREE PERINEAL TEARS

All women having a vaginal delivery should have a systematic examination of the perineum, vagina and rectum to assess the severity of damage prior to suturing.

Third-degree tears involve the external anal sphincter muscle. Fourth-degree tears also involve the rectal mucosa.

- They must be repaired in theatre under epidural or general anaesthesia by an experienced obstetrician.
- Give broad spectrum intra-operative and post-operative antibiotics to reduce infection risk and wound dehiscence.
- Use of stool softeners such as lactulose and a bulking agent such as Fybrogel for 10 days is recommended.
- If the repair breaks down eradicate local sepsis before attempting another repair.
- The prevalence of anal symptoms is reported to be 25–57%.
- Women should be followed up at 6 weeks and 6 months.

Subsequent delivery

Discuss the possibility of recurrence and deterioration of faecal symptoms. If symptomatic, offer elective caesarean section, as there is risk of deterioration in symptoms.

There is no evidence regarding the role of prophylactic episiotomy.

INSTRUMENTAL DELIVERY

Potential indications

- Failure to advance in the second stage, frequently due to failure of maternal effort, epidural analgesia and/or malposition of the fetal head
- Maternal conditions in which (prolonged) expulsive efforts may be detrimental e.g. cardiac and respiratory disease, severe pre-eclampsia or eclampsia
- 'Fetal distress' in the second stage
- Prolapse of the cord in the second stage

Delivery can be by the vacuum extractor (ventouse) or obstetric forceps.

The ventouse must not be considered as an easy way out when adverse features are present or the position of the fetal head is unknown.

Prior conditions for instrumental delivery
- A legitimate indication must be present.
- The presentation must be suitable, i.e. vertex, face (mento-anterior —not ventouse!) or after-coming head in a breech delivery.
- There must be no cephalo-pelvic disproportion. Moulding of the fetal skull must not be excessive.
- The head must be engaged. Ideally, no part of the fetal head should be palpable per abdomen, and if more than 1/5 can be palpated vaginal delivery must not be contemplated.
- The position of the head must be known.
- For forceps, the cervix must be fully dilated.
- The ventouse can, in some circumstances, be used before the cervix has reached full dilatation (see below).
- Analgesia must be adequate.
- The bladder must be empty.
- The uterus must be contracting.

Forceps to the after-coming head (ACH) in a breech delivery
This is the method of choice for delivery of the ACH because of the degree of control the operator can exercise.

Forceps in the delivery of low birthweight infants (<2500 g)
Lift-out forceps neither protects against nor induces birth trauma in LBW infants. Rotational forceps are best avoided for LBW infants. Ventouse should be avoided <34 weeks.

'Trial of forceps'
- This is justifiable when it is likely, but not entirely certain, that vaginal delivery by forceps will be successful. Otherwise the patient should be delivered by caesarean section.
- It should be carried out in a theatre by an experienced obstetrician, with the mother fully prepared for caesarean section to reduce delay in delivery if unable to deliver vaginally.

The use of the ventouse
Vaginal delivery is technically possible before full dilatation *but should not be attempted if there is any suspicion of cephalo-pelvic disproportion.*

The following points are a guide to its proper use:

- The patient's expulsive efforts are used to assist delivery.
- The fetal head must be at least at the level of the spines.
- The largest possible of the four cups should be used.
- If delivery is not imminent after pulling on the ventouse during three contractions the attempt must cease and the patient must be delivered by caesarean section.

Analgesia for instrumental delivery
- Perineal infiltration alone is suitable for episiotomy, and low outlet deliveries using the ventouse or 'outlet' forceps.

- Pudendal nerve block is useful for mid-cavity forceps and some ventouse deliveries. It does not provide adequate analgesia for rotational forceps. The transvaginal route is recommended for insertion of the block.
- Epidural anaesthesia is ideal particularly for rotational forceps; it is also suitable for emergency caesarean sections in which an existing epidural block is providing good analgesia.

CAESAREAN SECTION

Definition of classes of caesarean section adopted by the RCOG:

- *Emergency*—immediate threat to life of woman or fetus.
- *Urgent*—maternal or fetal compromise that is not immediately life threatening.
- *Scheduled*—needing early delivery but no maternal or fetal compromise.
- *Elective*—at a time to suit the patient and the maternity team.
- *Perimortem*—carried out in *extremis* while the mother is undergoing active resuscitation to save the fetus or the mother.
- *Postmortem*—carried out after the mother has died in order to try to save the fetus.

The overall caesarean rate in the UK is about 20%, but there are wide variations between regions and individual hospitals.

- It must not be carried out without good reasons.
- It is indicated when delivery must be effected rapidly for fetal and/ or maternal reasons and when it is not thought to be safe vaginally.
- The transperitoneal lower segment caesarean section accounts for virtually all of the operations in modern obstetrics.
- Classical caesarean section is very occasionally indicated, e.g. for transverse lie with PROM, or for caesarean section at 26 to 28 weeks. In this latter situation, the vertical incision starts in the lower segment but extends into the upper segment.

Epidural or spinal anaesthesia and caesarean section

Advantages
- It is safer for the mother.
- She is awake and sees the child at delivery.
- The father can usually be present.
- Consciousness is not impaired immediately post-operatively.
- Post-operative problems and pain are less than after general anaesthesia.
- Breast-feeding and mobilisation can start early.

Disadvantages
- The procedure takes longer.
- Occasionally anaesthesia is not complete. Therefore the patient should be fully prepared for general anaesthesia (GA).

- Contraindications to epidural/spinal anaesthesia are discussed on p. 144.

SOME IMPORTANT TECHNICAL POINTS ABOUT LOWER SEGMENT CAESAREAN SECTION (LSCS)

- H_2-receptor antagonists should be given pre-operatively to reduce the risk from aspiration of acid gastric contents.
- This also applies to procedures using epidural/spinal block lest conversion to GA becomes necessary.
- Induction of GA should take place at the last possible moment to reduce fetal exposure to the anaesthetic agents.
- The operation is carried out with a 10–15° left lateral tilt to prevent supine hypotension.
- A cuffed endotracheal tube must be used.
- Special care must be taken in Rh-negative women to remove residual blood from the peritoneal cavity because some of it may be Rh-D-positive fetal blood.
- Thrombo-prophylaxis must be considered (see also p. 75):
  - Low risk—early mobilisation and hydration.
  - Moderate risk—subcutaneous heparin and/or mechanical methods.
  - High risk—heparin prophylaxis and leg stockings.

DELIVERY IN SUBSEQUENT PREGNANCIES

- Elective caesarean section is advised if the cause is recurrent (e.g. CPD)
- If vaginal delivery is attempted, oxytocin must be used with extreme care and only with the strongest of indications. (It may be helpful to monitor intrauterine pressure).
- Epidural anaesthesia can be used; the pain of ruptured uterus will break through the epidural block.
- Significant increased risk of placenta accreta if placenta praevia.

MATERNAL MORTALITY AND CAESAREAN SECTION

See Further reading and Chapter 12.

- There were 40 *direct* and 51 *indirect* deaths in women who had a caesarean section in the UK in 1997–1999.
- The main associated causes of *direct* deaths (in order of frequency) were:
  - Hypertensive disease   12
  - Thrombosis   11
  - Sepsis   6
  - Haemorrhage   4
  - Amniotic fluid embolism   2
  - Trauma/other   1

- Surgical case fatality rates are a combination of the risk associated with the disorder for which the surgery is performed and that of the procedure itself (including anaesthesia and peri-operative care).
- The *direct* death case fatality rate for following caesarean section was:
  - About ×5 greater than for vaginal delivery.
  - ×12 greater for emergency caesarean section
  - ×2 greater for elective caesarean section.
- *Substandard care* was deemed to be a factor in a significant number of cases, the main criticisms being:
  - lack of facilities and staff for 'high risk' cases
  - failure to understand the severity of the woman's condition
  - misjudgement of fluid balance and transfusion requirements
  - inappropriate delegation or assumption of responsibility

Clear guidelines should be set for perimortem and postmortem caesarean sections and be made known in all Obstetric and Accident & Emergency Units.

FURTHER READING

Chamberlain G, Steer P (ed) 2001 Turnbull's Obstetrics, 3rd edn. Churchill Livingstone, Edinburgh

Creasy RK, Resnik R 1998 Maternal Fetal Medicine, 4th edn. Saunders, Philadelphia

Enkin M, Keirse MJNC, Neilson J, et al 2000 A guide to effective care in pregnancy and childbirth. Oxford University Press, Oxford

Hankins GDV, Clark SL, Gilstrap L, Cunningham G 1995 Operative Obstetrics. Appleton Lange

Iams JD, et al 1996 The length of the cervix and the risk of spontaneous premature delivery. New England Journal of Medicine 334: 567–72

James DK, Steer PJ, Weiner CP, Gonik B (eds) 1999 High Risk Pregnancy-Management Options, 2nd edn. Saunders, London

National Institute for Clinical Excellence. Clinical Guideline C 2001 The use of electronic fetal monitoring. NICE, London

National Institute for Clinical Excellence. Clinical Guideline D 2001 Induction of Labour. NICE, London

O'Driscoll K, Meagher D 1986 Active management of labour, 2nd edn. Saunders, London

RCOG, Greentop Guideline No.29. 2001. Management of third- and fourth-degree perineal tears following vaginal delivery. RCOG, London

RCOG, Greentop Guideline No.20. 2001. Breech presentation. RCOG, London

RCOG 2001 Why Mothers Die 1997–1999. The fifth report of the Confidential Enquiries into Maternal Deaths in the United Kingdom. RCOG Press, London

RCOG Clinical Guideline No. 1 (B) 2002. Tocolytic drugs for women in preterm labour. RCOG, London

RCOG Scientific Advisory Committee Opinion Paper 3, 2002 Intrauterine infection and perinatal brain injury RCOG, London

Stirrat GM, Taylor RW 2002. Mechanism of obstetric medial plexus palsy: a critical analysis. Clinical Risk 8: 218–222.

11. Third-stage problems and obstetric emergencies

THE NORMAL THIRD STAGE OF LABOUR

The third stage begins with delivery of the baby and ends with expulsion of the placenta.

Management
'Physiological' management *of the third stage involves:*

- division of the umbilical cord only when pulsation has ceased
- delivery of the placenta by maternal effort and aided by gravity without cord traction
- use of oxytocics only if haemorrhage occurs.

This policy allows blood volume to equilibrate between mother and baby and avoids side-effects of oxytocin.

'Active' management *of the third stage has become routine over the past 20 years in the UK and is associated with a 40% reduction in blood loss overall. This involves:*

- syntometrine (syntocinon 5 units; ergometrine 0.5 mg) with delivery of the anterior shoulder
- delivery of the placenta by *controlled cord traction (CCT)* after separation has occurred.

POSTPARTUM HAEMORRHAGE (PPH) AND RETAINED PLACENTA

Definition
Primary postpartum haemorrhage is the loss of 500 ml or more of blood within 24 hours of delivery.

Incidence
- Incidence 5%. Blood loss of >1000 mls is probably more significant and complicates 1–2% of deliveries.
- 0.5% of women require a blood transfusion of 2 units or more after a PPH.
- It accounted for 1 death in the UK in 1997–99; another 5 were associated with other problems such as hypertension, sepsis and anaesthesia.

Postpartum haemorrhage and retained placenta: associated factors	
• High multiparity (associated with uterine atony) • Polyhydramnios • Maternal age of 35 years or over • Delivery after an APH	• Past history of PPH (due to placenta praevia or abruptio placentae) • Multiple pregnancy • Coagulation disorders

Associated factors

These are listed in the information box.

Main causes

• Retained placenta (in part or whole)
• Uterine atony
• Soft tissue lacerations
• Coagulation Disorders

Management

Prevention

Proper management of the third stage, e.g. do not 'fiddle' with the uterine fundus while waiting for placental separation.

Treatment

• Rub up a uterine contraction.
• Correct hypovolaemia by intravenous fluids and screened Group O, Rh-D negative blood where necessary.
• Remove the placenta if it is retained or incomplete under general or epidural anaesthesia.
• Check for vaginal, cervical or uterine lacerations.
• Treat specific condition e.g. uterine atony:
  • *Conservative*: bimanual compression
  • *Medical*:
    • intravenous syntometrine 10 u bolus.
    • Intravenous Syntocinon Infusion—10 u/hour
    • Ergometrine bolus
    • IM or intramyometrial hemabate (PGF2α).
  • *Surgical*:
    • 'Brace suture'- see Further reading
    • Uterine packing inc. Sengstaken tube
    • Reduction of uterine vascularity, e.g. internal iliac artery ligation or uterine artery embolisation
    • Hysterectomy—neither too soon or too late
    • Repair trauma.
• Deal with coagulation failure as described on page 172.

Management of massive haemorrhage
(see Confidential enquiry 1997–99 in Further reading)

Prompt and decisive action is necessary: every labour ward must have a protocol for management with which all staff are familiar—ORDER.

O: Organisation—summon appropriate staff

R: Restoration of blood volume—2 large i.v. cannulae; crystalloid followed by O neg blood until cross-matched blood arrives.

D: Defective blood coagulation—baseline tests and correct clotting defects.

E: Evaluation of response—monitor BP, pulse and urine output. Titrate fluid replacement to pulse.

R: Remedy the cause of bleeding.

MORBID ADHERENCE OF THE PLACENTA (PLACENTA ACCRETA)

- This is a rare occurrence. Note increased rates of accreta with previous section (see p. 125).
- Remove as much placenta as possible under anaesthesia.
- Transfusion is often necessary.
- Placenta accreta often requires hysterectomy to secure haemostasis.

CORD PRESENTATION AND PROLAPSE

Cord prolapse complicates 0.2% of deliveries. It is associated with all factors maintaining the presenting part high above the pelvis or when it does not fit well into the pelvis at the time of rupture of the membranes, for example:

- transverse lie
- polyhydramnios
- cephalo pelvic disproportion (CPD)
- pre-term labour
- multiple pregnancy
- breech presentation.

Diagnosis
The cord is visible or palpable in the vagina. Consider if fetal distress occurs in association with spontaneous rupture of the membranes.

Management
Elevate the presenting part:

- Displace the presenting part with the examining hand.
- Fill the bladder with 750 ml of normal saline by indwelling catheter.
- Drop the end of the bed or stretcher.
- Keep the patient in the knee–elbow position until delivery can be effected.

Rapid delivery
- If the cervix is fully dilated, expedite delivery with forceps (or breech extraction perhaps).
- If the cervix is not fully dilated, arrange urgent caesarean section.

EMERGENCY PROCEDURES

UTERINE RUPTURE

Uterine rupture caused one maternal death in the UK from 1997–99. The main associated factors were:

- previous caesarean section scar
- the inappropriate use of oxytocin to augment labour (e.g. in multiparous women)
- failure to recognise obstructed labour.

Signs and symptoms
- Anything from lower abdominal discomfort to severe 'bursting' pain (which will even break through an epidural block)
- Unexplained maternal tachycardia
- Variable amounts of vaginal bleeding
- Fainting and ensuing shock
- Cessation of contractions
- Disappearance of the presenting part from the pelvis
- Fetal distress
- Possibility of an unrecognised rupture must be considered when bleeding continues after delivery despite well-retracted uterus, or there is unexplained shock (particularly if mother was delivered by forceps or has had a previous caesarean section).

Management
- Arrange immediate laparotomy.
- Replace circulating volume—as for major haemorrhage.
- Carry out the least extensive surgery compatible with the patient's immediate health and future welfare.
- Take great care to identify the ureters and exclude them from any sutures.

Future pregnancies
Close observation is required during any future pregnancy, and delivery should be by elective caesarean section at 38–39 weeks.

UTERINE INVERSION

- Complicates 1 in 2000 deliveries, even after appropriate management of the 3rd stage.
- Profound shock in 40% of cases.

- Haemorrhage in 90% of cases.
- The inversion may not be complete and, therefore, not immediately visible. Diagnosis is by vaginal examination, pelvic mass or sometimes protruding from vagina.

Management
- Try to reduce the inversion manually—successful in one third of cases.
- Initiate resuscitation.
- GA may be required for replacement.
- If the placenta is still attached and easy to remove, do so, once the shock has been corrected.
- The hydrostatic method for reduction is usually effective:
  - 2 litres of warm saline are infused rapidly into the vagina (use a silastic ventouse inside the vagina) and the even hydrostatic pressure exerted usually reduces the inverted uterus.

AMNIOTIC FLUID EMBOLISM

This caused 8 maternal deaths in the UK in 1997–99.

Associated factors
- Precipitate labour
- Polyhydramnios
- Hypertonic uterine action (with or without oxytocin)
- Induction or augmentation of labour in 5 of 8 maternal deaths in 1997–99.
- Increasing age—the rate begins to increase dramatically from 35 years of age.

Signs and symptoms
- Prodromal symptoms, e.g. shivering
- Maternal hypoxaemia, cyanosis and cardiovascular collapse
- Severe coagulation defect
- 'Fetal distress'.

Management
- General supportive measures as necessary in individual cases
- Endotracheal intubation and administration of oxygen and hydrocortisone (i.v.)
- Control coagulation defect.

COAGULATION FAILURE

Main causes in pregnancy
- Placental abruption
- Amniotic fluid embolism
- Endotoxic shock.

Diagnosis
- Clinical observation—including bleeding from abnormal sites
- Whole blood clotting time (normal 5–10 minutes)
- Thrombin clotting time—a sample of blood added to a tube containing a small amount of thrombin should clot within 10 seconds
- Reduction in platelet count
- Reduced fibrinogen titres
- Increased levels of fibrin degradation products.

Management
- The coagulation defect is usually self-limiting if the stimulus producing it is removed. Therefore, the uterus should be emptied as expeditiously as possible.
- Transfuse—see Management of massive haemorrhage (p. 170).

ACUTE ABDOMINAL PAIN IN PREGNANCY

The differential diagnosis of acute abdominal pain can be difficult in pregnancy.

CAUSES INCIDENTAL TO PREGNANCY

Examples include:

- appendicitis (see below)
- accident to ovarian cyst
- acute cholecystitis
- renal calculus
- intestinal obstruction
- volvulus
- perforated peptic ulcer
- rectus abdominis haematoma.

Appendicitis *can be difficult to diagnose in pregnancy because:*

- the appendix is displaced upward
- the site of pain is often atypical
- examination is made difficult by the pregnant uterus
- the body's reaction (e.g. leucocytosis) may be masked.

CAUSES RELATED TO PREGNANCY

Causes may be related to early or later pregnancy, as indicated in the information box.

Early pregnancy	Later pregnancy
• Abortion (including septic) • Cornual (or other ectopic) pregnancy • Acute retention of urine due to retroverted gravid uterus	• Abruptio placentae • Uterine rupture • Severe pre-eclampsia • Degeneration of fibroid • Pyelonephritis • Extrauterine pregnancy

FURTHER READING

American Academy of Family Physicians 1999. Advanced Life Support Course Manual. American Academy of Family Physicians, Missouri

Bonnar J 2000 Massive Obstetric Haemorrhage. Best Practice & Research in Obstetrics & Gynaecology—Obstetric Emergencies. Harcourt Publishers Ltd

Cox C, Grady K 1999 Managing Obstetric Emergencies. Bios, London

RCOG Green Top Guideline 2000 Placenta Praevia—Diagnosis & Management. London

RCOG 2001 Why Mothers Die CEMD 1997—1999. RCOG Press, London

RCOG Strat OG Programme 2001 Module 1 Perioperatice Obstetrics. RCOG, London

Steer P (ed) 1999 High Risk Pregnancy —Management Options. Saunders, Edinburgh

The Cochrane Collaboration 2001. www.cochrane.org

12. Perinatal and maternal mortality

Definitions

Livebirth: the complete expulsion or extraction from its mother of a product of conception, irrespective of gestational age, which then breathes or shows any evidence of life, such as beating of the heart, pulsation of the umbilical cord, or definite movement of voluntary muscles.

Stillbirth: birth of an infant who shows no evidence of life after birth.

Death, fetal (prenatal death): death of a fetus *in utero* which, at birth, weighs 500 g or more irrespective of gestational age.

Death, infant, early neonatal: death of a liveborn infant occurring less than 7 completed days (168 hours) from the time of birth.

Death, infant, late neonatal: death of a liveborn infant after 7 completed days of age but before 28 completed days.

The perinatal period: this commences when a fetus has developed to a weight of 1000 g (approximately equivalent to 28 weeks' gestation); it ends when the newborn baby has achieved an age of 7 completed days (168 hours) of life.

- In the absence of measured birthweight, a body length of 35 cm is considered equivalent to 1000 g birthweight
- When neither birthweight nor body length has been measured, a fetus is considered to have entered the perinatal period when the gestational age has reached 28 completed weeks (196 days).

PERINATAL MORTALITY

The perinatal mortality rate (PMR) is the number of stillbirths and first-week deaths occurring from 24 completed weeks of pregnancy to 7 days after birth per 1000 live and stillbirths.

- If an infant is born before 24 weeks' gestation and shows signs of life but then dies within 7 days it is included as a perinatal death.
- The RCOG recommends that births from 20 weeks' gestation (or fetal weight 300 g and above if gestation not known) should be notified.

- National perinatal statistics should include, as minima, infants with birthweight >500 g *or* at least 22 completed weeks *or* crown-heel length at least 25 cm
- For international statistics the minima should be birthweight 1000 g, gestational age 28 weeks or crown-heel length 35 cm.

The *post-neonatal mortality rate* is the number of infants who die between 28 completed days and 1 year after live birth per 1000 live births.

Mortality rates in the UK in 1999 are shown in the information box.

Mortality rates in the UK in 1999[#]

Perinatal mortality rate	8/1000 live & stillbirths
Stillbirth rate	5/1000 live & stillbirths
Neonatal mortality rate	4/1000 live births
Post-neonatal mortality rate	2/1000 live births

to the nearest whole number & excluding legal abortions

IMMEDIATE CAUSE OF PERINATAL AND POSTNEONATAL DEATH

The main determinants in 1998 are shown in Table 12.1:

Table 12.1   Main causes of perinatal and postnatal death in 1998

Stillbirth (SB)*	%	Neonatal death (NND)	%	Post-NND	%
Unexplained	49	Immaturity	49	Congenital malformations	28.5
Congenital malformations	12	Congenital malformations	23	SIDS[#]	25
Antepartum haemorrhage	11	Intrapartum events	10	Infection	20
Intrapartum related events	9	Infection	9	Immaturity	12
Maternal disorder	5			Accident	5
Pre-eclampsia	4			Intrapartum related events	1
Infection	3.5				

*excludes legal abortion
#Sudden infant death syndrome.

FACTORS INFLUENCING PMR

Birthweight
PMR and birthweight are closely related. In singleton pregnancies:

- The lowest PMR is in babies born with a birthweight of over 3000 g.
- 70% of perinatal deaths occur in the 6% of babies born weighing <2500 g
- 45% of SBs and 57% of NNDs occur in the 1% of babies <1500 g.

FGR is associated with a four-fold increase in PMR even when congenital anomalies are excluded.

Social class
The PMR rises as social class falls—from 6 for class I to about 11 for Class V. This may be partly explained by maternal smoking.

Maternal age and parity
- The PMR is still at its lowest in mothers between the ages of 25 and 29 years and highest for those under 20 or over 35 years of age.
- It is also at its lowest for the second child but increases from the fifth.
- These are influenced by social class and the association of congenital anomalies with age.

Mother's country of birth
The PMR varies with the mother's country of birth as shown in Table 12.2.

Multiple births
For multiple births the overall SB rate is 3–4 times and the NND rate 8–9 times that for singleton pregnancies. This is strongly associated with immaturity (see also p. 133).

Table 12.2 Perinatal mortality rate relating to the mother's origin

Mother's country of origin	PMR/1000 total births
UK	8
Bangladesh	9.5
India	11.3
Caribbean	11.5
E. Africa	12.4
Pakistan	15.8

Sub-optimal care

The fact that a stillbirth is unexplained does not mean that it was unavoidable. Up to 45% of stillbirths may be associated with sub-optimal care, for example:

- Failure to recognise and/or act on risk markers for adverse outcome
- Inappropriate grade of staff involved
- Poor documentation and communication (++).

Poor quality of post-mortem examination or failure to send appropriate samples was also frequent.

PERINATAL MORBIDITY

- There are still no national statistics available for perinatal morbidity or subsequent disability, neither is there any agreed definition of disability.
- It is not at all clear that the incidence of disability will fall as mortality is reduced.
- It is also still not clear what factors affect the developmental achievements of children, and why one child suffers while another does not.

PERINATAL PATHOLOGY

Good regional perinatal pathology services are fundamental to the practice of high standard obstetrics and neonatal medicine.

- *An autopsy should be requested in all cases of perinatal death even when the cause seems obvious* because it provides information that may be vital to understanding the cause of death and for future pregnancies. It is also an important clinical audit process.
- It is the right of each couple to have as much information as possible.

In 1999 the overall post-mortem examination rate was only 53% (range 42–69%).

PROCEDURES IN THE EVENT OF A PERINATAL DEATH

(see also Further reading)

Parental consent

Properly informed consent for post-mortem examination is vital. Parents must be given time for discussion and all questions must be answered accurately and honestly (if necessary by the pathologist).

Consent is required for:

- The post-mortem examination and retention of small samples of tissue for histology.
- The use of samples for teaching or research.
- Organ retention when this is advised for later and better detailed examination. The heart and brain are the most likely organs for which this may be requested.

The latter two points can be omitted according to the wishes of the parents.

Detailed inspection and measurement of the baby
The minimum requirements are:

- Measurement of weight, crown-heel, crown-rump, and foot lengths and occipito-frontal circumference.
- Look for malformations, deformations, state of maceration (if any) and evidence of trauma. Pay special attention to limbs, genitalia and facies.

Detailed clinical information
This must be supplied to the pathologist (preferably on a structured request form) who should also have access to the case notes.

- In the case of stillbirth, submit fetus and placenta together.
- The placenta of every baby born weighing less than 1500 g and/or less than the 3rd centile for gestational age and sex, and of all multiple pregnancies, should be sent for examination because these babies are at greatest risk of neonatal death

Maternal investigations
These are the responsibility of the obstetrician. The true value of some of those performed routinely is open to question (see information box).

Good practice
The parents must be treated with the utmost compassion and be encouraged (but not forced) to see their dead child even if disfiguring abnormalities are present.

- A polaroid photograph should be taken and kept for the parents to see and keep when they wish.
- Informed assistance should be given with registration and funeral arrangements.
- The GP and community midwife must be informed quickly.
- The couple should be seen by the obstetrician (and paediatrician in the case of a NND) when all the information on the case is available.

Investigation	Comment
TORCH screen	– of no demonstrable value routinely
Kleihauer test	– may reveal unexpected feto-maternal haemorrhage. Perform as routine
VDRL and Rh or other antibodies	– only if not checked antenatally
Random blood sugar	– of no proven value
Glycosylated Hb	– may be of value in screening for gestational diabetes (but see p. 89) Perform as routine
Thrombophilia screen	– may be of value in otherwise unexplained SB. Needs to be studied prospectively
Cytogenetics	– definitely indicated if baby is dysmorphic

Informing the legal authorities (see Further reading).
Among the circumstances in which a perinatal death should be reported to the coroner (or the equivalent legal authority) are if it:

- cannot readily be certified as being due to natural causes
- is linked to an accident
- is related to a medical procedure
- occurred in unusual or disturbing circumstances
- may be associated with medical mismanagement.

MATERNAL MORTALITY

Definitions
Maternal death: the death of a woman while pregnant or within 42 days of delivery or abortion from any cause related to or aggravated by the pregnancy or its management (excluding accidental or incidental causes).

Direct death: that resulting from obstetric complications of pregnancy, labour or the puerperium; from interventions, omissions, incorrect treatment, or from a chain of events resulting from any of these.

Indirect death: that resulting from pre-existing disease, or a condition arising during pregnancy not due to direct obstetric causes but aggravated by the physiological changes in pregnancy.

Late death: that occurring between 42 days and 1 year after abortion or delivery due to *direct* or *indirect* causes.

Coincidental (fortuitous) death: that due to causes unrelated to, but occurring in, pregnancy, labour or the puerperium.

Substandard care means that the care received (or made available to) the woman was deemed to fall below the 'contemporary standards of good practice'.

The maternal mortality rate is expressed per 100 000 'maternities', i.e. pregnancy, childbirth or abortion.

MATERNAL MORTALITY IN UK—1997–99

'Why Mothers Die 1997–99', the fifth Confidential Enquiry into Maternal Deaths (CEMD) in the United Kingdom was published in 2001 (see Further reading)

- The *direct* mortality rate was 5 per 100 000 maternities. This is the lowest ever recorded.
- The *indirect* mortality rate was 6.4 per 100 000 maternities. This is the highest recorded.
- Thus, for the first time, the number of *indirect* is greater than *direct* maternal deaths.

MAIN CAUSES OF MATERNAL DEATHS IN UK—1985–99

These are shown in Table 12.3 per million maternities (to nearest whole number or 0.5).

Each of the main causes is discussed in the relevant chapter.

The main 'Other' conditions (and number of deaths) associated with *indirect* maternal deaths were:

• Infectious disease (HIV 2)	13	• Central nervous system		34
		• Subarachnoid haemorrhage		11
• Diabetes	4	• Cerebral haemorrhage		
• SLE	2	& thrombosis		10
		• Epilepsy		9
• Haematological	4			
• Gastro-intestinal	7	• Respiratory system		9
		• Asthma		5
• Total 'Other' causes	75	• Cystic fibrosis		2

Key findings
- *Deaths associated with cardiac disease are now equal to thromboembolism (TE) as the commonest cause of maternal death.*
- One third (34%) of deaths occurred before delivery. The main causes in this group were ectopic pregnancy and thromboembolism.
- Among those factors significantly associated with a greater risk of maternal death are:
  - Social deprivation
    - ×20 in social classes III to VI compared with classes I & II
    - increased in travelling community.

Table 12.3

	1985–87	1988–90	1991–93	1994–96	1997–99
Direct					
Thrombosis and thrombo-embolism	14	14	15	22	16.5
Hypertensive disorders	12	11	9	9	7
Haemorrhage	4	9	6.5	5.5	3
Amniotic fluid embolism	4	5	4	8	4
Early pregnancy	8	8	5	7	8
Sepsis	4	5.5	6	6	7
Other direct deaths	12	7	6	3	3
• genital tract trauma	3	1	2	2	1
• other (e.g. acute fatty liver)	9	6	4	1	2
Anaesthesia	3	2	3.5	0.5	1
Indirect					
Cardiac	10	8	16	18	16.5
Psychiatric	–	–	–	4	7
Malignancies	–	–	–	–	5
Other	37	31	27	39	35
Total direct and indirect	98	100	98	122	114
Coincidental	11	16.5	20	16	11
Late	–	20	20	33	50

- Age, parity, obesity—increased in women <18 years of age and with increasing maternal age, parity and obesity
- Ethnicity—×2 in ethnic groups other than white
- Latebooking—20% of total deaths occurred in women who booked after 20 weeks'.
- Women with multiple pregnancies and those who had undergone IVF appear to be over-represented.
- In 1997–99 some degree of '**substandard care**' occurred in 60% of *direct* and 17% of *indirect* deaths. In 50% of *direct* deaths

'different treatment may have affected the outcome'. The main issues were:
- Lack of communication & teamwork
- Wrong diagnosis
- Failure to appreciate severity of condition leading to sub-optimal treatment
- Failure of GP or junior staff to diagnose or refer case to senior colleague
- Failure of consultant to attend
- Lack of clear policies for TE, eclampsia and massive haemorrhage
- Failure to diagnose ectopic pregnancy and TE in A&E department
- Intensive care unit full or distant
- Lack of blood products
- Inappropriate delegation of authority.

MATERNAL MORTALITY IN DEVELOPING COUNTRIES

WHO reports that in developing countries the lifetime risk of maternal death is 1 in 48 (rising to 1 in 16 in Africa) compared with 1800 in the developed world.

- The main causes overall are abortion, anaemia, eclampsia, haemorrhage, sepsis, and obstructed labour and its consequences.
- Most of the >500 000 maternal and 7.4 million infant deaths annually as well as millions of cases of maternal and childhood disease are easily preventable by access to antenatal care, trained personnel at birth, emergency obstetric care and modern contraception.

PERINATAL MORTALITY IN DEVELOPING COUNTRIES

Perinatal mortality rates (PMR) are said to range from 35 to 80/1000 births, but in most developing countries the true picture is unknown.

The commonest causes of *stillbirths* are intrapartum hypoxia, maternal infections (e.g. syphilis) and congenital anomalies.

Table 12.3 shows the four main causes of *neonatal death*.

- Early newborn mortality among girls is nearly double that in boys due to gender bias.

Remedies
Western-style medicine is inappropriate because its high cost technology cannot be properly maintained and it takes finances away from more locally appropriate care.

Table 12.3   Main causes of neonatal death in developing countries

Cause of NND	%	Comment
Infections	32	Mainly tetanus, pneumonia, diarrhoea and other sepsis
Complications of labour and delivery	29	Deaths mainly due to birth asphyxia and injuries
Low birthweight	24	Between 40 & 80% of NNDs occur among low birthweight (LBW) babies due to pre-term delivery, FGR or both. The health and nutrition of the mother are key factors
Congenital anomalies	10	Many of the deaths due to neural tube defects, cretinism and congenital rubella are now preventable.

Among the key features of appropriate care are:

• Monitor and treat pregnancy complications (e.g. anaemia, infections, pre-eclampsia).
• Set up immunisation programmes such as tetanus toxoid and rubella for mother; BCG, oral polio and Hep.B (if incidence of perinatal transmission is frequent) for the infant.
• Develop locally applicable strategies for LBW infants including 'kangaroo mother care'.
• Reduce the risk of mother-to-child transmission of HIV.
• Ensure skilled care at delivery and provide for clean delivery (e.g. soap, plastic sheet, a clean blade and a clean cord).
• Train attendants in resuscitation of asphyxiated babies (no more than bag and mask needed).
• Keep the newborn warm and initiate exclusive breast-feeding.

(See also Further reading).

FURTHER READING

Confidential Enquiry into Stillbirths and Deaths in Infancy (CESDI) 8th Annual Report The Maternal & Child Health Research Consortium, London (www.cesdi.org.uk)
CESDI The Fetal and Infant Postmortem. The Maternal & Child Health Research Consortium, London
RCOG 2001 Why Mothers Die 1997–9; Fifth Report on Confidential Enquiries into Maternal Deaths in the United Kingdom: RCOG Press
State of the World's Mothers & State of the World's Newborns 2001 Save the Children. www.savethechildren.org

13. The puerperium

The puerperium is the period of time over which the genital tract returns to normal after childbirth.

It is assumed to last 6 weeks.

The normal puerperium is characterised by:

- Lactation
- Lochia
- Involution of the uterus
- Return of the genital tract to normal.

Breast-feeding
Breast milk is every baby's birthright and every encouragement should be given to a woman to breast-feed. To do this:

- Inform all pregnant women about the technique and benefits of breast-feeding.
- Give new mothers encouragement and assistance as they begin.
- Give the baby no other food or drink than breast milk.

Among the benefits are:

- Passive immunity from immunoglobulins in breast milk
- Fewer gastro-intestinal symptoms
- Fewer neonatal seizures
- Lower incidence of auto-immune conditions (e.g. juvenile onset diabetes)
- Reduced risk of sudden infant death syndrome
- Psychological advantages for the baby
- Higher IQ (?).

Breast-feeding is an effective contraceptive as long as the baby is having at least 5 feeds/24 hours.

Suppression of lactation
This is seldom necessary now except, perhaps, after a perinatal death.

Bromocriptine can be used.

Management of breast engorgement
- Firm support of breasts with a good bra
- Adequate analgesia

- Warm bathing of breasts
- Expression should be avoided
- If necessary bromocriptine can be prescribed.

PUERPERAL PYREXIA

This is defined as a temperature of 38°C on any occasion in the first 14 days after delivery or miscarriage.

- A slight fever is not uncommon within the first 24 hours after delivery.
- Among the possible causes are:
  - Urinary tract infection
  - Genital tract infection
  - Breast infection
  - Deep vein thrombosis
  - Respiratory infection
  - Other non-obstetric causes.
- Carry out a full clinical investigation (including breasts and legs) as well as an MSU, cervical and high vaginal swabs, blood culture and sputum culture (if possible).
- After the investigations have been sent to the laboratory, and if the clinical situation warrants it, antibiotic therapy can be started.

MASTITIS

- *Acute intramammary mastitis* is due to failure of milk withdrawal from a lobule. Treatment involves getting the baby to empty the breast, cold compresses, and antibiotics if there is no improvement within 24 hours.
- *Infective mastitis* may be due to *Staph. aureus,* and treatment with an antibiotic to which that organism is sensitive may be necessary.
- *Breast abscess* formation is rare but preventable. Antibiotics are of value only if given early. An established abscess requires surgical drainage.

SECONDARY POSTPARTUM HAEMORRHAGE

This is defined as excessive (amount is not specified) blood loss from the genital tract more than 24 hours and less than 6 weeks after delivery.

- Among the commonest causes are retained placental fragments or blood clot (usually within a few days of delivery) or infection (often later).
- If the bleeding has been slight and there is no evidence of infection the patient needs no more than to be kept under observation.

- Careful evacuation of the uterus under general anaesthesia is indicated if:
  - An ultrasound scan suggests the presence of retained products
  - Heavy bleeding persists
  - The uterus is larger than expected and tender; the cervix is open.
- Any infection is treated appropriately.

PERINEAL PAIN

Prevention
- Avoidance of trauma at delivery
- Proper repair of tears or episiotomy.

Treatment
- Local anaesthetic sprays relieve pain in the immediate postpartum period. There is no evidence that ice, salt or other baths, or herbal remedies, produce lasting benefit. Local steroids should be avoided.
- Relief of pressure on perineum.
- Ultrasound or pulsed electromagnetic energy—controlled trials show no clear benefit.
- Analgesia—paracetamol or NSAIDs for mild pain; unfortunately no single analgesic seems to be of real value for severe pain.

EFFECTS OF CHILDBIRTH ON PELVIC FLOOR MUSCLES AND NERVES

- The pelvic floor muscles and nerves are affected to some degree even by a normal delivery. This is *not* a valid argument for increasing the rate of delivery by elective caesarean section.
- Ventouse extraction is usually less traumatic than forceps.
- Obstetric trauma predisposes to faecal incontinence.
- Division of the external anal sphincter at delivery is associated with long-term and sometimes severe effects on anal canal sensation and function. Prompt recognition and proper repair by an experienced operator are key factors in preventing long-term damage.

FURTHER READING

Chamberlain G and Steer P (eds) 2001 Turnbull's Obstetrics, 3rd edn. Churchill Livingstone, Edinburgh
James DK, Steer PJ, Weiner CP, Gonik B (eds) 1999 High Risk Pregnancy—Management Options, 2nd edn. Saunders, London

14. The newborn infant

Apgar score
This should be carried out on all babies at 1 and 5 minutes after birth.

Scores of zero to two are given for each of the following parameters:

• Heart rate
• Respiratory effort
• Muscle tone
• Response to catheter in nostril
• Colour.

A score of seven or less at 5 minutes suggests some degree of 'birth asphyxia'.

Clamping of the umbilical cord
If done before pulsation ceases, this can have serious haemodynamic effects on the baby. The balance between least haemodynamic disturbance and optimum distribution of blood between the baby and the placenta may be best achieved by clamping the cord 30 seconds after delivery of the baby.

Routine examination within 2 hours of birth
The object of the examination is to ask:

• Is the baby pre-term or small-for-dates?
• Are cyanosis, jaundice or anaemia apparent?
• Is there evidence of birth trauma? Even minor injuries should be shown and explained to and discussed with the parents (see Further reading).
• Are there any congenital anomalies (e.g. congenital dislocation of hips)?

Assessment of gestational age
Gestational age can be assessed independently of knowledge of menstrual age using a score from a series of physical criteria (the Farr score) that can be used alone or in combination with an assessment of neurological criteria (Dubowicz score).

The total score can be translated into an estimate of gestational age. For more information see Further reading.

RESUSCITATION

The priorities of resuscitation are:

• Maintenance of body temperature
• Clearance of airways
• Establishment of ventilation (with or without administration of oxygen).

Each obstetric unit should have:

• All staff trained in basic bag and mask resuscitation
• Staff available trained in advanced resuscitation
• Regular training sessions in immediate neonatal care and resuscitation.

More than 80% of babies requiring resuscitation will respond to bag and mask.

Of babies born with an Apgar score of zero known to have been alive shortly before birth 50% survive intact, 25% die and 25% survive with significant disabilities. It is, therefore, suggested, that active attempts should be made to establish circulation and resuscitate these babies.

RESUSCITATION AT THE THRESHOLD OF VIABILITY

Clear guidelines should be established for resuscitation of the extremely immature baby (<25 weeks) and, if at all possible, discussed with the parents before delivery:

• If possible a clear prospective decision should be made
• The presence of a very experienced neonatal paediatrician is required.

A decision not to commence, or to discontinue, resuscitation may be justified if the baby is extremely immature or in a poor condition at birth (e.g. due to asphyxia, birth trauma, infection, serious congenital malformation or failure to respond to resuscitation). (See Further reading)

INDICATIONS FOR THE PRESENCE OF NEONATAL PAEDIATRICIAN (OR EQUIVALENT) AT DELIVERY

• All caesarean sections
• All instrumental deliveries
save for simple 'lift out' forceps.

- Pre-term delivery
- Fetal growth restriction
- Significant APH
- Polyhydramnios
- 'Fetal distress'
- Any significant maternal condition known to affect fetus (e.g. diabetes, severe pre-eclampsia, ITP, thyrotoxicosis, drug abuse)
- Suspected amnionitis, membranes ruptured >24 h, maternal pyrexia
- Fetal anomaly
- Breech delivery
- Meconium staining of liquor
- Severe rhesus (or other) iso-immunisation

Multiple pregnancy.

ADMISSION TO SPECIAL CARE BABY UNIT (SCBU)

Babies should not be separated from their mothers without good cause.

All of the following babies usually need further special care on SCBU or transitional care ward:

- Gestational age less than 36 weeks
- Apgar score <3 at 1 minute and/or <5 at 5 minutes
- Birth weight less than 2000 g
- After prolonged resuscitation
- Some severe congenital anomalies
- Symptomatic hypoglycaemia, polycythaemia or anaemia
- All ill babies
- Persisting respiratory problem.

Most babies born with meconium below the vocal cords and those with drug-abusing mothers will also need admission.

The mother and father should be given an opportunity to see and hold the baby before transfer if at all possible.

NEONATAL SCREENING AND TREATMENT

PHENYLKETONURIA (PKU)

- The incidence is 1 in 10 000 live births.
- The Guthrie test or a chromatographic test should be carried out routinely within 7 to 14 days of delivery. If the Guthrie bacteriological test is used it should be postponed if the baby is on antibiotics.

CONGENITAL HYPOTHYROIDISM

- The incidence is about 1 in 4000 live births.
- Without a screening programme for its detection only 40% of cases will be diagnosed by 3 months of age.
- Hypothyroidism can lead to mental retardation unless treated early.

- Testing (on a dried blood filter-paper spot) can be carried out at the same time as for PKU. TSH alone or T_4 and TSH are measured.

CONGENITAL DISLOCATION OF THE HIP

If the hips are or can be dislocated, treat in an abduction splint (for 8–12 weeks) and refer to a paediatrician or orthopaedic surgeon.

BCG VACCINATION

BCG vaccination should be given under the following circumstances:

- Newborn children in families known to have had tuberculosis whatever the type and however long ago.
- Children of *all* Asian immigrant families (tuberculosis is still widespread in the Asian communities amongst those who have been in the country for some years).
- If the mother's sputum is positive for tuberculosis the baby should be given isoniazid-resistant BCG and treated with isoniazid. Baby and mother should be kept separate until the mother has been on anti-tuberculous treatment for 2 weeks.

OPHTHALMIA NEONATORUM

- This is defined as any purulent discharge from the eyes of an infant starting within 21 days of birth.
- It is still a notifiable disease and can cause severe damage if not treated promptly and adequately.
- Among the causes are:
  - *Neisseria gonorrhoeae*
  - Other bacteria
  - *Chlamydia trachomatis.*
- Treatment should be in consultation with an ophthalmologist and venereologist.

NEONATAL JAUNDICE

- If a term baby becomes jaundiced note date of onset, method of feeding, maternal blood group, history of perinatal trauma, and use of large volume of syntocinon containing fluid during labour.
- Investigate bilirubin level >200 μmol/l within 48 hours of birth. Check:
  - Proportion of direct bilirubin in blood
  - Blood group of mother and baby
  - Coombs' test and other antibodies
  - FBC, reticulocytes and differential white cell count
  - Urine for microscopy and reducing substances
  - Thyroid function tests
  - Glucose-6-phosphate dehydrogenase assay.

• Phototherapy will reduce the level and extent of the jaundice. It disrupts contact between baby and parents who may find it distressing. It is of no proven value for term infants over 48 hours of age with bilirubin levels <300 μmol/l.

DISCHARGE EXAMINATION

All babies should be examined in the presence of the mother before going home in order to:

• Assess his or her progress from birth
• Exclude malformations or traumatic lesions missed earlier
• Identify any superficial infections
• Reassure the mother.

The following should be checked:

• Baby's general appearance
• Superficial infections (and other lesions) for eyes, mouth, umbilicus, nails
• Heart for murmurs
• Male genitalia for hypospadias, undescended testes, herniae and hydrocoeles
• Female genitalia for vaginal discharge, fused labia, enlarged clitoris
• Abdomen (NB The liver is normally 1–2 cm palpable)
• Hips for congenital dislocation ⎫ Discuss with orthopaedic surgeon
• Feet for talipes equino varus ⎭ if present.

FURTHER READING

Dunn PM 2001 Neonatal resuscitation at the borderline of viability. Current Obstetrics & Gynaecology 11: 378–9
Speidel BD, Fleming PJ, Henderson J, et al 1998 A neonatal vade mecum, 3rd edn. Arnold, London

15. Ethics and law in obstetrics and gynaecology

ETHICS

WHAT ARE ETHICS AND MORALS?

Ethics is the system of thought by which we seek to understand the nature of moral judgement. It allows us to develop a set of core beliefs (or principles) that are clear, consistent and coherent as we try to move from the description of a particular situation to the analysis of universal principles and concepts.

Morals are codes of rules used by society, groups and individuals to guide their judgements and actions. They are heavily influenced by beliefs, attitudes and the kind of society in which one lives. In practice they should be comprehensive, clinically relevant and fully adequate to deal with the issues at hand.

A process of ethical reasoning is set out in Fig. 15.1.

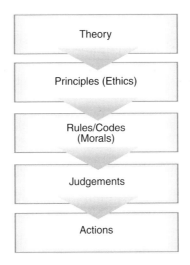

Fig 15.1   A process of ethical reasoning

DIVERSITY OF MORAL THEORY

The very essence of morality is that there is uncertainty and this leads to a diversity of moral theory. Only the briefest and necessarily incomplete overview is possible here. For fuller discussion see Further reading.

The two main theories are:

- *Deontology* or 'duties in action': In the 18th century, Immanuel Kant wrote a theory of ethics in which he described *categorical imperatives*. These had to be universally applicable, coherent (i.e. not contradictory) within 'a rational system of nature' and capable of being freely adopted by 'a community of rational beings'. Among the rules were 'do not kill, cause pain, disable, deprive of freedom or pleasure'; and 'do not deceive, break promises, cheat, break laws or neglect one's duty'.
  In his *Formula for the Dignity of Persons* he states, 'Act so that you treat humanity, whether in your own person or in that of any other, always as an end, and never as a means only'.
  The main problems with this theory are defining the meaning of 'rational' and agreeing on universally applicable rules.
- *Consequentialism or utilitarianism:* In the 19th century, Jeremy Bentham and John Stuart Mill developed a system in which 'rightness' and 'wrongness' were based on nothing more than consequences. For Bentham the main end was 'the maximum amount of happiness for the greatest number of people'. Mill modified this so that 'the common good' or 'benefit of the majority' were the moral arbiters rather than 'happiness'.
  In fact, this is the way most of us 'do ethics' in practice. However, although consequences are undoubtedly important in moral judgements and actions, consistent application of consequentialism leaves little room for the seriously disadvantaged in our society such as the severely disabled child, the terminally ill or the elderly with dementia.

Alternative/additional views

In trying to deal with the problems inherent in the above, several other views have been developed all of which provide valuable insights to allow theory to be translated into practice. (See Further reading).

Among them are:

- *Narrative ethics*—this takes account of the patient's context, emotions and relationships. Indeed whatever one's approach the patient's story must be part of the ethical relationship.
- *Virtue ethics*—Instead of asking, 'How should I act?' as in traditional ethics this asks 'How should I live?' This system tried to define 'excellences' of character or behaviour to which individuals or groups should aspire. It can be a useful approach particularly in

those faced with chronic and/or serious illness or disability. We may *care for* such people but do we *care about* them?

- *Feminist approaches to ethics*—this is characterised by the perspective that women have been and are oppressed and that this is morally unacceptable. The ethics is one of caring for individuals and, although caring resolutions may be different in their outcomes, they are linked by "personal regard and respect given to individuals". (see Cook in Further reading)

Four fundamental principles

These have been best expounded by Beauchamp and Childress (see Gillon in Further reading) and are shown in the box below.

Four fundamental principles	
• *Autonomy* ('self-rule')	Respecting the right of the individual to make choices about his or her own life *in the context of equal respect for all potentially affected.*
• *Beneficence*	Doing what is in the patient's best-interests
• *Non-maleficence*	Never causing harm and seeking to prevent it
• *Justice*	Treating all patients fairly and without unfair discrimination

Proponents of their use argue that they set out what our obligations are and provide a basis for practical solutions for particular situations.

Critics say that they are merely a checklist without an underlying theory; are often in conflict with one another (with no internal resolution); and do not deal with emotional aspects or relationships.

- *Autonomy* does *not* necessarily mean doing what someone requests or demands at one point in time. It implies a settled view of the individual reached by deliberation as to what is in his or her own long-term best interests. It is also to be balanced with the autonomy of others, including, in this context, medical staff.
- Dunstan (See Further reading) feels that autonomy has been wrongly 'exalted into an absolute claim over-riding other legitimate claims' and that the language of *rights* has over-ridden that of *duties*. The relationship between doctor and patient should be one of mutual obligation.

PROFESSIONAL OBLIGATIONS

The GMCs 'Duties of a Doctor' (see Further reading) sets out our obligations to our patients, our profession and ourselves. Patients must be able to trust doctors with their lives and well-being. To justify that trust, we as a profession have a duty to maintain a good standard of practice and care; to show respect for human life; and to 'always maintain the highest standards of professional conduct'. Among the key specific obligations are:

• being honest and trustworthy
• making the care of and respect for the patient our first concern
• recognising the limits of our professional competence
• keeping professional knowledge up to date
• respecting and protecting confidential information (unless with express permission or under exceptional circumstances).

THE LAW

The law does not, and is not intended to, express the ideal but rather the lowest common denominator of a code of ethics, by putting limits on what is and is not permissible.

LITIGATION IN OBSTETRICS AND GYNAECOLOGY

Those who practice in this specialty must, regrettably, expect to be faced by several claims during their professional life. The reasons for this are complex. Among them are:

• Patients' expectations are greater than ever before but resources are limited.
• The new NHS climate of health care encourages patients to complain assuming that this can improve the service provided. If things do not go as expected 'it must be someone's fault'.
• Unfortunately, when things do go wrong they are sometimes handled badly by poor communication.

It is, therefore, important that we manage and reduce this risk as much as is possible. This is dealt with comprehensively by Clements (see Further reading).

STANDARDS OF CARE

The traditionally accepted appropriate standard was defined in 1957 by the *Bolam* test in which patients were entitled to expect a degree of skill and care expected of an ordinary skilled doctor professing that skill. In 1993, the House of Lords in the *Bolitho* case determined that it was not sufficient to assert that others would have done or not done the same but that the practice under examination must be both reasonable and responsible. These are more fully discussed in Clements (Further reading).

RISK MANAGEMENT

This is defined as the identification, analysis and control of risk. Its primary aims are improving the quality of care and protecting patients. In this process there are some things that *must always be done* and some that *should never be done.*

Consequently, one should *always:*

- Maintain detailed, clear and legible records each time the patient is seen.
  - Write down specific reasons for policies and decisions.
  - Make these at the time of the observation whenever possible.
  - Obtain and note the results of any investigations.

Poor *note keeping* is the commonest cause of otherwise non-negligent cases being lost.

- Make sure that *drug prescriptions* are correctly recorded.
- Make sure *intravenous infusions* (including blood) are properly recorded.
- Recognise when you need to seek *advice from senior colleagues* and ask that they attend if you feel it necessary. *Record this in the notes.*
- Write comprehensive, clear and accurate *operation notes.* Include a check for swabs and instruments.
- Make sure that *pre-operative consent* is obtained well before surgery preferably by someone who has performed the procedure and understands the associated risks.
  - In the case of sterilisation make sure that the small risk of failure (even when the operation is done properly) is explained and recorded.
- Record patient hypersensitivity to drugs.
- Make particularly detailed records of any complications.
- Record if patients refuse, or act against, your advice.
- *Tell the truth at all times.*

Among those things that should *never* be done are:

- *Delete or revise a record* in the case notes after the event.
  - If a factual amendment is necessary write a full revised version giving the new time and date.
  - Do not strike out the old record.
  - If only a word needs to be changed annotate the change and initial it.
- *Remove* any part of the medical records.
- *Criticise* the work or conduct of a medical or nursing colleague in writing.
- Write *derogatory remarks* about a patient in the notes.
- *Delegate* a task to a junior colleague unless satisfied that he/she is competent to do it and understands fully what is required.

If a medical accident occurs
- Make sure that you and all involved write detailed notes of what happened and what has been said to the patient or the relatives.
- Inform the consultant in charge (if he or she is not already involved) who should involve the clinical director.

- Contact your medical defence society for advice.
- Be prepared to meet with the patient and/or family under the guidance of the clinical director.
  - Be open and honest with them
  - Never give the impression of 'covering up'.
- If you have to appear in a civil or coroner's court (or equivalent) as a witness make sure to obtain clear advice from your medical defence society.

FURTHER READING

Baron MW, Pettit P, Slote M 1997 Three Methods of Ethics. Blackwell, Oxford

Campbell A, Charlesworth M, Gillett G, Jones G 2001 Medical Ethics, 3rd edn. Oxford University Press, Oxford

Clements RJ 2001 Risk Management and Litigation in Obstetrics & Gynaecology. RSM/RCOG, London

Cook RJ (1994) in Principles of Health Care Ethics. R Gillon (ed). Wiley, London: pp 193–206

Dunstan G 1994 in Ethics in Obstetrics & Gynaecology. Bewley S, Ward RH (eds). RCOG, London

General Medical Council 2001 Duties of a Doctor: www.gmc-uk.org

Gillon R (ed) 1994 Principles of Health Care Ethics. Wiley, London

Jonsen A 1994 in Principles of Health Care Ethics. Gillon R (ed). Wiley, London: pp 13–21

McCullough LB, Chervenak FA 1994 Ethics in Obstetrics & Gynecology. Oxford University Press, New York

SECTION TWO
GYNAECOLOGY

16. Intersexes and congenital malformations of the genital tract

Gonadal differentiation into testis or ovary is dependent on the presence or absence of the Y chromosome. It begins during the fifth week of development.

The testis develops from the medulla of the primitive gonad whereas the ovary develops from the cortex. The development of the ovary is much slower than that of the testis.

Testicular development

The sex-determining region on the short arm of the Y chromosome (SRY) codes for the testicular determining factor (TDF) and is responsible for testicular differentiation.

This is dependent on the presence of H-Y antigen and TDF may regulate its expression (other autosomal genes are also involved).

Ovarian development
This depends on the presence of two X chromosomes associated with genes in the region p11.2 to p21 on the short arm of X.

- Deletion of the long arm in the region Xq13 usually leads to ovarian failure.
- Autosomal genes are involved in ovarian maintenance.

Development of genitalia
Both sexes develop two pairs of genital ducts—the Wolffian (or mesonephric) ducts and the Müllerian (or paramesonephric) ducts.

Male
- *Male development requires:*
  - Regression of the Müllerian ducts by an inhibitor produced mainly by Sertoli cells.
  - Growth of the Wolffian ducts stimulated by testosterone leading to development of the *epididymis, vas deferens* and *seminal vesicles.*

- The *penis* arises from the Müllerian tubercle; the *urethra* from elongation and fusion of the uro-genital folds and the *scrotum* from fusion of the labio-scrotal swellings.

Female
- In *female development* the open cranial ends of the Müllerian ducts form the *fallopian tubes*. The fused portions develop into the *epithelium* and *glands of the uterus*. The *myometrium* arises from the surrounding mesenchyme.
- The *vagina* is formed from both the vaginal plate and the utero-vaginal canal. It is fully formed by 20 weeks' gestation. The *clitoris* comes from the initial growth of the Müllerian tubercle the remnant of which forms the *hymen*.
- *External genitalia* arise from feminisation of the uro-genital sinus.

INTERSEX

Intersex is a condition in which there is discordance between chromosomal, gonadal, internal genital and phenotypic sex or the sex of rearing of the individual.

This may declare itself:

- At birth because of ambiguous external genitalia
- During childhood because of precocious puberty
- During adolescence because pubertal changes are inappropriate to presumed gender or because puberty fails to occur.

Some types of intersexuality may never become apparent (e.g. the XYY male or XXX female).

CLASSIFICATION
Chromosomal abnormalities
- *Turner's syndrome*—see p. 209.
- *Triple X female*—Some may have oligomenorrhoea and/or premature menopause but others go undetected.
- *Klinefelter's syndrome* (47 XXY)—Characterised by azoospermia, hypoplasia of seminiferous tubules, and perhaps gynaecomastia and eunochoidism.
- Aberration of H-Y antigen:
  - XX male—maleness is due to translocation of the H-Y antigens onto an autosome or one of the X chromosomes.
  - XY female—due to functional absence of H-Y. The clinical features are variable.

Gonadal aberrations
- *True hermaphrodite*—both testicular and ovarian tissue are present. External and internal genital sex vary widely. The commonest chromosomal structure is 46 XX.

- *Gonadal agenesis*—there is no gonadal tissue but no other congenital abnormality. The phenotype is female and the karyotype can be either 46 XX or 46 XY.
- *Absent anti-Müllerian factor*—noticeable at birth because of dubious genitalia. A normal vagina, uterus and tubes are present but with bilateral testes. The karyotype is 46 XY. The testis can produce androgen but not anti-Müllerian factor.

End-organ resistance
- Testicular feminisation—see p. 208.
- *Varying degree of hypospadias*—these may be due to relative cytosol receptor deficiency.
- Familial or sporadic *5α-reductase deficiency* will also result in the birth of children with dubious genitalia but who are genetically male. Virilisation occurs at puberty.

Female intersexuality
This may be due to:

- *Congenital adrenal hyperplasia* (CAH)—the commonest cause of intersex.
  - It is most frequently caused by a deficiency of 21-hydroxylase and therefore insufficient cortisol and aldosterone are produced. A female fetus will be exposed to an excess of adrenal androgens and virilisation will result.
  - Profound salt loss can be life-threatening in the neonate
- Ingestion of 19-norsteroid progestogens during pregnancy; or (rarely) excess maternal androgen production due, for example to the presence of an androgen secreting tumour.
  - A female fetus is born virilised to a greater or lesser extent.

MANAGEMENT
Early
- Check:
  - Buccal smear karyotype
  - Urinary 17-oxosteroids
  - Urinary pregnanetriol $\left.\right\}$ increased in CAH
  - Plasma 17α-hydroxyprogesterone
  - Plasma electrolytes.
- Treat salt-losing CAH with glucocorticoids (permanently).
- An X-ray after gastrografin instillation into the urogenital sinus will allow visualisation of the internal genitalia.
- In difficult cases, discuss with the parents assigning the sex of rearing to the sex which can be made adequate for coitus.

Later management

- Any corrective surgery to the external genitalia is best carried out before the age of 3 years.

- Exploratory laparotomy is rarely indicated and usually only in male intersexes and in true hermaphroditism.
- A male (XY) intersex showing virilism at birth will probably virilise at puberty. If the assigned sex is female the testes will need to be removed before virilisation begins at puberty.
- In *gonadal dysgenesis* advise removal of XY gonads because of the 25% risk of malignancy.
- In *testicular feminisation* removal of the testes should probably be advised shortly after puberty because of the up to 50% risk of testicular neoplasia.
- If an artificial vagina is required, it is best to wait until physical growth is complete before surgery is contemplated.
- In *gonadal agenesis* or after removal of gonads, oestrogens will be required to produce secondary sex characteristics at the appropriate time. Cyclical oestrogens and progestogens should be used if a uterus is present because of the risk of endometrial carcinoma if unopposed oestrogens are given over a long period of time.

CONGENITAL MALFORMATIONS OF THE GENITAL TRACT

EXTERNAL GENITALIA

- *Fusion of the labia*
- *Complete absence or duplication of the vulva* (both rare)
- *Persistence of the cloaca*—a serious problem. Urinary and faecal incontinence result
- *Defects of the posterior cloacal wall*—faecal continence is maintained by pelvic floor muscles
- *Defects in anterior cloacal wall*—affect urinary and genital tracts.

Minor abnormalities do not cause undue problems but major defects can result in bladder extrophy and deficient anterior abdominal wall.

LOWER GENITAL TRACT

- *Ectopic ureter*—usually an accessory ureter. The site of the orifice in relation to the bladder sphincter mechanism determines whether incontinence is present or not.
  - The orifice can be difficult to locate and may not show up on excretion urography.
- *Septate vagina*—not uncommon and only requires division if it poses mechanical problems for coitus or childbirth. It may accompany a uterine anomaly
- *Transverse vaginal membrane* (including imperforate hymen)—this will result in haematocolpos and cryptomenorrhoea (see p. 207)
- *Incomplete or absent vagina*—both are usually associated with absence of the uterus (and possible renal tract anomalies)

- Construction of an artificial vagina may have to be considered if the vagina is non-existent.
- Vulvo-vaginoplasty is a relatively simple and effective procedure (see Suggested further reading).

UTERINE ANOMALIES.

Agenesis or arrested development of one Müllerian duct will result in one of the following (see Fig. 16.1):

(i) Unicornuate uterus (with tube)
(ii) Unicornuate uterus plus some form of rudimentary horn
(iii) The rudimentary horn may not be joined to the unicornuate uterus.

Failure of, or incomplete, fusion of Müllerian duct may produce the following:

(iv) Double uterus (didelphys) with septate vagina
(v) Double uterus (didelphys) with normal vagina
(vi) Arcuate deformity
(vii, viii) Septate or sub-septate uterus

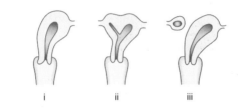

i ii iii

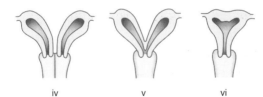

iv v vi

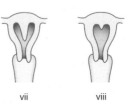

vii viii

Fig 16.1

These anomalies may be associated with dysmenorrhoea, dyspareunia, miscarriage, pre-term labour, intrauterine growth retardation or fetal malpresentation.

Surgical correction is only indicated for more severe anomalies, which have already produced problems.

A uterine septum can be removed hysteroscopically.

FURTHER READING

Shaw RW, Soutter WP, Stanton SL (eds) 1997 Gynaecology, 2nd edn. Churchill Livingstone, Edinburgh

Tindall V R 1990 Jeffcoate's principles of gynaecology, 5th edn. Butterworths, London

17. Disorders of menstruation and associated problems

AMENORRHOEA

Definitions
- *Primary amenorrhoea*—no menstruation by the age of 14 years accompanied by failure to grow properly or develop secondary sexual characteristics;
  or no menstruation by the age of 16 when growth and sexual development are normal.
- *Secondary amenorrhoea*—the absence of menses for 6 months (or greater than three times the previous cycle intervals) in a woman who has menstruated before.

When diagnoses are being considered, these 'primary' and 'secondary' categories must not be adhered to too rigidly.

Causes
If the amenorrhoea is not physiological (pre-pubertal, pregnancy, post-menopausal) it may be due to:

- Disorders of outflow tract and/or uterus
- Disorders of ovary
- Disorders of hypothalamo-pituitary axis.

DISORDERS OF THE OUTFLOW TRACT AND/OR UTERUS

Cryptomenorrhoea
Vaginal atresia or an imperforate hymen prevents menstrual loss from escaping.

Features
Primary amenorrhoea in a teenage girl with normal sexual development complaining of:

- Intermittent abdominal pain
- Possible difficulty with micturition
- Palpable lower abdominal swelling
- Bulging, bluish membrane at lower end of vagina.

Management
Incise membrane under anaesthesia and aseptic conditions.

Absence or hypoplasia of vagina

Features
Growth, development and ovarian function are usually normal.

The uterus is usually absent if only the lower third of the vagina has developed but may be normal or rudimentary.

Renal anomalies (in 30%) or skeletal defects (in 10%) may be present also.

Chromosome anomalies should be excluded.

Management
A functional vagina can be created by surgery or by dilators. Surgery should be carried out in specialised centres.

Testicular feminisation
The phenotype is female but the genotype is XY, and testes are present. It is inherited by an X-linked recessive gene resulting in absence of cytosol androgen receptors.

Features
- Growth and development are normal (may be taller than average and eunochoid).
- Breasts are large but with sparse glandular tissue, nipples and pale areolae.
- Inguinal herniae occur in 50% of cases (usually bilateral).
- There is little or no axillary and pubic hair.
- Labia minora are underdeveloped.
- The vagina is blind ending, the uterus absent and the fallopian tubes rudimentary.
- The testes are in the abdomen or inguinal canals.
- Normal levels of testosterone are produced but there is no response to androgens (endogenous or exogenous).
- There is no spermatogenesis.

Consider the diagnosis in a female child:

- With bilateral inguinal herniae
- With primary amenorrhoea and absent uterus
- When body hair is absent.

Management
- Treat as female.
- There is a 50% risk of testicular neoplasia if the testes are not removed shortly after puberty. Their removal is, therefore, advised after puberty and oestrogen replacement therapy started.
- Rare cases of incomplete testicular feminisation do occur. They have a variable degree of masculinisation.

Asherman's syndrome

Secondary amenorrhoea following destruction of the endometrium by overzealous curettage. Multiple synechiae show up on hysterosalpingography.

Management
Break down intrauterine adhesions through a hysteroscope and insert an intrauterine device (IUD) for 10–12 months to deter reformation.

Infection
For example: tuberculosis and uterine schistosomiasis can lead to secondary amenorrhoea.

DISORDERS OF THE OVARY

Chromosomal abnormalities
Turner's syndrome (45X)—gonadal dysgenesis.

Features
Most constant features:

- Amenorrhoea (primary but rarely secondary)
- Short stature
- Failure of secondary sexual development
- Webbing of the neck.

Less common features:

- Increasing carrying angle
- Shield chest
- Coarctation of aorta
- Renal collecting system defects.

Streak ovaries are present; gonadotrophins are high and oestrogens low.

A mosaic chromosome pattern (e.g. XX/X0) will lead to various degrees of gonadal dysgenesis, secondary amenorrhoea and premature menopause.

Management
- Short stature may be treated if the diagnosis is made early by use of oxandrolone and/or growth hormone before commencing oestrogen replacement therapy.
  - If a Y chromosome is present in the genotype the risk of gonadal malignancy makes gonadectomy advisable

Failure of gonadal development
- Gonadal agenesis (see p. 203).

Resistant ovary syndrome
This is a rare condition in which follicle-stimulating hormone (FSH) is elevated despite normal ovarian development and potential.

- It may resolve spontaneously or intermittently.
- In rare cases ovulation may be induced by a combination of ethinyl estradiol (to try to induce ovarian gonadotrophin receptors) and exogenous gonadotrophin therapy.
- Otherwise no treatment is possible except hormone replacement therapy (see p. 259).
- In young women needing contraception the combined oral contraceptive pill is advised as unexpected ovulation may occur.

Premature menopause
See p. 258.

DISORDERS OF THE HYPOTHALAMO-PITUITARY AXIS

Hyperprolactinaemia

Features
- Prolactin is controlled primarily by inhibition by dopamine from the hypothalamus. It is not subject to negative feedback by peripheral hormones.
- Hyperprolactinaemia is defined as levels of >800 mU/l. It is only clinically significant if accompanied by oligo-amenorrhoea.
- It accounts for 20% of women with amenorrhoea and 2% with oligomenorrhoea. Hyperprolactinaemia interferes with the menstrual cycle by indirect suppression of the pulsatility of luteinising hormone (LH) secretion.
- Women with prolonged hyperprolactinaemic amenorrhoea are at risk of osteoporosis.
- Galactorrhoea occurs in <50% of women with hyperprolactinaemia.

Causes
Among the potential causes are:

- 'Idiopathic' (about 40% of cases)—levels are usually <2500 mU/l. (Beware spurious diagnosis due to misinterpretation of results! Stress may cause modest increased prolactin levels).
- Prolactin secreting 'tumours' (40–50%); most are 'microadenomas' (i.e <10 mm diameter)—it is arguable whether these are true neoplasms.
  A macroadenoma is to be expected if prolactin levels exceed 2500–3000 mU/l
- Other tumours compressing the pituitary stalk (rare—e.g. craniopharyingioma).
- Primary hypothyroidism (3–5%)
- Drugs (1–2%)—metoclopramide and phenothiazines are the commonest; among the others are cimetidine, haloperidol, methyldopa, pimozide and reserpine.
- Chronic renal failure and polycystic ovary syndrome may lead to mild elevations of prolactin.

Investigation

- *Slight to moderate elevation*—repeat the estimation, and if it is still elevated, screen for gross abnormality by lateral skull X-ray. If this shows enlargement of the pituitary fossa or erosion of the clinoid processes proceed to CT scan to detect a macroadenoma. CT scans are increasingly used in preference to skull X-ray.
- *Marked elevation*—repeat the test but arrange X-ray and CT scan for as soon as possible. The patient who has headaches or a visual field defect requires urgent investigation.
  - MRI scanning offers better resolution of small microadenomas but this is of little additional practical value unless surgery is being considered.
  - An abnormal pituitary fossa may not be caused by a pituitary tumour but can be due to the *empty sella syndrome*. This is a benign condition due to a congenital defect in the roof of the fossa into which the subarachnoid space then extends.

Treatment

Microadenomas tend to grow slowly if at all. In up to 30% of patients spontaneous regression will occur.

- The treatment of choice is a dopamine agonist (e.g. bromocriptine, or cabergoline). This will suppress prolactin secretion (aim at levels of 200–300 mU/l), correct oestrogen deficiency, permit ovulation and reduce the size of most prolactinomas.
- Surgery and radiotherapy are usually reserved for patients with very large tumours with extrasellar manifestations (e.g. pressure on the optic chiasma).

If pregnancy ensues, check visual field perimetry every 2 months and prescribe a dopamine agonist and seek specialist help if there is evidence of tumour re-growth. Measurement of prolactin levels in pregnancy is of no value as levels are raised in normal pregnancy.

Weight loss-associated amenorrhoea

- A loss of more than 10 kg is frequently associated with amenorrhoea. It usually occurs in young women (frequently teenagers); they become obsessed with their body image and starve themselves. Anorexia nervosa is a misnomer because there is no loss of appetite.
- Oestrogen levels can be profoundly suppressed. If a progestogen challenge test (see below) is negative, there is a significant risk of osteoporosis, and hormone replacement therapy should be given.
- Hypothalamo-pituitary-ovarian function is usually restored when the lost weight is regained but occasionally may take many months for normal cyclical activity to return and for amenorrhoea to resolve.
- Ovulation induction is only indicated if the patient wishes to become pregnant.

Kallman's syndrome

- A rare cause of hypogonadotrophic hypogonadism in which anosmia is associated with primary amenorrhoea. The underlying cause is an absence of LHRH.
- Treatment with ethinyl oestradiol will induce normal secondary sexual development but the initial dosage should be low (<5 µg daily) to prevent premature epiphyseal fusion of long bones and arrest of breast development.
- Pulsatile LHRH therapy is a specific and reliable treatment for later ovulation induction.

'Post-pill amenorrhoea'

- The oestrogen/progestogen contraceptive pill does not predispose to amenorrhoea once pill-taking ceases.
- An assumption that amenorrhoea is merely an after-effect of pill-taking means that hyperprolactinaemia will be missed in one in five cases and premature ovarian failure in one in ten cases.
- Once other underlying causes are excluded this type of amenorrhoea usually responds well to ovulation induction with clomiphene if pregnancy is desired.

BASIC INVESTIGATION OF AMENORRHOEA

- Full history and examination.
- Pelvic ultrasound scan if amenorrhoea primary.
- Check serum prolactin level and thyroid function.
- If a chromosomal anomaly is likely on clinical grounds (e.g. short stature) check the karyotype.
- Carry out a progestogen challenge test (e.g. medroxyprogesterone acetate 5 mg daily for 5 days) to check endogenous oestrogen levels. The occurrence of withdrawal bleeding shows that the endometrium is reactive and the outflow tract patent.

If the prolactin level is normal, and there is no galactorrhoea, further investigation for a pituitary tumour is unnecessary. Galactorrhoea requires evaluation of the pituitary regardless of prolactin levels or menstrual pattern.

If the prolactin level is significantly elevated a pituitary tumour must be excluded as described above.

Measure FSH and LH.

- A low LH (<5 i.u./l) suggests hypogonadotrophic hypogonadism.
- A high FSH (>40 i.u./l) on successive readings indicates ovarian failure. If the woman is under 35 years of age check her karyotype. (The presence of a Y chromosome suggests that the risk of gonadal malignancy is high.)
- A low FSH and LH (<3 i.u./l) suggests constitutionally delayed puberty or hypothalamic amenorrhoea.

- A raised LH (>10 i.u./l), raised testosterone and normal FSH suggests polycystic ovary syndrome (see below).

OLIGOMENORRHOEA

Definition
The occurrence of menses on only five or fewer occasions per year.

Causes
Its causes are the same as those for secondary amenorrhoea, and if investigation is needed it should follow the same plan.

POLYCYSTIC OVARY SYNDROME (PCOS)

Definition
The association of hyperandrogenism with chronic anovulation in women without specific underlying diseases of the adrenal or pituitary glands.

Causes
There is evidence of an autosomal dominant mode of inheritance. The male phenotype may be premature balding.

Prevalence
PCOS is present in:

- 30–40% of women with amenorrhoea
- 75–90 % of women with oligomenorrhoea
- >70% of women with anovulatory infertility.

Polycystic ovaries may also be found in:

- 20% of asymptomatic women (although the incidence of irregular menses and slight hirsutism was greater in this group—see Further reading)
- up to 90% of hirsute women with regular menses.

Pathogenesis
- Insulin resistance may be the primary defect inherited or acquired due to insulin receptor antibodies. A small proportion may be due to primary abnormalities of adrenal androgen production (e.g. 21-hydroxylase deficiency).
- The resulting hyperinsulinaemia leads to amplification of the stromatrophic effect of LH on the ovary, a small effect at the pituitary level increasing the production of LH, and a direct hepatic action which reduces sex hormone binding globulin (SHBG) production.

- The enhanced LH activity leads to an imbalance in ovarian steroidogenesis, with increased production of androgen (predominantly androstenedione and testosterone) by theca cells.
- Conversion of androgen to oestrogen within the follicle by granulosa cells is greatly reduced because of a *relative* deficiency of FSH and the excess androgen enters the circulation.
- Aromatisation of the androgen surplus occurs peripherally in adipose tissue independently of FSH. This leads to a relatively constant oestrogen production with a larger than usual proportion of oestrone.
- Acyclic formation of oestrogen, particularly when unopposed by progesterone, results in abnormal feedback on the pituitary. FSH is suppressed and LH secretion promoted.
- The altered gonadotrophin profile distorts ovarian steroidogenesis further by accentuating theca cell hyperfunction and suppressing granulosa cell aromatase activity.

The extent to which hirsutism occurs depends on the intracellular conversion of androgens to the active dihydrotestosterone by 5-alpha reductase.

Oligomenorrhoea may occur, but otherwise the unopposed action of oestrogen leads to dysfunctional bleeding.

Clinical features (roughly in order of frequency)
- Subfertility
- Hirsutism
- Oligomenorrhoea

- Obesity

- Dysfunctional uterine bleeding
- Acne/male pattern alopecia
- Family history of maturity onset diabetes
- Recurrent miscarriage.

The menstrual disturbance often begins at the menarche which may be delayed.

The presence of pigmented velvety patches in the skin flexures and on the neck (*acanthosis nigricans*) in women with PCOS is associated with insulin resistance.

Diagnosis and differential diagnosis

- The diagnosis is usually based on a combination of clinical, ultrasonographic and biochemical criteria.
- High-resolution transvaginal ultrasound will show the morphological feature of polycystic ovaries (multiple peripheral follicles <8 mm diameter and increased prominent echo-dense stroma) in up to 80% of anovulatory women.
- If a woman has oligomenorrhoea, PCOS is likely in the presence of hirsutism, polycystic ovaries on ultrasound and excess circulating androgens.
- The differential diagnosis includes hyperprolactinaemia, acromegaly, congenital adrenal hyperplasia or androgen secreting tumours of the ovary.

ENDOCRINE ABNORMALITIES

- Mean serum LH levels are usually increased (>10 i.u.), though normal concentrations do not exclude PCOS as LH release is pulsatile; FSH levels are normal.
- Serum concentrations of testosterone and androstenedione are raised in over 90% of cases.
- Serum concentrations of oestradiol (total and free) are within normal limits in early and mid-follicular phases. However the pattern of secretion is abnormal with no preovulatory or midluteal increase. These effects may be compounded in obese women due to peripheral conversion of androgens by adipose tissue.

METABOLIC ABNORMALITIES

- Women with PCOS have a greater frequency and degree of hyperinsulinaemia and insulin resistance.

MANAGEMENT OF ANOVULATION

- If the woman is obese, loss of weight may be all that is necessary.
- Cycle control can be achieved by a low-dose combined oral contraceptive pill if she does not wish to conceive.
- Ovulation can usually be induced with clomiphene but 20–25% of women do not respond. A 'low dose' schedule of gonadotrophins may be successful in these women (see p. 236). They are at increased risk of multiple follicular development and ovarian hyper-stimulation.
- Treatment with HMG or pulsatile LHRH have been disappointing, but HMG following pituitary suppression with an LHRH analogue may be more successful.
- Low-dose FSH given subcutaneously by infusion pump may allow follicular maturation and, therefore, ovulation.
- Laparoscopic ovarian diathermy or laser 'drilling' should be reserved for cases which have not responded to drug treatment or in which the size of the ovaries is causing symptoms (see p. 235).
- Metformin, sometimes combined with clomiphene, has been reported as a successful treatment for ovulation induction in PCOS. Metformin is not licensed for ovulation induction. Its use should be closely audited, usually as part of a research programme.
- Dysfunctional bleeding will usually respond to the combined oestrogen–progestogen pill or a progestogen only. This treatment will also reduce the increased risk of endometrial carcinoma occurring in these women due to prolonged unopposed oestrogen action.

MANAGEMENT OF HYPERANDROGENISM

See under 'Hirsutism' below.

MANAGEMENT OF METABOLIC DISORDERS

- Because of the increased risk of type II diabetes and cardiovascular disease:
  - Carry out a glucose tolerance test, lipid profile in obese young women with PCOS
  - Encourage weight reduction
  - Also commence surveillance of blood pressure.
- These should be considered even in non-obese women with PCOS although there is, as yet, no evidence of benefit.

HIRSUTISM

Definition
Excessive and inappropriate growth of facial and body hair usually with a male pattern of distribution.

Causes:
The most important are:

- Idiopathic/constitutional
- Endocrine—PCOS; adrenal hyperplasia/Cushing's syndrome; hypothyroidism; acromegaly
- Androgen-secreting tumours of adrenal or ovary
- Drugs—e.g. androgens, anabolic steroids, danazol, diazoxide, phenytoin.

Investigations
Aim to differentiate among the above potential causes and include testosterone, LH (day 4–6 in cycle), thyroid function and pelvic ultrasound scan.

Treatment
- Sympathetic handling and reassurance are necessary at all times.
- Treat specific underlying conditions.
- Cosmetic treatments include bleaching, depilatory preparations, electrolysis, shaving and laser (if dark haired): may be sufficient if hirsutism is moderate or localised

Antiandrogens:

- A combination of ethinyloestradiol 35 µg with cyproterone acetate (CPA) 2 mg ('Dianette') is effective. It also provides contraception.
- Potency is increased by adding CPA 25–50 mg/day for the first 10 days of each packet (NB This may reduce libido).
- Improvement in hirsutes is slow with maximal effect around 18 months. Treatment should be continued for at least 6 months.
- *Liver dysfunction is a rare but serious complication.*

- Spironolactone (with a low-dose oral contraceptive pill) is a less effective alternative used in the US where CPA is not generally available.
- Finasteride 5 mg daily, a 5-alpha reductase inhibitor is effective treatment for hirsutism, but is currently unlicensed.
- Dexamethasone (also combined with an oral contraceptive pill) can be used for women with excess adrenal androgens.

EXCESSIVE MENSTRUAL LOSS

Definitions
Normal menstruation is defined as that occurring every 21–35 days, lasting 2–7 days and resulting in the loss of between 35 and 40 ml of blood.

Excessive loss can be due to menses which are too long, too frequent, too heavy, and/or too irregular.

'Menorrhagia' is defined as 'excessive' (80 ml or more) regular menstrual loss over several consecutive cycles. It is the commonest cause of iron deficiency anaemia in women of reproductive age in the UK.

Objective measurement of loss is not routinely practicable.

CAUSES
Physiological
Menorrhagia is a subjective complaint which may not be confirmed if blood loss were to be measured in all cases. About 30% of women describe their menstrual loss as heavy. In a study measuring menstrual loss:

- 25% of women with loss <60 ml considered that they had heavy menses.
- 40% of women with loss >80 ml considered that they had normal menses.

Dysfunctional uterine bleeding (DUB—60% of cases)
Definition
Excessive menstrual loss not due to organic disease.

- DUB can occur during *anovulatory cycles* in which a prolonged cycle usually ends in heavy, persistent vaginal bleeding.
  - Anovulation is commonest at the extremes of menstrual life.
  - The older women who develop it are often obese (see below) and it is commoner when carbohydrate intolerance (e.g. maturity onset diabetes) is present.
  - It can occur as part of the polycystic ovary syndrome.

- It may be associated with other endocrine disorders, e.g. hypothyroidism, adrenal hyperplasia, acromegaly.
- The proliferative effects of oestrogen are unopposed by progesterone.
  - The hyperplastic endometrium is shed when the ovarian follicle begins to degenerate or the endometrium outgrows its blood supply.
  - In its most severe form there is *cystic glandular hyperplasia* of the endometrium and the clinical result is known as *metropathia haemorrhagica*.
- DUB occurring during *ovulatory cycles* is related to local disorders of prostaglandins and their receptors in the endometrium.
- Characteristically heavy regular menses occur in a 35 to 45-year-old woman, often accompanied by lower abdominal discomfort, dysmenorrhoea and dyspareunia. The uterus is slightly enlarged and can be markedly tender to palpation.
- The endometrium is normal.

Other gynaecological causes (35% of cases)
- *Endometriosis*—see p. 222
- *Chronic pelvic inflammatory disease*—see p. 267
- *Uterine tumours*—e.g. submucous leiomyomas (see p. 301); carcinoma of the endometrium (see p. 304) may develop in cases of pre-existing endometrial hyperplasia.
- *Ovarian theca cell and granulosa cell tumours* often produce oestrogen (see p. 311) and cause menorrhagia.
- *Intrauterine devices* (IUDs). The menstrual loss doubles in up to 50% of IUD users, although it is reduced in the levonorgestrel releasing IUD.

Endocrine and haematological causes (<5% of cases)
- Thyroid disorders
- Bleeding disorders—*von Willebrand's disease* and *idiopathic thrombocytopenia* (or rarely *leukaemia*) may present with menstrual disorders. Women on long-term anticoagulant therapy may have menorrhagia.

Post-sterilisation—there is no consistent evidence that menstrual loss increases after sterilisation. It is usually related to stopping the combined contraceptive pill.

- Psychological factors can play an important part.

MANAGEMENT OF EXCESSIVE MENSTRUAL LOSS
Investigation
- A comprehensive history and examination is vital (take the opportunity to perform cervical cytology if it is due).
- A menstrual diary collected over several months can be helpful.

- Take blood for full blood count and check thyroid function if symptoms of hypothyroidism are present.
- The uterine cavity may initially be investigated using transvaginal ultrasound.
- Endometrial sampling should be carried out in women of 40 years of age or over if inter-menstrual bleeding or menorrhagia persists. It is rarely necessary (or useful) in younger women. If possible it should be carried out as an outpatient procedure.

General management
- Specific organic disorders must be treated appropriately.
- The obese woman must be strongly advised to lose weight.
- Reassurance should be offered about normal levels of blood loss, particularly if haemoglobin is normal.

Drug treatment
Irregular *anovulatory cycles* will usually respond to progestogen therapy from day 15 (or earlier) to 25 of the cycle. The combined oestrogen/progestogen pill is usually effective in young women.

Dysfunctional bleeding associated with ovulatory cycles is much more difficult to manage in the long term:

- The evidence suggests that *antifibrinolytic* therapy using tranexamic acid taken during menstruation is the most effective drug treatment. No increased risk of thrombo-embolism has been observed. Treatment may be continued indefinitely.
- *Prostaglandin synthetase inhibitors* (e.g. mefenamic and flufenamic acids or naproxen sodium) are also effective.
- It is suggested that either of the above types of drug be considered as first line treatment.
- The *progestogen-releasing intrauterine device* is an effective treatment for menorrhagia.
- *Progestogen* therapy is ineffective and has side-effects (e.g. nausea, breast tenderness, water retention).
- Second line drugs include danazol, gestrinone, and gonadotrophin releasing hormone analogues. They are effective in reducing heavy menstrual blood loss but side effects limit their long-term use.

Surgical treatment
It is essential that the operator has the appropriate training, skills and supervision.

- Diagnostic curettage or other endometrial sampling are NOT therapeutic for menorrhagia.
- Sub-mucous fibroids or polyps can be removed hysteroscopically.
- *Endometrial ablation* by Nd-YAG laser, resection under hysteroscopic control, microwave ablation or fluid thermal ablation are all effective treatments. The short term advantages are not necessarily sustained in the long term. Table 17.1 compares them with hysterectomy (see Lethaby et al in Further reading).

Table 17.1 Endometrial ablation/resection compared with hysterectomy

Outcome measure	Hysterectomy	Endometrial Ablation/Resection
Post-operative complications	Up to 45% for abdo. hyst—e.g. pain, haemorrhage, wound infection, urinary infection: (less for vag. hyst?); mortality—0.4 to 2/1000 operations	<15%—uterine perforation, fluid overload, haemorrhage, urinary infection; mortality—anecdotal reports only
Effectiveness	100% have amenorrhoea	Amenorrhoea in 15–25%; light loss in further 60–75%
Return to normal activities (weeks)	From 4 to 12 weeks	From 1 to 4 weeks
Re-operation rate	Nil	About 15% and 25% at 1 and 2 years, respectively
'Satisfaction'	Better in the medium to long term	No significant difference between ablation and hysterectomy after 4 months
Comparative cost	Higher initially	About 50% saving at 4 months but only 30% at 2 years

- *Hysterectomy* is a common surgical remedy:
  - About 80% are performed abdominally although the proportion carried out vaginally is increasing.
  - Laparascopically assisted hysterectomy may be appropriate for some women but this needs to be evaluated further (see p. 329).
  - Although there is no evidence of a need to remove healthy ovaries as a matter of routine (in women who are not at high risk of ovarian cancer—see p. 313), oophorectomy (often bilateral) is carried out in up to 50% of abdominal hysterectomies.
  - Antibiotic prophylaxis should be given.
  - Appropriate thrombo-embolic prophylaxis should be given.

Endometrial hyperplasia
- If the glands and stroma increase together and there are no atypical cells the risk of developing malignancy is under 2%.
- If hysterectomy is not carried out initially such women should be kept under observation by annual outpatient endometrial sampling.

- If the hyperplasia is 'atypical' (with abnormal cells in irregular glands) the risk of endometrial adenocarcinoma is increased and hysterectomy is indicated (see p. 305).

DYSMENORRHOEA AND THE PREMENSTRUAL SYNDROME

PRIMARY DYSMENORRHOEA

Definition
Painful periods for which no organic or psychological cause can be found.

Features
- It usually occurs in teenage girls.
- The pain is colicky and usually begins shortly after or at the onset of menses.
- It tends to last for only 24 to 48 hours.
- There is often an exacerbating psychological element.
- There may be an increased production of prostaglandins. It occurs only in ovulatory cycles.

Management
Exclude organic causes by history and examination.

- Suppression of ovulation using the combined oestrogen/ progestogen pill may be helpful, or progestogens alone in the second half of the cycle.
- Symptomatic relief can often be obtained by prostaglandin synthetase inhibitors such as mefenamic and flufenamic acids or naproxen sodium.
- Procedures such as forced dilatation of the cervix or pre-sacral neurectomy are never indicated.

SECONDARY DYSMENORRHOEA

Definition
Painful periods for which an organic or psychosexual cause can be demonstrated.

Features
- It usually commences in adult life.
- It begins several days before the menses and gradually increases in severity as menses approach.
- The commonest associations are with pelvic inflammatory disease, endometriosis, fibroids or psychosexual problems.

Management
Laparoscopy can be helpful in ascertaining the cause which can then be treated.

PREMENSTRUAL SYNDROME

Definition
A symptom complex of unknown aetiology occurring in the week before menstruation.

Features
It is most frequent around the age of 35 years.

Tension, irritability and depression can be marked. 'Fluid retention' causes a bloated feeling in the abdomen, breast tenderness and swollen clumsy fingers.

Management
- Treatment is empirical because the cause is unknown. Placebo response is high (50–90%).
- Sympathetic handling and understanding are of paramount importance.
- There have been few properly controlled trials of any of the many proposed remedies. Among them are the following:
  - *Pyridoxine* (vitamin B_6) may provide some relief but this has not been clearly demonstrated in good trials.
  - *Evening primrose oil* (240 mg b.d) contains gamolenic acid and may be of benefit.
  - The *combined oral contraceptive pill* may help some women, though this has yet to be tested properly!
  - Trials of *progestogen* therapy (e.g. dydrogesterone or progesterone) from mid-cycle have not shown clear benefit.
  - *Mefenamic acid* (500 mg t.d.s) started mid-cycle for 2 weeks has been shown to be effective in some cases.
  - *Bromocriptine* (1 mg t.d.s) may alleviate pre-menstrual breast tenderness and swelling.
  - Empirical use of *diuretics* is not justified. They can be of benefit in some women who have oedema or measured weight increase (not merely bloating).
  - *LHRH agonists plus oestrogen* may be useful for short-term treatment of severe cases.
- *Hysterectomy and bilateral salpingo-oophorectomy* may be necessary for a small group of women who are particularly severely affected.

ENDOMETRIOSIS

Definition
The presence of endometrial tissue in sites other than the uterine cavity.

- In *internal endometriosis (adenomyosis)* the ectopic endometrium is confined to the myometrium.

- *External endometriosis*, with deposits occurring in a variety of ectopic sites, is more common but is seldom found together with adenomyosis. This argues for different aetiological factors.

EXTERNAL ENDOMETRIOSIS

Features
The more 'endometriosis' is recognised the less well we seem to understand it!

- It is found in over 20% of asymptomatic women undergoing sterilisation (in whom it may be a normal physiological variant).
- Clinically it presents most commonly in nulliparous women or those of low parity at between 30 and 45 years of age.

The 'characteristic' symptoms are:

- Heavy, often irregular menses
- Secondary dysmenorrhoea (25–30%)
- Dyspareunia (30–40%)
- Pelvic pain between menses (40–60%)
- Subfertility—found in 15–60% of women undergoing diagnostic laparoscopy.

There may also be symptoms relating to organs contiguous with the uterus.

However, the frequency and severity of symptoms presumed to be caused by endometriosis do not correlate well with the extent or site of lesions: many women are asymptomatic.

The American Fertility Society revised classification and scoring system for endometriosis is given in Table 17.2.

Pathogenesis
There are several theories for its development:

- *Retrograde menstruation* and implantation of viable cells on, for example, the ovaries and peritoneum of the pouch of Douglas
- *Metaplasia*—both epithelial and stromal cells of the endometrium have a common precursor in the coelomic epithelium and adjacent mesenchyme. This could account for all abdominal and pelvic endometriosis, and the rare cases in the rectovaginal septum, umbilicus and canal of Nuck
- *Mechanical transplantation* into scars at the time of surgery, e.g. hysterectomy or hysterotomy. It very rarely follows caesarean section
- *Venous or lymphatic 'metastasis'*—this (or metaplasia) could account for the rare pulmonary endometriosis.

It seems probable that all cases do not arise in the same way.

Table 17.2   The American Fertility Society revised classification of endometriosis

ENDOMETRIOSIS		<1 cm	1–3 cm	>3 cm
Peritoneum:	superficial	1	2	4
	deep	2	4	6
Ovary: R	superficial	1	2	4
	deep	4	16	20
Ovary: L	superficial	1	2	4
	deep	4	16	20

POSTERIOR CUL-DE-SAC OBLITERATION	Partial	Complete
	4	40

ADHESIONS		<1/3 enclosure	1/3–2/3 enclosure	>2/3 enclosure
Ovary: R	filmy	1	2	4
	dense	4	8	16
Ovary: L	filmy	1	2	4
	dense	4	8	16
Tube: R	filmy	1	2	4
	dense	1*	8*	16
Tube: L	filmy	1	2	4
	dense	1*	8*	16

*If the fimbriated end of the fallopian tube is completely enclosed, change the point assignment to 16.

Stage I	Minimal	Score 1–5
Stage II	Mild	Score 6–15
Stage III	Moderate	Score 16–40
Stage IV	Severe	Score >40

Pathology

The appearances of endometriosis may develop gradually from non-pigmented, 'atypical' lesions to the typical black 'powder-burn' lesions. The former may also be more active 'biochemically'.

The ectopic endometrium menstruates causing severe irritation, a sterile inflammatory reaction, and dense adhesions.

The commonest sites in order of frequency are:

- both ovaries (55%), which may show merely surface deposits or contain 'chocolate' cysts (containing old menstrual blood) of various sizes. These may arise by invagination of surface deposits or metaplasia of follicular or luteal cells.
- the posterior leaf of the broad ligament (35%).
- the pouch of Douglas (35%) and uterosacral ligaments (30%).
- the rectum, urinary tract or lungs may occasionally be involved.

Fertility can be compromised by tubal and ovarian damage and pelvic adhesions. High concentrations of prostaglandins and macrophages in the peritoneal fluid of affected women may also affect oocyte quality. However, the association between mild endometriosis and subfertility is not fully explained.

Diagnosis
The presentation is variable and there is considerable overlap with other conditions such as irritable bowel syndrome and pelvic inflammatory disease.

* It is often suspected after a careful history is taken.
* The presence of tender nodules on the uterosacral ligaments is also suggestive.
* Laparoscopy is the 'gold standard' diagnostic test. The significance of the occasional tiny deposits on, for example, the ovaries or pouch of Douglas is disputed.
* For histological diagnosis both glandular and stromal tissue must be present.

Medical treatment
* Non-steroidal anti-inflammatory drugs (NSAIDs) may be effective in reducing pain.
* Hormonal manipulation is given to suppress endogenous cyclical changes in oestrogen and progesterone to prevent menses. This can be achieved using:
  * Continuous therapy with progestogen or the oral contraceptive pill for 6 to 9 months
  * Danazol or gestrinone for 4 to 6 months—these have androgenic side-effects and must be discontinued if signs of virilisation develop
  * Gonadotrophin-releasing hormone (GnRH) agonist—for no more than 6 months due to bone loss during therapy. The loss is restored almost completely 2 years after stopping treatment. Longer term treatment with 'add-back' therapy with hormone replacement therapy (HRT) can be used to prevent menopausal symptoms and prevent mineral bone loss.

There is no role for medical therapy with hormonal drugs in the treatment of endometriosis-associated infertility.

Surgical treatment
* *Conservative surgery* by laparoscopy or laparotomy: small deposits can be diathermied, excised or vaporised using a CO_2 laser. Large chocolate cysts require excision.
* *'Radical' surgery* is reserved for women with severe symptoms that have failed to respond to conservative remedies or when continuing fertility is not an issue.
  * The preferred operation is *hysterectomy and bilateral salpingo-oophorectomy* with excision of as many other endometriotic lesions as possible.

- Prior treatment with danazol or GnRH agonists may be worthwhile in severe cases.
- Continuous combined HRT should be given post-operatively due to the theoretical risk of un-opposed oestrogen therapy stimulating endometriotic deposits.

INTERNAL ENDOMETRIOSIS/ADENOMYOSIS

Definition
Islets of endometrial tissue, glands and stroma deep in the uterine wall which responds by hyperplasia of muscle and fibrous tissue.

Features
It tends to occur in older, multiparous women, in contrast to external endometriosis.

- The clinical presentation is:
  - Increasingly severe menorrhagia
  - Secondary dysmenorrhoea
  - Gradually enlarging tender uterus.
- Symptomatically it is difficult to differentiate from uterine fibroids or dysfunctional bleeding.
- The uterus may be diffusely thickened or there may be localised swellings closely resembling leiomyomas.
- It may be suspected with pelvic ultrasonography although it is virtually impossible to diagnose it definitely other than by histology after hysterectomy

Treatment
Treatment is by hysterectomy with conservation of ovaries (unless there are other indications for their removal).

STROMAL ENDOMETRIOSIS

- This rare condition acts more like a neoplasm than do other forms of endometriosis.
- Histologically, solid masses of cells resembling endometrial stroma are found in the endometrial wall, but other features of neoplasm are uncommon (e.g. mitoses are few and pleomorphism slight). It may be a form of a low-grade sarcoma.

Features
- The peak incidence is between the ages of 35 and 50 years.
- It does not regress on removal of the ovaries.
- Metastases do occur, but rarely.
- Clinically it may present with menorrhagia or postmenopausal bleeding and pelvic pain.
- It is usually diagnosed only after hysterectomy. The prognosis is usually good.

FURTHER READING

Eden JA 1991 Hirsutism. In Studd J (ed) Progress in Obstetrics and Gynaecology. 9:319–334. Churchill Livingstone, Edinburgh

Fox R 1994 In Studd J (ed) Polycystic ovarian disease and insulin resistance: pathophysiology and wider health issues. Progress in Obstetrics and Gynaecology 11: 351–370. Churchill Livingstone, Edinburgh

Franks S 1995 Polycystic Ovary Syndrome. New England Journal of Medicine 333: 853–861

Lethaby A, Shepperd S, Cooke I et al, 2000 Endometrial resection and ablation versus hysterectomy for heavy menstrual bleeding. Cochrane Library Issue 2 Oxford: Update software

RCOG 1998 RCOG Guideline Summary. The Initial Management of Menorrhagia. RCOG Press, London

RCOG 1999 RCOG Guideline Summary. The Management of Menorrhagia in Secondary Care. RCOG Press, London

RCOG 2000 RCOG Guideline. The investigation and management of endometriosis. RCOG Press, London

Shaw RW 1991 In Studd J (ed) Treatment of endometriosis. Progress in Obstetrics & Gynaecology; 9: 273–287 Churchill Livingstone Edinburgh

Wardle PG, Hull MG 1993 Is endometriosis a disease? Clinical Obstetrics & Gynaecology 7(4) 673–85. Bailliere Tindall, London

18. Fertility and subfertility

FERTILITY IN THE FEMALE

THE HYPOTHALAMUS

Controls anterior pituitary function by substances secreted by cells within it and transported to the pituitary via the portal circulation.

- A single decapeptide neurotransmitter controls FSH and LH-gonadotrophin-releasing hormone (GnRH). Its half-life is only a few minutes, and a continuous but pulsatile release occurs. Release is controlled by:
  - A long feedback loop due to circulating target gland hormones
  - A short feedback loop due to the effect of gonadotrophins on the hypothalamus
  - An ultrashort feedback by which it inhibits its own synthesis
  - A series of neurotransmitters such as serotonin (5-hydroxytryptamine), melatonin, noradrenaline and dopamine (see below)
- The hypothalamus exerts a tonic negative control on prolactin through the major *prolactin inhibitory factor*, dopamine.

THE PITUITARY GLAND

It is influenced by the hypothalamus via:

- Tonic and cyclic centres for the secretion of GnRH:
  - The tonic centre is situated in the medial basal hypothalamus.
  - It is responsible for basal levels of gonadotrophin.
  - Oestradiol has a negative feedback effect on it, and it is also dopamine-dependent.
  - The cyclic centre lies in the pre-optic area in the anterior part of the hypothalamus.
  - It is responsive to positive feedback by oestradiol and produces the mid-cycle surge of gonadotrophins.
- The posterior pituitary pathway:
  - Cells in the supraoptic and paraventricular nuclei secrete vasopressin, oxytocin and neurophysin.
  - They are transported along the pituitary stalk to the posterior pituitary where they are stored in axonal terminals.

- They also pass into the CSF and then to the portal system of the anterior pituitary.
- Oxytocin is involved in gonadotrophin secretion.

GONADOTROPHIN RELEASE

- There are two pools of gonadotrophin, one released immediately it is synthesised and the other held in reserve.
- The rate of storage exceeds release, which makes the mid-cycle surge possible. (This is also the time when sensitivity to GnRH is greatest.)
- Oestradiol inhibits immediate release and increases storage. The effect is overcome by the positive feedback action of oestradiol on the cyclic centre.
- Low levels of progesterone increase release and storage after oestrogen priming. High levels of progesterone increase GnRH pulse frequency.
- The release of LH is pulsatile, and of FSH non-pulsatile.

REGULATION OF THE MENSTRUAL CYCLE

Recruitment of follicles (days 2–6)
- Initiation of follicular growth is independent of gonadotrophin stimulation.
- Follicles grow during infancy, ovulation, periods of anovulation, pregnancy and the menopause until the numbers are exhausted. For the vast majority of follicles, growth is limited and atresia inevitable.
- As FSH levels increase, a group of follicles begins to grow further but the mechanism by which these follicles are chosen is unknown.
- The period of initial growth ends as oestrogen levels rise 7–8 days before the pre-ovulatory LH surge.

Selection of follicles (days 7–10)
- FSH stimulates follicular growth but also facilitates steroidogenesis by increasing the activity or number of LH receptors.
- Changes in hormonal levels are regulated by feedback mechanisms:
  - Oestradiol inhibits FSH (negative feedback)
  - Low levels of oestradiol inhibit LH
  - High levels of oestradiol stimulate LH (positive feedback) and FSH.

Dominant follicle selection (days 10–14)
- Oestrogens rise slowly, then rapidly, to peak just before ovulation.
- FSH falls due to negative feedback.
- LH increases steadily to its mid-cycle surge.
- The follicle destined to ovulate protects itself by its own hormone production.

• Ovarian stromal cell production of androgens (androstenedione and testosterone) increases enhancing the atresia of non-ovulatory follicles and stimulating libido.

Ovulation
• The rapid rise in oestrogen triggers an LH and FSH surge.
• The LH surge triggers resumption of meiosis by the oocyte.
• Degeneration of the collagen in the follicular wall allows it to rupture.
• Expulsion of the oocyte is brought about by prostaglandins induced by LH, and hormones such as noradrenaline and relaxin.
• The LH surge also triggers breakdown of the basement membrane between the theca and granulosa cell layers of the follicle wall.
• The granulosa layer is invaded by new blood vessels, exposing the cells to cholesterol for the first time in the cycle. This allows them to synthesise and secret progesterone.

Luteal phase
• Days 1–3 post-ovulation—granulosa cells increase in size, accumulate lutein (a yellow pigment) and secrete progesterone (see above).
• Days 8–9 post-ovulation—peak level of progesterone is reached. (A plasma level of progesterone over 30 nmol/l (10 ng/ml) is good presumptive evidence of ovulation.)
• Days 9–11 post-ovulation—the corpus luteum begins to decline unless pregnancy supervenes. Regression may be due to a local luteolytic effect or to oestradiol production by the corpus luteum (CL). In pregnancy it is maintained by human chorionic gonadotrophin (hCG) until 6 to 8 weeks gestation.
• In the absence of pregnancy the time from the LH surge to the onset of menstrual flow is usually 14 days.

FERTILITY IN THE MALE

The testes have two functions: *steroidogenesis* (mainly androgens) by the interstitial cells of Leydig between the seminiferous tubules; and *spermatogenesis*, which begins in the germinal epithelium of the tubules.

The seminiferous tubules and interstitial cells are controlled by:

• GnRH and gonadotrophins.
• Positive and negative feedback signals—testicular steroids (particularly oestrogen) inhibit GnRH. Androgens diminish the LH-releasing effect of GnRH without affecting FSH. Oestrogen potentiates FSH and LH secretion by GnRH. Seminiferous tubules secrete *inhibin*, a non-steroid substance, which specifically inhibits FSH release.

The effects of androgens are:

- Spermatogenesis
- Development of accessory glands
- Development of secondary sex characteristics
- Metabolic and psychic effects determining 'maleness'
- Increasing libido
- Feedback on the hypothalamus and pituitary (see above).

ERECTION

Erection is due to tumescence of the penile cavernous bodies. It is mediated through the parasympathetic nervi erigentes (S2–4).

EJACULATION

Ejaculation is a reflex action involving a complex co-ordinated autonomic stimulation of the genital tract. It has two stages:

- *Stage 1.* Contractions of the epididymis, vas deferens and seminal vesicle pump sperm from the epididymis and seminal fluid from the prostate and seminal vesicles into the posterior urethra. As the seminal fluid arrives in the prostatic urethra contraction of the internal urethral sphincter closes the bladder neck (this prevents retrograde ejaculation). The second stage is triggered.
- *Stage 2.* The semen is expelled due to relaxation of the external sphincter and rhythmic contractions of ischiocavernous, bulbocavernous and perineal muscles.

TESTICULAR FUNCTION AND AGE

- Gonadal function in men is preserved well into old age and any decline is gradual.
- Although FSH and LH levels remain normal, testosterone levels tend to fall, suggesting decreased sensitivity to gonadotrophin.
- The so-called 'male climacteric' is more likely to be related to psychological, cardiovascular and neurological effects of ageing than to diminished production of androgens.

SUBFERTILITY

Definition
The involuntary failure to conceive within 12 months of commencing unprotected intercourse.

- *Primary subfertility*—no previous pregnancy
- *Secondary subfertility*—previous pregnancy (whatever the outcome).

The incidence of primary subfertility alone is at least 12% of couples.

Causes (and approximate incidence)
- Idiopathic   25%
- Sperm defects or functional disorder   25%
- Ovulation failure   20%
- Tubal damage   15%
- Endometriosis   5%
- Coital failure   5%
- Cervical mucus defect   3%
- Azoospermia   2%

Principles of management
- Deal with the infertile couple together.
- No one is 'at fault' or 'to blame'; it is a shared problem.
- Carry out investigations and treatments consistently in proper sequence.

INVESTIGATIONS

Aims of investigation

- An explanation for the infertility
- A prognosis
- A basis for treatment.

History
Check past medical, surgical and family histories.

Subfertility: history	
Both partners	Previous abdominal or pelvic surgery
	Sexually transmitted disease
	Coital history
	Smoking
	Drug history
	Previous pregnancies
Female	Menstrual history
	Galactorrhoea
	Hirsutism
Male	Mumps orchitis
	Occupation—excess heat, radiation, toxic chemicals?

Examination
Female: Look for signs of endocrine or other systemic diseases, hirsutism, tumours and genital abnormalities. Carry out general, abdominal and pelvic examination.

Male: Look for signs of endocrine or other systemic diseases, lack of virilisation and genital abnormalities including testicular size, epididymal cysts and varicocoeles

ROUTINE INVESTIGATIONS IN THE FEMALE

General
- Check for *Chlamydia* and Rubella antibody levels. If the latter is negative, immunise and advise against pregnancy for 1 month.
- Treat any possible chlamydia infection (see p. 264) especially *before* testing tubal patency/uterine instrumentation.

Investigation of ovulation
- There is no evidence that the use of temperature charts and LH detection methods to time intercourse improves outcome.
- Regular menstruation is strongly suggestive of ovulation, but this should be checked by mid-luteal serum progesterone measurement (7 days before predicted menses).

Ovulation patterns vary between cycles and it may therefore be necessary to repeat tests on more than one occasion.

An endometrial biopsy to evaluate the luteal phase is not recommended as part of routine investigations. It may be used to exclude tuberculosis where the disease is common.

There is no value in measuring thyroid function or prolactin in women with a regular menstrual cycle, in the absence of galactorrhoea or symptoms of thyroid disease.

Hysterosalpingography (HSG)

Indications:
- History/examination suggest tubal damage or if chlamydial antibody titres are elevated
- Other investigations abnormal or infertility persists despite treatment
- Previous surgery on uterus or tubes

The woman must avoid pregnancy in HSG cycle. General anaesthetic is seldom necessary. Oral mefenamic acid for analgesia and buscopan i.v. can be given to counteract tubal spasm.

ROUTINE INVESTIGATIONS IN THE MALE

Semenalysis
Test after 3 days abstinence from intercourse. Two readings a month apart are necessary to confirm abnormality.

Normal values:

- Volume 2–6 ml
- Density 20–250 $\times 10^6$ ml

- Motility > 50% with forward motion within 2 hours
- Morphology > 50% normal sperm

Other features to be noted are:

- Viscosity
- Sperm clumping
- Liquefaction
- Presence of inflammatory cells

Routine testing for antisperm antibodies is not indicated in the initial investigation of seminal fluid analysis. If indicated, anti-sperm antibodies can be tested for using the mixed erythrocyte-spermatozoa antiglobulin reaction (MAR test). Anti-Rh antibodies and semen are mixed with Rh-positive erythrocytes. If spermatozoa carry antisperm antibodies they are caught up in the agglutination reaction.

Postcoital test

This is not recommended as part of the routine assessment of the infertile couple. It may be useful if the male has problems in producing a sample for semen analysis or where there is concern about sperm function or sperm/cervical mucous interaction.

Timing: About 12 hours after intercourse after 3 to 5 days abstinence.

Normal (positive): more than 5 sperms with progressive motion per high-power field (HPF).

Inconclusive: 1 to 5 sperms with good motility.

Abnormal (negative): no sperm *or* all immobile/non-progressive *or* sperm agglutination.

For an inconclusive or abnormal result to be valid the cervical mucus must be pre-ovulatory—i.e. clear, copious (>0.3 ml), ductile (>10 cm) and pH >6.5.

MANAGEMENT IN THE FEMALE

General

- Folic acid 0.4 mg daily (4 mg if previous neural tube defect or medication for epilepsy).
- Avoidance of smoking and heavy alcohol consumption.
- Supervised weight reduction where appropriate.

Induction of ovulation

Defective ovulation can be due to:

- Non-specific hypothalamo-pituitary dysfunction
- Hyperprolactinaemia
- Polycystic ovarian disease (see p. 213)
- Other endocrine disorders.

The cumulative conception rate with ovulation induction after 2 years is 95% for amenorrhoeic women and 80% for those with oligomenorrhoea (when these are the sole disorders).

Amenorrhoeic women
If the patient has amenorrhoea with normal prolactin and gonadotrophin levels, carry out a progestogen challenge test.

- If no withdrawal bleeding follows Provera 5 mg daily for 5 days, gonadotrophin or pulsatile GnRH therapy is likely to be necessary.
- If withdrawal bleeding occurs, therapy with oral fertility agents is indicated (see below).

Women having menstrual cycles (however irregular)
- If mid-luteal progesterone levels are low prescribe clomiphene or tamoxifen (see below).
- Check progesterone levels again in the second treatment cycle. If normal ovulation is still not occurring, the dose of clomiphene or tamoxifen can be increased.
- If there is still no ovulation check plasma oestrogen levels and/or follicular growth using ultrasound in the follicular phase.
- A good rise in oestrogen or follicular growth without ovulation or failure of any oestrogen response or follicular growth suggests that gonadotrophin therapy is likely to be necessary.
- If pregnancy does not occur within six treatment cycles despite good ovulation, review other factors critically. Ovulation induction with clomiphene may be continued for up to 12 months.

Oral fertility agents
These compete with natural oestrogens by blocking receptors in target organs, including the pituitary, leading to increased FSH levels. Follicles develop and ovulation follows in 85% of well-oestrogenised women.

Clomiphene. The dose is 50–150 mg daily from days 2 to 6 of the cycle. Side-effects are few but include: hot flushes, abdominal discomfort and visual disturbances may occur.

Tamoxifen. The dose is 20–40 mg twice daily from days 2 to 5. Side-effects are as above.

- The incidence of miscarriage and twins (up to 10%) is slightly increased.
- Ovarian hyperstimulation is rare and usually resolves spontaneously.

Laparoscopic ovarian diathermy
This is the minimal access surgical equivalent of ovarian wedge resection. The mechanism of action is not well understood.

- It is appropriate only for women with polycystic ovarian syndrome (see p. 213) and who are unresponsive to clomiphene, have early follicular phase serum LH levels >10 i.u./l or who recurrently respond excessively to gonadotrophin therapy.

- With laser, the multiple small subcapsular follicles are ruptured giving a 'pepperpot' appearance to the ovarian surface.
- With diathermy, the central stromal tissue of the ovary is partially destroyed by inserting the diathermy needle at several sites.
- LH levels fall after treatment and ovulation will occur spontaneously in about 75–80% of treated women for up to 9 months. This offers the chance of natural conception.
- The remaining 20–25% of women will either become responsive to clomiphene or have a more predictable response to gonadotrophins.
- About 15% of patients may develop peri-ovarian adhesions.

More research is needed into the sequelae of causing ovarian damage in this way.

Gonadotrophin therapy
This is indicated in women with hypogonadotrophic hypogonadism who are resistant to oral agents or pulsatile GnRH.

Occasional and casual use is dangerous because:

- Ovarian sensitivity varies between cycles and patients
- The difference in dose between normal ovulation and hyperstimulation is small
- The rate of high multiple conceptions and miscarriage is high unless control is meticulous

Human menopausal gonadotrophin (hMG) or purified FSH is used to stimulate follicular development.

- Women who have hypothalamic or hypopituitary causes of ovulation failure (e.g. Kallman's syndrome) will require hMG for an adequate response because it contains both LH and FSH.
- After follicular development has been stimulated, human chorionic gonadotrophin (hCG) induces ovulation.
- Treatment should be monitored by serial serum oestradiol assays and ultrasound measurement of follicular growth (number and size).
- Cycles should be abandoned and intercourse avoided if multiple mature follicles develop.

Multiple pregnancy rates are between 12 and 45% depending on the degree of control. If good, 75% of the multiple pregnancies are twins. *Anything higher is a failure of treatment.*

Hyperstimulation
Mild in 6% of cases. Severe in 2% of cases.

- *Mild*—excess oestrogen output with ovarian enlargement; no cysts; some abdominal pain. No active treatment is needed.

- *Moderate*—detectable but not large ovarian cysts; abdominal pain, nausea, vomiting, diarrhoea and ascites. Admit for observation, rehydration and symptomatic treatment. Infusion of colloid (intravenous albumin) may be necessary.
- *Severe*—large ovarian cysts, massive ascites (possibly with hydrothorax). Severe abdominal pain and distension. There is a risk of DIC and thromboembolism if the woman has an underlying thrombophilic tendency (see p. 331). On rare occasions this may be life threatening.

Management—correct fluid and electrolyte imbalance (avoid diuretics). Intravenous colloid should be used for infusion rather than crystalloid. Screen for early evidence of DIC. Laparotomy should be avoided unless there is a cyst accident or active bleeding.

Gonadotrophin releasing hormone (GnRH or LHRH)
- Pulsatile subcutaneous (or intravenous) infusion of GnRH by miniaturised automatic infusion systems is indicated mainly for ovulation induction in women with hypothalamic or hypopituitary causes of ovulation failure.
- It can also be successful in treatment resistant hyperprolactinaemia and clomiphene-resistant anovulation.
- Endocrine events in the normal cycle are mimicked and the multiple pregnancy rate is low.
- Treatment is monitored using ultrasound measurement of follicular development.
- After ovulation the pulsatile infusion may be discontinued and luteal phase support may be given by a single injection of hCG.
- It is usually ineffective in women with polycystic ovary syndrome (PCOS—see p. 213).

TUBAL FACTORS

- HSG and laparoscopy (with or without hysteroscopy) are complementary investigations of tubal function.
- Ultrasound assessment of tubal patency is now possible but gives no information about damage to the endosalpinx. As this is an important predictor for success of tubal microsurgery, HSG is preferred.

Indications for laparoscopy
- Abnormal HSG
- History or examination suggest need for direct investigation, e.g. endometriosis, previous PID, etc.
- All other investigations normal or abnormal but corrected (in such cases unsuspected problems can be found in up to 30% of cases).

Peritubal adhesions—avascular adhesions can be divided at laparoscopy or laparotomy (salpingolysis). Treatment of thick vascular adhesions gives poor results.

Tubal blockage—micro-surgery for mild/moderate damage; IVF if severe.

Salpingostomy (surgical opening of ostia)—conception rate no more than 20%.

Excision of block and re-anastomosis—conception rate 10 to 15%.

• The incidence of ectopic pregnancies is increased in treated cases.

MANAGEMENT IN THE MALE

General
• Avoid smoking and excess alcohol.
• If poor quality sperm wear loose fitting underwear and trousers, and avoid environmental situations that might cause testicular hyperthermia.

Erectile impotence
Among the causes are psycho-sexual problems, vascular disease (e.g. secondary to smoking) and hyperprolactinaemia.

Causes of azoospermia

Ejaculatory failure
• Exclude retrograde ejaculation by examining urine postcoitally (especially if ejaculate volume <2 ml).
• If psychogenic impotence is present refer for psychosexual counselling.
• Consider neurological disorders (e.g. multiple sclerosis or diabetic neuropathy), urological factors and drug side-effects (e.g. antihypertensive therapy).

Failure of spermatogenesis
• Assess testicular size—this diagnosis is more likely if volume <15 ml by orchidometer.
• Check FSH levels. Significant elevation is found in:
  • Klinefelter's syndrome (therefore check karyotype)
  • Spermatogenic arrest
  • Sertoli cell only syndrome
  • Testicular atrophy.
• In selected cases intracytoplasmic sperm injection (ICSI) may be possible (see p. 240), but there is no remedy in the majority of cases.

Obstruction
• If testicular size and consistency and FSH are normal consider congenital or acquired block of the vas deferens. Investigate by semen biochemistry (see below) and/or vasography.

Hypogonadotrophism
• This is indicated by lack of virilisation, impotence and reduced testosterone level with normal or low FSH and LH levels.

Table 18.1   Seminal biochemistry

Acid phosphatase, zinc	Fructose	Carnitine	Possible site of defect
Absent	Present	Present	Prostate
Present	Absent	Present	Seminal vesicles
Present	Present	Absent	Epididymis

- It is the only treatable cause of azoospermia using hMG. Because spermatogenesis takes over 70 days, treatment must be prolonged. Once spermatogenesis has been stimulated hCG alone will maintain sperm counts.

Oligospermia
- This is often accompanied by seminal plasma of high viscosity and/or low volume which fails to liquefy.
- Low sperm density and poor motility frequently related.
- Seminal biochemistry may indicate the source of the problem (Table 18.1).
- Elevated FSH levels (>8 i.u./l) suggest irreversible sterility. Low levels of testosterone and high LH levels are frequently secondary to severe testicular damage which is irreversible.
- Testicular biopsy is of little diagnostic value.
- Cytogenetic studies. Karyotype will reveal abnormalities in up to 6% of infertile males and 20% when azoospermia is present. No treatment is available apart from donor insemination (DI).
- Therapy for oligospermia. There is no proven effective drug treatment. All claims for success using clomiphene or mesterolone must be compared with the spontaneous pregnancy rate in oligospermic men.
- High ligation of a varicocoele improves semenalysis in 60% of cases of oligospermia and pregnancy rates may improve.

ARTIFICIAL INSEMINATION

Husband artificial insemination (AIH)—only when intercourse is impossible due to male impotence or anatomical defects but a normal ejaculate can be obtained.

Donor insemination (DI)

- The greatest care must be taken to protect the identity of the donors
- Counselling is vital to ascertain that both husband and wife are sure they wish this form of treatment. Inseminations are usually carried out twice in the peri-ovulatory phase. Prior investigation of female infertility is mandatory. Checking for stress-induced

ovulatory dysfunction during the initial 2–3 treatment cycles is advisable.

• Following 12 unsuccessful cycles of DI other treatment options should be considered.

ASSISTED CONCEPTION

These procedures are carefully controlled in the UK by the statutory Human Fertilisation and Embryo Authority (HFEA).

Intracytoplasmic sperm injection (ICSI)

• Individually selected sperm are injected into oocytes by microscopic manipulation before *in vitro* fertilisation (IVF, see below).
• It is appropriate for men with severe oligospermia or significant sperm dysfunction.
• Where a specific gene defect associated with male infertility is known or suspected (e.g. congenital bilateral absence of the vas deferens) appropriate genetic counselling and testing should be offered.
• In conjunction with surgical recovery of sperm from the epididymis or testis, it can also by-pass the problem for men with:
  • congenital absence of the vas deferens (exclude an association with carriage of the cystic fibrosis gene)
  • failed reversal of vasectomy
  • failed surgery for bilateral obstruction of the vas deferens.
• Follicular stimulation and oocyte collection from the woman is as for standard IVF. Only morphologically mature oocytes are suitable for micro-injection.
• Technique
  • Under an operating microscope, the cumulus cells are removed chemically from the oocyte, which is then held gently by a micro-pipette.
  • A fine micro-pipette is used to draw up a single motile sperm (tail first). This is then advanced through the zona pellucida and vitelline membrane.
  • The sperm is deposited (head first) into the cytoplasm of the oocyte nucleus.
  • About 10% of sperm will be damaged by the procedure, but fertilisation rates of 60–75% are now being reported.
• ICSI is likely to reduce the demand for DI, currently the only alternative for many couples suffering from severe male subfertility.
• Long term longitudinal follow-up of children born after ICSI is important and should ideally be co-ordinated on a national basis.

In vitro fertilisation (IVF)

• It is now estimated that up to 35% of subfertile couples could benefit from IVF.

- It is most suitable for women with tubal blockage or damage, endometriosis or those with prolonged unexplained subfertility.
- The advent of ICSI now makes IVF appropriate for treatment of male subfertility.
- IVF (or GIFT, see below) may be used for egg donation and may optimise the chances of pregnancy for women over 35 years of age who have ovulatory disorders but have failed to conceive with gonadotrophin therapy.
- It is expensive and requires sophisticated laboratory facilities and highly skilled medical, nursing, scientific and technical personnel.

SUGGESTED GUIDELINES FOR PROCEEDING WITH ASSISTED CONCEPTION

- Clear positive recommendation from GP.
- No more than one previous child.
- A continuing stable heterosexual relationship of at least 2 years' duration (although this has been challenged).
- Treatment is technically feasible with a good chance of success. Women over 40 years of age have a reduced chance of success.
- Couples in good health such that both can be reasonably expected to bring up the child together.
- Appropriate domestic and social circumstances.
- An understanding by all parties of the statutory responsibility to consider the welfare of any child born as a result of treatment.

(These guidelines could be applied to the whole problem of infertility)

OUTLINE PROTOCOL FOR IVF

- Multiple ovulation is induced with hMG or purified FSH after pituitary down-regulation with an GnRH analogue to inhibit any endogenous LH rise. Follicular maturation is monitored ultrasonically and by serum oestradiol levels.
- Mature oocytes are recovered just before ovulation (following an injection of hCG) by transvaginal aspiration of follicles under ultrasound guidance using i.v. sedation. Alternatively, laparoscopy may be used. The aim is to collect at least four eggs.
- Fertilisation of ovum by sperm occurs within 24 hours in a fluid culture medium at physiological temperature and atmospheric conditions. There is a 70% chance of each mature egg being fertilised.
- A legal maximum of three embryos are transferred to the uterus through the cervical canal after 2 to 3 days (i.e. around the eight-cell stage). In women under 40, usually a maximum of two embryos should be transferred.

Gamete intra-fallopian transfer (GIFT)
- GIFT is suitable for all women who are candidates for IVF except those with blocked or damaged fallopian tubes, or when ICSI is used.

- Oocytes are collected as above, mixed with 2–5×10^5 sperm in buffered medium and transferred into the fimbrial end of the tube by laparoscopy.
- GIFT is theoretically superior to IVF because fertilisation occurs in the normal site and implantation at the normal time (5–6 days) after ovulation (cf. IVF at 2 days). This is reflected in a slightly greater number of pregnancies and births with GIFT than in IVF (see below). However it is more invasive as a laparoscopy and general anaesthesia is needed. It too is expensive, and the conditions for setting it up should be as for IVF.

Intrauterine insemination (IUI)
- IUI using husband's semen after superovulation of the woman is an effective treatment in selected cases.
- As with GIFT, it is only suitable for women with patent, healthy fallopian tubes.

Ovum donation followed by IVF
This can be used with the same considerations as for DI (p. 239) in women who:

- Have had their ovaries removed.
- Have experienced premature menopause.
- Have gonadal dysgenesis including Turner's syndrome.
- Have ovarian failure following chemotherapy or radiotherapy.
- Carry a serious genetic defect.

Appropriate hormonal support is required for the first four of these.

RESULTS OF IVF AND GIFT

- Transfer of a single embryo results in a pregnancy in approximately 10% of cases.
- It is therefore usual to transfer two (or a legal maximum of three if reduced chance of success) embryos if possible. This gives a 25–30% chance of a single pregnancy, a 5% chance of twins, and a 1–2% chance of triplets (if three embryos transferred).
- There is an increased risk of ectopic pregnancy, particularly in cases of tubal damage.
- The overall efficiency of the method (the 'take-home baby rate') is between 15 and 20% for each cycle. This probably does not differ significantly from conception rates in normal couples.
- HFEA data suggest that transfer of 2 embryos rather then 3 does not reduce the overall success rate while virtually eliminating the chance of triplets.
- About 20% of women will have a child per cycle of IVF treatment compared with about 25% for GIFT.
- In ICSI pregnancy rates of up to 35% per cycle can be achieved after transfer of up to 3 embryos.

OUTCOMES AFTER ASSISTED CONCEPTION

Pregnancies after **standard IVF** are at increased risk of *pre-term delivery* and *low-birth weight infants.*

* This cannot be fully explained by multiple pregnancies as the risk is still present in singletons. It may be due to the process itself, maternal factors or both.
* Singleton pregnancies following **ICSI** or **frozen embryos** may not share these risks.

The incidence of *congenital and chromosomal anomalies* after:

* **Standard IVF** is generally similar to that found in the general population though some increased risk of NTD, gut atresias and exomphalos has been reported from Sweden (see Further reading)
* **ICSI** may be associated with an increased risk of paternally derived chromosomal and other new mainly sex chromosome defects. There may also be an increased risk of hypospadias in male infants.

Postnatal growth and development of children born after **assisted conception** seem to be within normal range.

The overall safety of **embryo freezing** remains to be established.

FURTHER READING

Behrman SJ, Patton GW, Holtz G (eds) 1994 Progress in infertility, 4th edn. Little Brown & Co, Boston

Ericson A, Kallen B 2001 Congenital malformations in infants born after IVF: a population based study. Human Reproduction 16: 504–9

Fishel S (ed) 1994 Clinical Obstetrics and Gynaecology 8: Micromanipulation techniques. Bailliere Tindal, London

RCOG Guideline 1998 The Initial Investigation and Management of the Infertile Couple. RCOG Press, London

RCOG Guideline 1998 The Management of Infertility in Secondary Care. RCOG Press, London

RCOG Guideline 2000 The Management of Infertility in Tertiary Care. RCOG Press, London

19. Contraception and sterilisation

Human fertility can be measured in several ways, for example:

- *General fertility rate*—the number of births during a year per 1000 women of childbearing age
- *Age-specific fertility rate*—the number of births during a year per 1000 women of a specified 5-year age range
- *Total fertility rate*—the average size of a completed family.

The 'Pearl index' is a measure of contraceptive effectiveness using the numbers of pregnancies occurring per 100 woman-years (w.y.) of exposure.

STEROIDAL CONTRACEPTION

Steroidal contraception has, as its basis, synthetic oestrogens and progestogens. The effect of any one *combined oral contraceptive* (COC) will depend on the balance of the oestrogen and progestogen it contains.

- The oestrogen in most pills is now *ethinyl estradiol* using the lowest possible effective dose.
- The 'traditional' progestogens have been *ethynodiol, levonorgestrel* and *norethisterone.*
- The newer progestogens *desogestrel* (DSG), *gestodene* (GSD) and *norgestimate* bind more specifically to progesterone receptors and have less effect on sex hormone-binding globulin (SHBG) and high-density lipoprotein (HDL). They are thus less anti-oestrogenic and may reduce the risk of arterial disease. There is, however, some evidence that the risk of venous thromboembolism with DSG and GSD is 1.7× that using 'traditional' progestogens (information about norgestimate is insufficient). This is discussed further below.

Modes of action
- Inhibition of ovulation due to negative feedback on the hypothalamo-pituitary-ovarian axis
- Induction of changes in cervical mucus, endometrium, myometrium and fallopian tubes, which makes them hostile to sperm and unfavourable for ovum transplant and implantation.

Types of steroidal contraceptives

Combined oral contraceptives (*COC*) are the most widely used:

- *monophasic* (fixed dose) pills—oestrogen and progestogen are taken in constant doses for 21 days followed by an interval of 7 days
- *biphasic* and *triphasic* preparations—contain phased doses of oestrogen and progestogen which make it possible to titrate the dose to the individual woman in order to find the lowest dose of both hormones that will provide good cycle control, and fewest side-effects.

Continuous low-dose oral *progestogens* (*POP*) have a good contraceptive effect provided they are taken regularly 3–4 hours before expected intercourse.

- Ovulation is only inhibited in 40% of women, and the anti-fertility effect on cervical mucus (which wears off after 16–20 hours) is important.
- Irregular menstruation is frequent but improves as use continues. Some patients develop amenorrhoea.
- An association with ectopic pregnancies is still in dispute. The POP may produce a genuine increase because of its effect on the fallopian tube, or it may be less effective in preventing ectopic than intrauterine pregnancies. Where possible the COC or injectable progestogen (which inhibits ovulation) should be used in those with a past history of ectopic pregnancy.
- Lactation is not inhibited by POP and there does not appear to be an effect on blood pressure. They are particularly suitable for lactating women, diabetics, those with contraindications or intolerance to oestrogen, and possibly those with a past history of venous thrombosis.

Injectable progestogens e.g. *medroxyprogesterone acetate* (Depo-Provera™) 150 mg i.m. every 3 months or *norethisterone oenanthate* 200 mg i.m. every 8 weeks.

- They are highly effective.
- Menstruation tends to be irregular and may be prolonged: amenorrhoea will supervene in about one third of users within 1 year.
- Effects on glucose tolerance and plasma lipids are markedly less than those caused by COC. Occasionally there is some weight gain. There appears to be no effect on blood pressure or blood coagulability. No increased risk of carcinoma of breast, endometrium or cervix has been noted.
- Menstrual cycles and fertility usually return to normal within 6 months of the last injection but with Depo-provera the 'hangover' effect can last up to 2 years.
- If used during lactation the quality and quantity of milk are improved. Only a tiny quantity of steroid is ingested by the infant and as yet no adverse effects have been noted.
- Do not use in an already pregnant woman.

Implants avoid the 'first-pass' effect of the oral route. *Norplant*™ delivered levonorgestrel in six subdermal capsules, but these could be difficult to remove; a new version *Implanon*™, which is a single, matchstick-sized implant has now superseded it.

• Training in insertion and removal is required.
• If inserted within 24 hours of the start of menstruation, no additional contraception is required.
• Implanon™ should be removed before the end of 3 years.

(See below for progestogen-containing IUDs.)

Efficacy
Failure can be due to the method or the patient.

• With older medium-dose COC the Pearl index was <1/100 w.y.
• With modern low-dose COC the rate is about 3/100 w.y.
• The POP has a failure rate of 2–3/100 w.y. (in older women it can be as low as 0.9)
• Injectable progestogens have a Pearl index of 0–0.4/100 w.y.

Non-contraceptive benefits of COC
• Less dysmenorrhoea and menorrhagia (and therefore less anaemia)
• Reduced risk of carcinoma of endometrium and ovary (by at least 50%); pelvic inflammatory disease; and benign breast disease
• Possible protective effect against fibroids and rheumatoid arthritis.

Possible adverse effects of COC
The risk/benefit balance must be weighed for each woman, taking into account the presence of risk markers.

Thrombotic and Cardiovascular risks are shown in Table 19.1

Table 19.1 Thrombotic and cardiovascular risks

Condition	Relative risk	Associated risk markers
Venous thrombosis	<2 with low-dose COC containing levonorgestrel, norethisterone or ethynodiol Pills containing DSG and GSD may increase that risk further ×2	Close family history; marked obesity (BMI >30 kg/m^2); immobility (e.g. plaster cast or in a wheelchair); prominent varicose veins; presence of factor V Leiden mutation
Haemorrhagic stroke	1.5–2	Smoking; hypertension
Thrombotic stroke:	5	Close family history; smoking; diabetes; marked obesity
non-fatal	in 1/10 000 w.y.	
fatal	in 2–4/10 000 w.y.	

Table 19.1 (*Cont'd*)

Condition	Relative risk	Associated risk markers
Hypertension	Develops in about 5% of women within 5 years of commencing COC: *stop if BP rises to 160/95 mmHg or more*	Age, family or personal history of hypertension; obesity and previous hypertension in pregnancy are not associated risks
Myocardial infarction:	3–5	Smoking, age, hypertension, hyperlipidaemia
fatal	in 1/10 000 w.y.	

Metabolic changes
- Weight gain—associated with pills containing levonorgestrel but not desogestrel (DSG) or gestodene (GSD).
- Carbohydrate metabolism—modern low-oestrogen and progestogen preparations produce minor effects on insulin secretion and little or no change in glucose tolerance. Significant glucose intolerance occasionally occurs in susceptible individuals, and insulin-dependent diabetics may need to increase their dose.
- Lipid metabolism—the effect on the ratios of total and low density lipoprotein (LDL) cholesterol to high density lipoprotein (HDL) cholesterol (important indicators of risk of cardiovascular disease) depends on the relative doses of oestrogen/ progestogen and the type of progestogen. The aim of modern pills is to have a near-neutral effect.

Effects on gastrointestinal tract
Reports of an increased incidence of cholelithiasis and cholecystitis were associated with higher doses of oestrogen. The risk is not significantly increased with low-dose COC. A slight increased risk of ulcerative colitis and Crohn's disease is associated with COC use and smoking.

Cancer and COC use
Breast cancer—COC use reduces the risk of benign breast disease but the question of an increased risk of breast cancer remains unresolved. Further studies are necessary on women at increased genetic risk of breast cancer and who use COC.

- Studies suggesting an increased risk among young women (particularly if used before a first pregnancy) were conflicting and confusing. If such a risk exists in these women it can be minimised by using the lowest effective doses of oestrogen and progestogen.

Cervical neoplasia—an increased incidence of cervical intraepithelial neoplasia is likely to be due to greater sexual activity in women on COC, but there is evidence that oestrogen may have a direct stimulating effect on HPV.

- Long-term use of oral contraceptives may be a co-factor in the 4-fold risk of cervical carcinoma in women with HPV (see Further reading)
- This has to be set against the strongly protective effect against carcinoma of endometrium and ovary.

Ovarian cancer—there is a >50% reduction and this effect persists for many years after stopping COC.

Endometrial cancer—similarly reduced by at least 50%.

Drug interactions
- Enzyme-inducing drugs may reduce the effect of oestrogens and progestogens. They include most anticonvulsants (not sodium valproate), rifampicin and griseofulvin.
- Interference with gut flora and the enterohepatic circulation of ethinyl oestradiol can be caused by broad spectrum antibiotics (also by a vegetarian diet). Progestogens are not affected in this way.
- Advice depends on the length of therapy:
  - *short-term*—use barrier method during and for 7 days after stopping drug
  - *long-term*—use monophasic 50 µg ethinyl oestradiol COC (can be taken as four packs without a break then a 'tablet-free' interval); contraceptive efficacy can be judged by the occurrence of irregular bleeding.

Contraindications to combined oral contraceptive pill
Absolute and relative contraindications are shown in the information boxes

Prescribing COC
The following guidelines have been suggested (see Guillebaud in Further reading)

- *Which oestrogen?* Use the lowest acceptable dose of *ethinyl oestradiol*.
- *Which progestogen?* Because of the suggested increased risk of venous thromboembolism (TE) and despite a possible lesser risk of arterial disease (heart attack or stroke—see over), in 1995 the Committee on Safety of Medicines (CSM) in the UK advised that:
  - COC containing *desogestrel* (DSG) or *gestodene* (GSD) should not be used in women with risk markers for TE (see p. 76) including obesity or varicose veins. (*Note: A previous history of TE is an absolute contraindication to COC use.*)
  - COC containing DSG or GSD should only be used by women who are 'intolerant of other COCs' and who make a fully informed choice about the possible risk of TE.
- Intolerance of other COCs' includes irregular bleeding, weight gain, acne or headaches.

COC: Absolute contraindications

Cardiovascular
- Previous arterial or venous thrombosis
- Ischaemic or other severe heart disease; pulmonary hypertension
- Thrombophilia (see p. 80) or blood dyscrasias
- Previous cerebral haemorrhage
- Severe hypertension
- Focal migraine
- Transient ischaemic attacks
- Hyperlipidaemia
- Combination of any of above risk markers

Hepatic
- Chronic liver disease, and following acute disease until liver function tests have been normal for 3 months
- Cholestatic jaundice of pregnancy
- Chronic idiopathic jaundice (e.g. due to Dubin–Johnson or Rotor syndromes)
- Liver adenoma; porphyria

Other
- Oestrogen-dependent neoplasms (particularly breast cancer)
- History of serious condition affected by sex steroids (e.g. pemphigoid gestationis; haemolytic uraemic syndrome)
- Undiagnosed abnormal genital tract bleeding
- Pregnancy

COC: Relative contraindications
- Oligomenorrhoea (investigate first and may then be prescribed if no other contraindication)
- Women over 35 years of age who smoke
- Latent or established diabetes
- Cholelithiasis (but can be used after cholecystectomy)
- First-degree relative with breast cancer
- Obesity, if associated with other risk factors
- Non-focal migraine when ergotamine is not required for treatment
- Sickle cell disease (injectable progestogen better). Sickle cell trait is not a contraindication
- Crohn's disease

- Among the other women for whom a DSG/GSD pill might be more suitable are:
  - those with a single risk marker for arterial disease (see above)
  - those aged 35 up to the menopause in the absence of all risk markers for venous or arterial disease.
- If a DSG/GSD pill is to be used:
  - it must be the patient's informed choice
  - all counselling and discussion must be clearly recorded in the case-notes.

Surgery and the COC pill
Whether or not to stop the pill before major surgery is controversial (see Further reading).

- With low-dose oestrogen pills the risk of postoperative TE is about 1% for pill users and 0.5% for non-pill users.
- This must be balanced against the risks of stopping the pill 4–6 weeks before surgery, the most important of which is unwanted pregnancy.
- The woman must be made aware of the above and, if the COC is stopped, adequate alternative contraception must be provided
- THRIFT (see Further reading) suggest that without other risk markers there is insufficient evidence either to routinely stop the pill before elective major surgery or use specific thrombo-prophylaxis.
- Thrombo-prophylaxis is advised for emergency surgery.

INTRAUTERINE DEVICES (IUDs)

This is now the second most common reliable and reversible method of preventing pregnancy. The ideal IUD must be effective; easy to fit (with minimal discomfort); and should remain in the uterine cavity until the woman wishes it removed.

Types of IUD in common use
- Copper (Cu)-containing with surface areas of 200–375 mm^2
- Progestogen-releasing.

Modes of action
- 'Foreign body' reaction
- Copper ions affect tubal fluid, sperm transport and oocytes
- Progestogens make cervical mucus 'hostile' and thin the endometrium.

Efficacy
- The Pearl index of the Cu devices (200 mm^2) is 2–4/100 w.y.
- For the newest devices with 375 mm^2 of copper or progestogen-releasing, this falls to <1/100 w.y., which is as effective as sterilisation.

Timing of insertion
- The best time is towards the end of menstruation but, if necessary, fitting can take place at any point in the cycle.
- Post-pregnancy side-effects, expulsion or perforation rates are no higher if inserted at 3–4 weeks than at 6 weeks.
- An IUD can be fitted at the time of suction termination of pregnancy but the optimum time may be 1–2 weeks later because the risk of perforation is less.
- Insertion of an IUD within 5 days of unprotected intercourse will act as a post-coital contraceptive.

POSSIBLE COMPLICATIONS AND SIDE-EFFECTS OF IUDs

- Vaginal bleeding—this is the commonest reason for removal.
  - With Cu-releasing devices menstrual loss may increase by 40–50%.
  - With progestogen-releasing devices loss is reduced by 40–50% but intermenstrual spotting/bleeding occurs in up to 80% of women.
  - Pain—some low abdominal pain or backache may follow insertion.
  - Rarely it is severe and the device may need to be removed.
  - Dysmenorrhoea can be increased particularly if the woman is nulliparous.
- Vaginal discharge—may be temporary or persistent.
  - It arises from the endometrium as it reacts to the presence of a foreign body but symptomatic discharges must be investigated.
- Ectopic pregnancy—the rate for modem IUDs is <1.5/1000 w.y.
  - Cu-releasing devices are protective against ectopic pregnancy.
  - The progestogen releasing IUDs are associated with an increase in the rate of ectopic pregnancy. Another form of contraception is advised in a woman who has previously had an ectopic pregnancy.
- Expulsion is most likely during the first month.
  - About 50% of all expulsions take place within 3 months of insertion; after the first year very few are expelled.
  - Among the associated factors are:
    - the skill and experience of the person fitting the device
    - use of an inappropriate size or type of IUD
    - use in young nulliparous women.
- Uterine perforation occurs in about 1/1000 insertions.
  - Most devices can be removed from the peritoneal cavity by laparoscopy but laparotomy is sometimes necessary.
  - Cu-bearing devices tend to form omental masses and adhesions, and should be removed promptly.
- Pelvic infection—the risk is increased 2-fold but only for the first few weeks after insertion.
  - The major risk factor is the number of sexual partners of the woman and her partner.
  - Monogamous women using a copper device have no increased risk.
  - The progestogen releasing devices are associated with a

reduction in the rate of infection.
- Lost threads may be due to unrecognised expulsion; perforation of the uterus (see above); or a normally-sited device with the threads above the external os.
  - The site of the IUD can be checked by ultrasound.
  - Threads may be retrieved using a thread retrieval device.

Pregnancy with an IUD in place
- The risk of miscarriage is increased 5-fold particularly if the IUD is left *in situ*; a major associated complication is second trimester septic abortion.
- Intrauterine candidal infection resulting in fetal death can rarely occur.
- The device should therefore be removed if the threads are accessible; if threads are not visible, counsel about risk of miscarriage and later intrauterine infection.
- Exclude ectopic pregnancy.

CONTRAINDICATIONS TO THE USE OF IUDs

Table 19.2   Contraindications to the use of an IUD

Contraindication	Nulliparous women	Parous women
Pregnancy	absolute	absolute
Serious pregnancy-related pelvic infection within previous year	absolute	absolute
Active pelvic inflammatory disease	absolute	absolute
Significant congenital uterine anomaly	absolute	absolute
Undiagnosed uterine bleeding	absolute	absolute
Carcinoma of cervix or endometrium	absolute	absolute
Previous ectopic pregnancy	absolute	absolute
Risk from bacteraemia, e.g. valvular heart disease, renal dialysis or transplant, or immunosuppressive drugs	absolute	absolute
Multiple sexual partners	relative	relative
Past history of STD	absolute	relative
Menorrhagia	relative	relative
Copper allergy or Wilson'sdisease	Avoid Cu bearing devices	

BARRIER CONTRACEPTION

Table 19.2 lists contraindications for parous/nulliparous women. Barrier contraceptives prevent live sperm from entering the cervical canal either by mechanical occlusion (caps and condoms) or by killing sperm (spermicides).

• Condoms are the most popular.
• Caps include vaginal diaphragms, cervical caps, vault caps and vimules (see Further reading). The most commonly used is the diaphragm, which should be:
  • used in conjunction with spermicides
  • fitted before intercourse and removed 6 hours afterwards.
• The use-effectiveness of these methods varies widely depending on the motivation of the couple, but the theoretical effectiveness of caps and condoms is high, with pregnancy rates as low as 2/100 w.y.
• Barrier methods have assumed great importance in the battle against the spread of HIV infection. They should therefore be discussed with *all* couples seeking contraceptive advice, even if they are using another method in addition.

POSTCOITAL CONTRACEPTION

The most commonly used is the Yutzpe method—*ethinyl oestradiol* 100 μg and *levonorgestrel* 500 μg taken within 72 hours of unprotected intercourse, repeated 12 hours later. However, nausea and vomiting are common. The pregnancy rate is 3% among women at risk.

Large doses of *levonorgestrol* (750 μg twice (Levonelle-2™) have a 1% pregnancy rate with significantly reduced side-effects.

• It is not recommended as a routine method but is useful as an emergency method, including following rape.

SAFE-PERIOD METHODS

Several methods may be used to detect the fertile and infertile phases in the cycle.

Rhythm method
The lengths of the previous 12 cycles are recorded and the time during which intercourse is to be avoided is between 18 and 11 days before the next period is due to begin. This method is not applicable if the cycle is very irregular, or after recent pregnancy, and may be affected by illness or emotional upset.

Cyclical temperature changes

These can be used in two main ways:

- The couple abstain from sexual intercourse until 3 days after the temperature has risen.
- Intercourse can take place in the early follicular phase, and time of abstinence is determined by use of the calendar and timing of the temperature rise.

Cervical mucus

Cervical mucus becomes profuse and watery with a good spinnbarkeit at ovulation. The popular 'sympto-thermal' method combines observation of cyclical temperature and cervical mucus changes.

These methods are effective when used consistently by highly-motivated couples, but even then it is reported that accidental pregnancy may occur in up to 14% of women using the 'sympto-thermal' method for 2 years.

Lactational amenorrhoea

This can provide up to 98% (protection) but only if used under the following conditions:

- Within 6 months of delivery
- Amenorrhoeic
- Fully (or almost fully) breast-feeding.

COITUS INTERRUPTUS

Male withdrawal is the oldest and most widely used method of contraception. It is simple, moderately effective and without serious side-effects (excluding pregnancy).

MALE AND FEMALE STERILISATION

Sterilisation in either partner is increasingly popular for birth control, with 23% of women of reproductive age in the UK having chosen sterilisation as their preferred method. The peak age in women is between 30 and 34 years. The popularity of this irreversible approach is due to the limitations of other, reversible, methods.

In counselling couples requesting sterilisation the following general points must be borne in mind, as detailed in the RCOG Guideline on sterilisation (www.rcog.org.uk):

- *Awareness of alternative long-term contraceptive methods* to the one requested:

- Men and women requesting sterilisation should have their knowledge of and access to alternative methods of long-term contraception confirmed, including comparative failure rates and advantages and disadvantages of each method.
- Non-operative methods of long-term contraception should have been specifically rejected before proceeding with sterilisation.
- Both vasectomy and tubal occlusion should be discussed with all patients requesting sterilisation. Women in particular should be aware that vasectomy carries a lower failure rate in terms of post-procedure pregnancies and less risk related to the procedure.
- *Reversibility:*
  - Men and women seeking sterilisation should be advised that the procedure is intended to be permanent. However, they should also be given information on the success rates associated with reversal should this procedure ever be required, particularly those related to the different methods of tubal occlusion.
- *Post-procedure pregnancy rate*—the failure rate (i.e. the risk of pregnancy following the procedure) should be explicitly mentioned:
  - For women this averages approximately one in 200 in her lifetime and pregnancy can occur several years after the procedure.
  - It will be lower in older women and maybe higher when the procedure immediately follows the end of pregnancy.
  - The rate for men should be quoted as 1 in 2000 after two azoospermic samples 2–4 weeks apart at least 8 weeks after the procedure.
- *Risk of ectopic pregnancy*
  - Women should be explicitly informed that post-procedure pregnancies are often ectopic and, therefore, a threat to their health.
  - They should be advised to seek medical advice promptly if they think they are pregnant, or have abnormal abdominal pain or vaginal bleeding.
- *Intended method and alternative methods*—Women should be informed of:
  - the method of access and tubal occlusion being recommended in their case,
  - the reasons for preferring it over other methods,
  - the procedure to be used if the intended method cannot be completed successfully.
- *Risk of operative complications:*
  - Women should be informed of the risks of laparoscopy and the chances of requiring laparotomy if there are problems with laparoscopy, particularly those at increased risk from conditions such as previous abdominal surgery or obesity.
- *Need for contraception before and after operation:*
  - Women must be advised to continue to use effective contraception until their next (post-procedure) period. No

precautions can be guaranteed to avoid pre-procedure fertilisation, which may be undetectable.
  • Men should be advised to use effective contraception until they have had two consecutive semen analyses showing azoospermia 2–4 weeks apart at least 8 weeks after the procedure.
• *Effect on long-term health*:
  • Both men and women can be reassured that there is no substantial long-term health risk from sterilisation procedures.
  • Women should be reassured that tubal occlusion is not associated with an increased risk of heavier or irregular periods when performed after 30 years of age.
  • Men should be informed about the possibility of chronic testicular pain after vasectomy.
• *Post-procedure information:*
  • Women should be advised post-operatively about the final method of tubal occlusion and of any complications that occurred during the procedure.

FEMALE STERILISATION

Current techniques
Laparoscopy—this is the most popular technique. The fallopian tubes are occluded by clips or bands or, if there are technical difficulties, bipolar diathermy. There is no need to stop oral contraception beforehand.

Mini-laparotomy—this can be used in women not suitable for laparoscopy. Access to the tubes can be, for example, via a proctoscope inserted through a small suprapubic incision.

Hysteroscopic techniques (e.g. using diathermy or tubal plugs)—these require further development but look promising in that they do not require general anaesthesia.

Posterior colpotomy—the tubes are approached through a small incision in the pouch of Douglas; complication rates are higher than for above methods and the RCOG has recommended it be discontinued.

Failure rates
The overall failure rate is quoted as 1 in 200 and depends on the type of operation and experience of the operator.

Pregnancy can result from:

• true method failure
• surgical error—e.g. misidentification of tubes
• woman in luteal phase and pregnant at time of operation.

Technical failure is associated with obesity; history of pelvic inflammatory disease; previous abdominal or pelvic surgery; and the skill/experience of the operator.

Reversibility

Tubal re-anastomosis will restore fertility in 50–70% of women (depending on the method of sterilisation and the experience of the operator).

- Ectopic pregnancy can be expected in about 8% of conceptions.

MALE STERILISATION (VASECTOMY)

- This can be performed as an outpatient procedure under local anaesthetic.
- The *vas deferens* is approached through small bilateral scrotal incisions, cut and ligated or diathermied. Two sperm-free specimens at 3 and 4 months post-operation should be obtained before the patient can be deemed to be sterile.
- The **failure rate** is 1–4/1000 procedures (see p. 255).

Reversibility

If the technique used for vasectomy is amenable to reversal, sperm will return to the ejaculate in 70–90% of men, and about 30% of their partners will become pregnant.

FURTHER READING

Chief Medical Officer Statement on risks of oral contraceptive pill. www.doh.gov.uk

Chief Medical Officer Statement on risks of OCP and HPV. www.doh.gov.uk

Glasier A and Gebbie A. 2001 Handbook of Family Planning and Reproductive Health Care, Churchill Livingstone, Edinburgh

Guillebaud J 2000 Contraception Today, 4th edn. Dunnitz, London

Gupta S, Kirkman R 2002 Intrauterine Devices—update on clinical performance. The Obstetrician & Gynaecologist 1: 37–41

Kemmeren JM, Algra A, and Grobbee DE 2001 Third generation oral contraceptives and risk of venous thrombosis: meta-analysis. British Medical Journal 323: 131–32

Moreno V, Bosch FX, Munoz N, et al. 2002 Effect of oral contraceptives on risk of cervical cancer in women with HPV infection: the IARC multicentric case-control study Lancet 359: 1085–192

RCOG National Evidence-Based Clinical Guidelines Male and Female Sterilisation. RCOG, London www.rcog.org.uk/guidelines

THRIFT Consensus Group 1992 Risk of and prophylaxis for venous thromboembolism in hospital patients. British Medical Journal 305: 567–574

20. The climacteric

Definitions
- The *menopause* is the time at which menstruation ceases.
  - The average age at which the menopause occurs is 51 years.
- The *climacteric* is the transitional period during which a woman's reproductive capacity ceases.
- A *premature menopause* is one which occurs before 45 years of age. It affects about 1% of women. Among the causes are:
  - genetic
  - metabolic
  - infection
  - auto-immune
  - iatrogenic (surgery, chemotherapy, radiation)
  - idiopathic.

PHYSICAL CHANGES OCCURRING FROM THE MENOPAUSE

- Low oestrogen levels after the menopause cause symptoms and changes in oestrogen target tissues.
- Differences in symptoms may reflect differences in genetics and general constitution that effect remaining androgen production and consequently, after peripheral conversion, circulating oestrogen levels.

OESTROGEN TARGET TISSUES

- The vaginal epithelium becomes thinner and less vascular.
- Deterioration in collagen reduces the support available to the pelvic floor and, therefore, there is an increased risk of utero-vaginal prolapse.

Uterus
This is reduced in size:

- myometrial cells are partly replaced by fibrous tissue
- endometrium becomes atrophic.

Bladder and urethra
- The urogenital epithelium atrophies especially in the urethra and the trigone.

- There is an increase in stress incontinence, urethral syndrome (see p. 276) and risk of infection.

Skin and breasts
- The epidermis and dermis become thinner and less elastic; sebaceous and sweat gland secretion decreases.
- The glandular tissue of the breast atrophies, being replaced by fat.

Cardiovascular systems
- The levels of cholesterol, phospholipids and triglycerides rise.
- The risk of coronary artery disease gradually increases to the extent that it is the major cause of death in this group of women.

Skeleton
- Calcium and the collagen matrix are both lost from the bone at about 1% per year; resulting in osteoporosis.

SYMPTOMS ASSOCIATED WITH THE CLIMACTERIC

Symptoms frequently begin before the menopause. There are five groups of interlinked symptoms:

- *Vasomotor*—over 75% of menopausal women will have hot flushes and night sweats; the aetiology is not understood; it is not merely lack of oestrogen.
- *Emotional*—between 25 and 50% will complain of lethargy, lack of concentration, irritability, aggressiveness, depression, lability of mood, or anxiety.
- *Sexual*—decreased libido; dyspareunia—often due to atrophic vaginitis.
- *Urinary*, e.g. urgency and frequency of micturition—usually due to atrophic trigonitis and urethritis.
- *Musculo-skeletal*—laxity of ligaments and decreasing muscular strength may give rise to a variety of joint-related aches and pains.

Management
General medical disorders (e.g. hyperthyroidism) need to be excluded.

Therapy is of three main types:

- treatment of related disorders e.g. obesity, hypertension
- psychological support
- hormones and other drugs.

HORMONE REPLACEMENT THERAPY (HRT)

Aims:

- To reduce symptoms of oestrogen deficiency

- To prevent disorders associated with oestrogen deficiency (e.g. osteoporotic fractures)
- To minimise the risk of disorders associated with HRT (e.g. endometrial and breast cancer).

TYPES OF HRT

Oestrogens
- Conjugated equine oestrogens are still the most common oestrogen used in HRT, although the use of synthetic oestrogens is increasing.
- Oestrogens can be administered orally, transdermally (by patches and gels); subcutaneously (by implant) and vaginally. A nasal spray has recently become available.

Progestogens
- Because unopposed oestrogen increases the risk of endometrial carcinoma an adequate dose of progestogen must be added to the HRT in women who still have a uterus to protect the endometrium.
- Most commonly synthetic progestogens are added to oestrogen in tablets and patches in the second half of the cycle.
- Continuous low dose progestogens are also used and reduce the pre-menstrual syndrome-like side effects of cyclical progestogens.
- Continuous combined 'no bleed' preparations should only be used in women who are at least 12 months post-menopausal.
- The levonorgestrol releasing Mirena™ intrauterine system (IUS) has also been used to protect the endometrium and appears to be effective. It is not yet licensed in the UK for this use (in contrast to many other European countries).

Selective oestrogen receptor modulators
Raloxifene is an oestrogen agonist to bone, but it is anti-oestrogenic to breast (c.f. Tamoxifen) and endometrial tissue. It may, however, exacerbate vasomotor symptoms.

Non-oestrogen based HRT
Tibolone is a synthetic hormone with weak oestrogenic, progestogenic and androgenic effects that provides 'bleed free' bone protection and appears to be particularly beneficial for libido and mood (androgenic effects). It is unsuitable for use within 12 months of the last menstrual period.

Phyto-oestrogens
There is little good evidence, but soya extracts and black kahoosh may alleviate some menopausal symptoms.

BENEFITS OF HRT

Symptoms
- Vasomotor symptoms and vaginal dryness respond extremely well to oestrogen therapy.

- Intravaginal oestrogens can also reduce the risk of recurrent UTIs and the symptoms of urethral syndrome.
- Stress incontinence is not generally significantly improved by HRT.

Coronary heart disease
Oestrogen is an antioxidant and calcium channel blocker, and alters high- and low-density lipoproteins favourably. It might, therefore, be expected to reduce the risk of coronary heart disease (CHD).

- Initial observational studies demonstrated a 30% reduction but this may have been due to bias, i.e. women taking HRT were also better educated, thinner, less likely to smoke, etc.
- More recent RCTs have failed to show any overall benefit in CHD. There was a slight increase in rates of CHD in the first year or two of treatment with HRT, with a possible decrease in later years, both in women with previous CHD and in those without. The results of further large long term RCTs will not be available for several years. (See Further reading)

Osteoporosis
- Oestrogens reduce the risk of hip fracture by 30% and spine fractures by 50%. However, the risks increase after cessation of treatment such that at 10 years after stopping HRT, the risks of fracture return to the untreated levels.
- Calcium supplementation potentiates the beneficial effect of oestrogen on bone.

CNS
HRT does not decrease the incidence of stroke.

It tends to protect against memory loss (by up to one third) and Alzheimer's disease (O.R. 0.7).

Miscellaneous
- Colon cancer—several epidemiological studies report a reduction in the incidence of colonic cancer of up to 33% in women taking HRT.
- Cataracts may also be reduced by one third.
- Use of oestrogen improves wellbeing in symptomatic women and is also associated with longer survival.

DISADVANTAGES OF HRT
Endometrial cancer
- The risk of endometrial cancer is low as long as there is adequate protection with progestogens.
- Observational studies suggest a slight increased risk, even with oestrogen–progestogen combination, after 5 to 10 years use of HRT.

Breast cancer
• There is no excess risk of breast cancer with up to 5 years HRT. However, after 5 years, 10 years and 15 years the excess number of women with breast cancer was 2, 6 and 12 cases/1000 women, respectively
• The addition of a progestogen does not confer protection against the increased risk and, indeed, might increase it.
• The Mirena IUS has been proposed as a useful alternative.

Venous thromboembolism
Oestrogen may double the risk of DVT and pulmonary embolism though the absolute risk is small—4 extra cases per 100 women years in the 'HERS' trial (see Further reading).

Miscelleneous
• Oestrogen doubles the risk of requiring cholecystectomy.
• Breast tenderness is increased by oestrogens and may be helped by evening primrose oil.
• Abnormal bleeding is common, particularly with continuous progestogen regimes and should always be investigated (see below).

CONTRAINDICATIONS TO HRT

Absolute
• Endometrial cancer
• Receptor +ve breast cancer
• Undiagnosed vaginal bleeding
• Undiagnosed breast lump
• Suspected pregnancy
• Severe active liver disease.

Relative
• Hypertension
• Past history of thromboembolism
• Diabetes mellitus
• Gallstones
• Uterine fibroids
• Endometrial hyperplasia
• Otosclerosis
• Migraine
• Malignant melanoma
• Benign breast disease.

OTHER DRUGS FOR VASOMOTOR SYMPTOMS

• Clonidine improves vasomotor symptoms for some patients.
• Propranolol does not reduce hot flushes but may help tachycardia or palpitations.
• Psychotropic drugs are not appropriate for purely menopausal symptoms.

DURATION OF TREATMENT

• This depends on informed choice for each woman.
• The risk/benefit ratio is less clear than was previously thought.

- In balance the benefits of HRT use outweighs the risks, but care in prescribing must always be taken, particularly with long-term (over 5 years) use.

POSTMENOPAUSAL BLEEDING (PMB)

All cases must be thoroughly investigated (except for the withdrawal bleeding which occurs at the expected time in menopausal women taking HRT).

Investigations must include:

- complete pelvic examination
- cervical smear
- endometrial biopsy.

Optional investigations:

- Hysteroscopy
- Transvaginal scan for endometrial thickness.

FURTHER READING

Barrett-Connor E 1998 Clinical Review: Hormone Replacement Therapy. British Medical Journal 317: 457–461
Collins J 2001 Benefits and Risks of Hormone Replacement Therapy. Medicine 10: 5–11
Dixon J 2001 Hormone Replacement Therapy and the Breast. British Medical Journal 323: 1381–1382
Herrington DM, Reboussin DM, Brosnihan KB, et al. 2000 Effects of estrogen replacement on the progression of coronary artery atherosclerosis. New England Journal of Medicine 343: 522–9
Hulley S, Grady D, Bush T, et al. 1998 Randomized trial of estrogen plus progestin for secondary prevention of coronary heart disease in postmenopausal women. Heart and Estrogen/progestin Replacement Study (HERS) Research Group. Journal of the American Medical Association 280: 605–13
New Zealand Guidelines Group. 2001 Guidelines for Hormone Replacement Therapy. www.nzgg.org.nz
Shaw R W, Soutter W P, Stanton S L (eds) 1996 Gynaecology, 2nd edn. Churchill Livingstone, Edinburgh
Studd J. 2000 Management of the menopause: Millennium Review. Parthenon, London

21. Pelvic infections

PELVIC INFLAMMATORY DISEASE (PID)

Definition
Inflammation and infection of the upper genital tract in women, typically involving the fallopian tubes, ovaries and surrounding structures.

Primary—an infection which ascends from the lower genital tract due to:

- Sexually transmitted diseases (STDs) caused by organisms such as *Chlamydia trachomatis* and *Neisseria gonorrhoeae*. PID is the most common serious complication of STDs, and these organisms cause at least 70% of all cases.
  - Up to 60% of women with gonorrhoea are asymptomatic for months or even years and up to 10% of men may be symptomless carriers.
  - Chlamydial antibodies can be found in up to 70% of infertile women with tubal damage.
  - There is no history of clinically recognised PID in 30–80% of infertile women with blocked tubes.
- *Escherichia coli* and other gut organisms.
- Replacement of normal vaginal flora (primarily lactobacilli) with organisms associated with 'bacterial vaginosis' (see p. 324), e.g. bacteroides, anaerobes, *Mycoplasma hominis* and *Ureaplasma urealyticum*.
- Iatrogenic—about 15% of all cases: due, for example, to D & C, HSG, termination of pregnancy (0.5% post-TOP), insertion of an IUD.
- After delivery or miscarriage.

Secondary—less than 1% of all cases:

- An infection caused by direct spread from nearby pelvic organs (most often the appendix *or* other diseases (e.g. schistosomiasis or filariasis).
- A minority of women with PID are HIV positive.

PREVALENCE AND RISK MARKERS

- The overall incidence is approx 10–13/1000 women of reproductive age, with a peak of 20/1000 in the 15–24 year age group.

- Exact incidence is however unknown because the disease cannot be diagnosed reliably from clinical symptoms and signs and furthermore many cases are asymptomatic.
- Pelvic inflammatory disease is rare in women who are not sexually active.

It is one of the commonest reasons for emergency admission to a gynaecology ward.

Risk markers include:

- young age at intercourse
- recent new sexual partner
- reduced socioeconomic circumstances
- multiple sexual partners
- smoking
- vaginal douching.
- use of IUD (barrier methods and COC protect—see p. 246)

CLINICAL FEATURES OF ACUTE PID

- Lower abdominal pain (usually bilateral) is the commonest presenting symptom, which may be accompanied by:
  - abnormal vaginal discharge
  - irregular vaginal bleeding
  - dysuria
  - dyspareunia
  - nausea and/or vomiting
  - fever
  - general malaise.
- Diagnostic accuracy using the above criteria is 35–65%. They can be present in up to 20% of women with no pelvic pathology.
- Among the conditions most frequently causing false-positive or false-negative errors in differential diagnosis are:
  - acute appendicitis
  - endometriosis
  - ectopic pregnancy
  - corpus luteum haemorrhage
  - ovarian cysts
  - inflammatory conditions of other organs.
- Lower abdominal and adnexal tenderness, and pain on moving the cervix ('cervical excitation') are found in >90% of women with proven PID.

DIAGNOSIS

- Consider PID in any woman of reproductive age with acute pelvic pain.
- Send triple swabs: high vaginal swab and air-dried slide for microscopy and culture; endocervical and urethral swabs for *C. trachomatis* and *N. gonorrhoeae*.
- Raised C-reactive protein (CRP) and white-cell count.
- *Laparoscopy* is the gold standard for diagnosis (but it is invasive and not used in most hospitals as a routine first line investigation). For positive diagnosis all of the following features must be present:
  - erythema of fallopian tubes

- oedema and swelling of tubes
- seropurulent exudate on the surface of the tube from the fimbriated end.
- The inflammation is usually but not invariably bilateral.
- The degrees of severity are:
  - *mild* if these criteria are present but the tubes are mobile and patent
  - *moderate* if the findings are more florid, the tubes are not mobile and their patency is uncertain
  - *severe* if a tubo-ovarian mass or masses are present.
- Swabs can be taken for culture at laparoscopy from the fallopian tubes or the pouch of Douglas; peritoneal fluid can also be cultured

TREATMENT OF ACUTE PID

- Early empirical treatment is common, due to a lack of reliable clinical diagnostic criteria for PID.
- The absence of infection from the lower genital tract, where samples are usually taken, does not exclude PID, and so may not influence the decision to treat. However, swabs must be taken to check for STDs.
- Most women can be treated as out-patients. Among those for whom in-patient treatment may be necessary are the following:
  - failure to respond to or tolerate treatment as outpatient: patient cannot or will not attend for clinical follow-up within 72 hours
  - severe disease
  - suspected pelvic abscess
  - woman is HIV-positive
  - patient is adolescent (because of importance of adequate therapy to reduce chances of long-term sequelae)
  - patient is pregnant
  - uncertain diagnosis or other cause of 'acute abdomen' cannot be excluded.

Antibiotic therapy

- There is no good evidence on the optimal duration of treatment, or on oral versus parenteral treatment. Treatment is usually recommended for 14 days.
- Treatment with single agents such as penicillins or tetracyclines is inadequate; cephalosporins do not deal with chlamydia.
- A multiple regimen is required to cover gonococci, chlamydia, Gram-negative organisms and anaerobes. Table 21.1 gives regimens suggested by the Centers for Disease Control and Prevention (CDC) in the USA. For details of dosage see BNF and Further reading.

Surgery

The main role of surgery in the management of acute PID is after rupture of a tubo-ovarian abscess and to drain a pyosalpinx.

Table 21.1 **Antibiotic regimens for acute PID. Source: www.cdc.gov, USA.**

	Regimen 1	Regimen 2
In-patient	Cefoxitin i.v. plus doxycycline i.v. or orally. Continue for at least 48 hrs after clinical condition is significantly improved then give oral doxycycline for a total of 14 days	Clindamycin i.v. plus gentamicin i.v. or i.m. Then as for regimen 1 with oral clindamycin as an alternative to doxycycline
Out-patient	Cefoxitin i.m. (plus probenecid) or other third-generation cephalosporin and oral doxycycline for 14 days	Oral ofloxacin plus clindamycin or metronidazole for 14 days

CONTACT TRACING

If an STD is diagnosed, contact tracing is mandatory and is best carried out by specialised genito-urinary/sexual health clinics. Male partners should be examined for STDs and treated as appropriate.

SEQUELAE

- *Chronic pelvic pain* will follow in 20% of affected women: of these, 60–70% will be infertile and/or have dyspareunia.
- *Subfertility* due to tubal damage and occlusion occurs in:
  - 10% of women after a single episode of PID
  - 20% after two episodes
  - 40% after 3 or more episodes.
- *Ectopic pregnancy*—PID increases the risk 7- 10-fold (10% of those who conceive have an ectopic pregnancy).
- *Recurrent PID*—The patient classically complains of:
  - heavy and irregular menses
  - dysmenorrhoea
  - dyspareunia
  - chronic pelvic pain
  - infertility.

There may also be chronic vaginal discharge. The uterus and adnexae are tender; the former is often fixed in retroversion. The condition which most closely mimics chronic PID is endometriosis.

FURTHER READING

Clinical Evidence. Issue 5. June 2001. Pelvic inflammatory disease. Pages 1123–1127. BMJ Publishing Group, London. www.ClinicalEvidence.org
Edmonds DK 1999 Dewhurst's Textbook of Obstetrics and Gynaecology for Postgraduates, 6th edn. Blackwell Publications,

22. Disorders of micturition

Urinary incontinence has been defined by the International Continence Society (ICS) as 'a condition of involuntary urine loss that is a social or hygienic problem, and is objectively demonstrable.'

- It has been estimated that at least 14% of women over 30 years of age suffer from urinary incontinence.
- 2% of the total health budget is spent on incontinence services alone.
- Many women will not seek advice because of embarrassment.
- In addition to the great distress and social inconvenience it causes, in a small proportion of cases incontinence is the presenting feature of a serious pelvic pathology or degenerative neurological diseases.

Definitions
- *Genuine stress incontinence (GSI)* is the involuntary loss of a small amount of urine when the intravesical pressure exceeds the maximum urethral pressure, in the absence of detrusor activity.
- *Detrusor instability (DI)* is a condition in which the bladder is shown objectively to contract, either spontaneously or on provocation, during bladder filling, while the subject is attempting to inhibit micturition.
- *Reflex incontinence* is the involuntary loss of urine due to abnormal spinal reflex activity in the absence of the sensation to micturate.
- *Overflow incontinence* is the involuntary loss of urine when the intravesical pressure exceeds maximum urethral pressure due to bladder distension and in the absence of detrusor activity.
- *True incontinence* is the involuntary loss of urine due to a defect in the anatomical integrity of the urinary tract (i.e. fistula).

Genuine stress incontinence and detrusor instability are by far the two commonest diagnoses in women under the age of 70. In many women the two conditions exist together.

MAKING DIAGNOSIS

The pattern of incontinence may give some indication of the cause of the problem, but, in the vast majority of women, this can only be accurately defined at urodynamic studies. The real importance of the history is to gain some idea of the nature and severity of the woman's symptoms and to try to detect any serious underlying pathology.

HISTORY

Urinary symptoms
- *Stress incontinence*—its severity is indicated by the activity required to cause it; leakage during very strenuous exercise would not be as significant as from walking, coughing or laughing. It usually reflects bladder neck weakness (GSI) but it is also a common feature of detrusor instability.
- *Urge incontinence*—the leakage of urine associated with urinary urgency, is more typical of DI but may be present in women with pure genuine stress incontinence.
- *Urgency*—this is a sudden desire to void (with fear of leakage) and again is a feature of DI.
- *Frequency*—the voluntary passage of urine more than seven times in a day; it may reflect a reduced bladder capacity (interstitial cystitis or pelvic tumours), bladder hypersensitivity (bladder calculi, tumours or infection), increased urine production (diabetes, diuretics or excess intake) or detrusor instability. In some women, frequency indicates nothing more than the desire to keep the bladder empty to avoid incontinence. Increased frequency may or may not be associated with nocturia, which is defined as waking more than twice in the night to pass urine. In isolation in elderly women, nocturia is often a feature of congestive cardiac failure with dependent oedema returning to the circulation during recumbency. Nocturia is a particularly serious symptom in elderly women because of the risk of falls and bone fracture.
- *Dribbling incontinence*—this is suggestive of a fistula or retention with overflow.
- *Dysuria and/or haematuria*—this may be caused by bladder infection, calculi or tumour.
- *Poor stream*—this may indicate some form of bladder outlet obstruction, which can sometimes be overcome by temporarily returning their prolapse into the vagina. Sensation of prolapse may be a significant symptom that requires separate consideration. It does not necessarily indicate genuine stress incontinence.

Neurological symptoms
Leg weakness or paraesthesia, for example, may reflect an upper or lower motor neurone problem such as multiple sclerosis.

Fluid intake

The volume, nature and timing of fluid intake will effect bladder function. A high intake of caffeine-containing drinks cause increased frequency. The risk of nocturia is increased if a drink is taken near to bedtime.

Other considerations

- Past medical and surgical history—e.g. STD; polio; surgery to spine or genitourinary tract; cerebrovascular accident; cerebral, spinal or pelvic trauma.
- Gynaecological and obstetric history—particularly of rapid or slow labours, 'difficult' delivery (especially with forceps) or large infants.
- Previous urological complaints—e.g. enuresis, urinary infections, haematuria.
- Family history—e.g. enuresis, diabetes.
- Concurrent disease—e.g. multiple sclerosis, Parkinson's disease.

PELVIC EXAMINATION

The purpose is to:

- demonstrate incontinence and/or utero-vaginal prolapse
- detect any other pelvic pathology
- note other features such as oestrogenisation of the vaginal wall, the ability to contract the pelvic floor and scarring from any previous surgery.

INVESTIGATIONS

- *Urine microscopy and culture* are compulsory as urinary infections can mimic many of the symptoms of DI especially.
- *Urinary cytology* should be performed if haematuria, sensory urgency or bladder pain are present.
- Measure *blood sugar* levels (noting how long after food) if there is increased frequency or other risk markers for diabetes.

Frequency and volume chart

A 7-day record is useful; women with DI classically void small amounts, frequently, whereas women with GSI void larger volumes and not overnight. It can also help exclude an excessive fluid intake.

Pad test

Over a 1-hour period, a series of standard exercises are performed to provoke incontinence and this allows an objective measure of the severity of the incontinence.

Urodynamic studies

These are a group of tests that look in detail at bladder and urethral function.

Uroflowmetry

A cheap and non-invasive test of urinary function. The patient is asked to pass urine into a vessel with a measuring device. It calculates the rate of flow and the total volume voided. In a female the minimum flow rate should be 15 ml/s and voided volume over 150 ml. Straining can lead to abnormal flow patterns with interrupted flow.

Residual volume

A guide to the adequacy of bladder emptying. Women who cannot empty their bladder completely are at increased risk of urinary tract infections and are more likely to be unable to micturate after surgery for GSI. It can be measured by ultrasonography or by catheterisation.

Filling cystometry

This tests bladder function by examining the relationship between the bladder pressure and volume during filling and voiding. It is a particularly useful test of detrusor function. Urinary and rectal catheters measure the intra-vesical and intra-abdominal pressures, respectively, and subtraction of these calculates the detrusor pressure. Warm saline is slowly infused into the bladder at between 10 and 100 ml/min, and the patient is asked to signal when she feels the first desire to void. The detrusor pressure is monitored as the bladder fills and any increase in detrusor pressure noted. At the end of filling, the patient is asked to stand to provoke an increase in detrusor pressure and the patient is asked to cough. Any leakage of urine is recorded on the pressure profile to determine whether or not it coincides with detrusor activity. Finally, during voiding the woman is asked to interrupt the flow by contracting (squeezing) her levator floor.

Normal cystometry

- Residual volume less than 50 ml
- First desire to void between 150 and 200 ml
- Capacity of greater than 400 ml
- Slow steady detrusor pressure rise
- Absence of abnormal detrusor contractions
- No leaking on coughing
- Maximum detrusor pressure of 70 cmH$_2$O while voiding
- The patient should be able to stop voiding.

Abnormal cystometry

- If leakage of urine occurs without a rise in detrusor pressure, genuine stress incontinence can be diagnosed.
- Involuntary detrusor activity during filling confirms detrusor instability.
- Small bladder capacity suggests interstitial cystitis.
- High residual indicates incomplete bladder emptying.
- High detrusor pressure during voiding indicates outflow obstruction.

Micturating cystourethrography and videocystourethrography
These are even more specialised tests, allowing the functional anatomical relationship of the urethra, urethro-vesical junction and bladder base to be visualised, facilitating the diagnosis of stress incontinence in complex cases.

Among the indications for urodynamic investigations are:

- anyone being considered for surgery because DI is diagnosed in 10–15% of women whose symptoms and signs suggest GSI
- irritative symptoms which do not respond to treatment
- all complicated cases (e.g. women with neuropathy or suspected obstruction).

An *intravenous urogram* will help to exclude congenital anomalies, calculi or ureteric fistulae.

Cystoscopy should be carried out if there is sensory urgency with a small-capacity bladder to exclude interstitial cystitis or malignancy.

GENUINE STRESS INCONTINENCE (GSI)

AETIOLOGY

There are two mechanisms for the development of GSI:

- Prolapse of the proximal urethra and bladder neck out of the abdominal cavity means that a rise of abdominal pressure does not compress the bladder neck and, therefore, increases the vesical pressure but not the urethral pressure.
- Secondly a reduction in resting urethral closure pressure, below that of the bladder, will lead to incontinence.

These changes may or may not be accompanied by a cystocele.

- *Vaginal delivery* leads to stretching of supporting tissues around the bladder neck and, more importantly, denervation of the levator muscles that form part of the sphincter mechanism.
- *Menopause* is associated with a large increase in the incidence of GSI and is thought to be due to loss of collagen from the supporting tissues secondary to oestrogen deficiency.
- *Congenital weakness* of connective tissues plays a part in a small proportion of cases.
- *Fibrosis* secondary to surgery resulting in a rigid (drainpipe) urethra occasionally plays a part.

TREATMENT OF GSI

Reassurance
Women may be referred with very mild symptoms and reassurance that no underlying pathological process exists is all that some require.

Change of lifestyle/diet
Weight loss and cessation of smoking may reduce abdominal pressure. Fluid restriction (<1.5 l/day) and timed voiding may make the incontinence less of a problem.

Physiotherapy
Pelvic floor exercises (PFE) are intended to build up the muscles of the levator floor. They are best taught by a specialist physiotherapist and up to 60% of women may benefit. Patients should be warned that it may take 4 months before any improvement is noticed. Weighted cones that the woman has to retain in the vagina by clenching her levator muscles are said to lead to improved results. Many women like the idea of active therapy but PFE demands a continuing programme of exercises and so compliance is often poor and relapse rates are moderately high. Electrical stimulation (inferential therapy) is a passive method of strengthening the pelvic floor.

Continence devices
These act by occluding the urethra to urine leakage in women with GSI. They are particularly useful for very elderly women in whom surgery is contraindicated and for younger women who only get incontinence during extreme exercise.

Surgery
There have been two meta analyses of surgical procedures (see Jarvis, 1994 and Black and Downs, 1996 in Further reading).

* *Anterior vaginal repair with bladder neck buttress* cures about 50% of women and significant complications are relatively rare.
* *Burch colposuspension* involves elevation of the vagina (and bladder neck) through a suprapubic incision. This is the 'gold standard' with a 90% objective cure rate:
  * Sutures run through the vagina to the iliopectineal ligament at the pelvic brim.
  * Laparoscopic colposuspension offers similar initial efficacy and early return to work, but poorer longterm results and an increased frequency of urinary tract injuries suggest that an open approach may be preferable.
* *Tension free vaginal tape* appears to offer a new surgical option with up to 85% success rates. Long term follow up is required to ensure that there are no long term complications (e.g. urethral erosion) but it remains a valid technique.
* In *Marshall–Marchetti–Krantz colposuspension* sutures are attached to the periosteum just lateral to and behind the symphysis pubis. Up to 5% of women develop *osteitis pubis* following this procedure.
* *Stamey bladder neck suspension* procedure involves the passage of non-absorbable suture from the para-urethral tissue to the rectus

sheath. It is done under cystoscopic control to ensure that the bladder is not perforated and determine the degree of elevation. It is a useful procedure for women with a narrow or rigid vagina that will not elevate with a standard colposuspension.

• *Paraurethral injection of collagen or silicon* into the side walls of bladder neck, thus narrowing the proximal urethra. The relapse rate is high but the procedure can be repeated with ease.

• For women with persistent GSI after several surgical failures, *insertion of artifical sphincters* may be possible but only by those well trained in this technique.

DETRUSOR INSTABILITY (DI)

AETIOLOGY

The cause of primary instability of the detrusor remains unknown. It may be a variant of normal bladder function because:

• It is the natural state in all infants.
• About 10% of the population never develop stable bladder function.
• Urodynamic studies suggest that it may be present in 60–70% of 'normal' women.
• It may rarely be secondary to an upper motor neurone lesion (e.g. multiple sclerosis leading to detrusor hyperreflexia).

TREATMENT OF DI

Reassurance
For some women, reassurance that it can just be a variant of normal bladder function may be all that is required.

Change of lifestyle/diet
The frequency described by these women is due to them voiding before they get severe urgency and leak. From the frequency volume chart it can be shown that if large volumes are being passed (i.e. >300 ml), and the women should be encouraged to drink less, especially drinks containing caffeine such as coffee and tea. Incontinence aids such as pads and nappies may be appropriate.

Behavioural therapy—bladder drill
This is a form of self-training. The woman is advised to hold on to urine for 1 hour even if leaking occurs. When this is reached with continence maintained the period is increased gradually up to 2 hours. Success rates of up to 80% have been achieved with inpatient therapy. Hypnotherapy and acupuncture have had some success but, as with most behavioural therapies, there is a high relapse rate.

Drug therapy

Drugs are the mainstay of treatment for severe symptoms, though possibly drug treatment in association with behavioural therapy is most effective.

- Anticholinergic drugs oxybutinin and a more selective M3 receptor antagonist, tolterodine, can both substantially improve symptoms even if the incontinence is not completely cured, and they appear similarly effective (70% improvement). Unwanted antimuscarinic effects, particularly dry mouth, are less common with both tolterodine and modified-release oxybutinin.
- Tricyclic antidepressants (imipramine) have an anticholinergic effect and may be particularly useful for nocturia symptoms.
- Trospium and propiverine are newer agents that are well tolerated, but more data on their efficacy are needed.

Surgery

There is little place for surgery apart from exceptional cases. Small bowel may be used to increase the bladder capacity (**clam cystoplasty**) or the ureters may be implanted into an isolated loop of small bowel connected with the abdominal surface (**ileal conduit**).

GENITOURINARY FISTULAE

- *Uretero-vaginal fistulae* usually follow hysterectomy (particularly radical surgery).
- *High vesico-vaginal fistulae* can follow lower segment caesarean section, uterine rupture, hysterectomy or radiotherapy for cervical carcinoma. The ureteric orifices may be near the edge.
- *Mid-vaginal vesico-vaginal fistulae* may be caused by pressure necrosis after prolonged obstructed labour or colporrhaphy fistulae. These are the commonest and are mostly due either to pressure necrosis or trauma by rotational forceps.
- *Urethral fistulae* may occasionally be so large as to virtually destroy the whole urethra and the bladder neck.

MANAGEMENT

Some defects will close spontaneously and all will heal to some extent if given enough time. Even if spontaneous closure does not occur, surgery should be deferred to allow maximum tissue healing. If secondary to radiation this may take up to a year or more.

Pre-operative management

In addition to attending to the patient's general health, among the pre-operative investigations which should be carried out are urine culture and sensitivity, intravenous urography, cystoscopy and assessment under anaesthesia.

If the fistula is associated with radiotherapy for neoplasm a biopsy of the edge should be taken to exclude residual tumour activity.

Operative closure
- All but the simplest cases should be referred to centres or surgeons with special expertise.
- Most urethro-vaginal and vesico-vaginal fistulae can be repaired vaginally by dissection and repair in layers.
- The bladder wall closure must be watertight.
- Over 70% of fistulae can be closed at the first attempt, falling to about 30% if three or more repairs have previously been attempted.
- Continuous catheter drainage is necessary for a minimum of 10 days (up to 3 weeks for radiation fistulae). The drainage system should be closed.
- In any subsequent pregnancy all deliveries should be by elective caesarean section.

THE URETHRAL SYNDROME

Definition
Recurrent attacks of frequent and painful micturition not associated with any significant abnormality in the urinary tract and irrespective of the presence or absence of bacteriuria.

Used synonymously with 'recurrent cystitis'.

AETIOLOGY

- *Infective*—significant bacteriuria (>106 organisms/ml) is present in only about half of the cases. The commonest infective agents are normal bowel flora. Among the others are *T. vaginalis, N. gonorrhoeae* and *C. trachomatis*. Tuberculosis of the bladder is a rare cause.
- *Gynaecological*—e.g. postmenopausal oestrogen deficiency.
- *Chemical or allergic reactions*—may be due to soaps, douches, deodorants, contraceptive foam or anti-oxidants in condoms. It can also arise by wearing nylon underwear or tights.
- *Sexual*—its occasional association with first intercourse has led to the term 'honeymoon cystitis'.
- *Psychological*—anxiety and neuroticism are not infrequent associations. Which is cause and which effect is not always entirely clear.
- *Bladder problems*—DI is present in over 25% of cases. A bladder tumour is a rare cause but it must be suspected if there is haematuria.
- *Other causes*—multiple sclerosis may rarely present in this fashion.

MANAGEMENT

- A full history is vital. Haematuria requires full investigation. A full gynaecological assessment is essential.
- Routinely test urine for protein, glucose, blood and infection.
- An optimistic attitude and positive approach to treatment is important because there is often an understandably large functional overlay in these patients.
- Simple remedies may be the most effective (e.g. perineal and introital hygiene; potassium citrate and sodium bicarbonate with a high fluid intake).
- Start antibiotic therapy if symptoms do not subside within 48 hours of commencing a high fluid intake.
- Try hormone replacement therapy in menopausal women.

FURTHER READING

Cardozo L (ed) 2000 Urinary Incontinence. Bailliere's Best Practice & Research. Clinical Obstetrics & Gynaecology. 14; 2
Managing incontinence due to detrusor instability. Drugs and Therapeutics Bulletin. August 2001; Vol 39, 8
Shaw RW, Soutter WP, Stanton SL (eds) 1997 Gynaecology, 2nd edn. Churchill Livingstone, Edinburgh
Tindall VR 1990 Jeffcoate's Principles of Gynaecology, 5th edn. Butterworths, London

23. Uterine displacement and utero-vaginal prolapse

- Mobile retroversion of the uterus is a variant of normal, occurring in over 20% of women.
- It is usually asymptomatic and too many gynaecological symptoms have been attributed to it in the past. Backache is more frequently due to other conditions.
- An associated positioning of the ovaries in the pouch of Douglas may be a cause of dyspareunia.
- Retroversion is not a cause of subfertility.
- An acutely retroverted gravid uterus may become 'impacted' in the pelvis as the uterus enlarges. Acute retention of urine may result.
- Mobile retroversion does not need treatment. The use of Hodge pessaries or ventrosuspension cannot be justified.
- Fixed retroversion is most frequently due to pelvic inflammatory disease (p. 264) or endometriosis (p. 222). The associated symptoms and signs and the management depend on the underlying disease.

UTERO-VAGINAL PROLAPSE

Definition
The protrusion of the uterus and/or the vagina beyond normal anatomical confines. The bladder, urethra, rectum and bowel may be secondarily involved.

Prolapse typically has been described with three degrees of severity:

- First degree—descent of the cervix to the introitus
- Second degree—descent of the cervix, but not the whole uterus, through the introitus
- Third degree (procidentia)—descent of the cervix and the whole uterus through the introitus.

This classification is very subjective and makes no assessment of coexistent cystoceles, rectoceles and enteroceles. The International Continence Society has recommended a series of more objective parameters for the assessment for prolapse, the 'POPQ' system, which assesses all of the components of prolapse, see Jackson and Smith in 'Further reading'.

Support of the pelvic floor

- The cervix and upper vagina are supported by the uterosacral and cardinal ligaments.
- The midportion of the vagina is attached by endofascial condensations to the pelvic side walls.
- The lower third of the vagina is supported by the levator ani muscles and the perineal body.
- The axis of the vagina may also be important; normally it lies in a horizontal plane, flat on the levator muscles. This protects it during coughing and other activities that increase the intra-abdominal pressure. If the axis is disrupted, for example after vaginal delivery, this may predispose to prolapse.

AETIOLOGY

Attenuation of the support mechanisms may occur as a result of:

- *Vaginal delivery and pregnancy*—prolapse is uncommon in nulliparous women. Vaginal delivery may cause mechanical injury and denervation of the pelvic floor, which contribute to subsequent prolapse. These risks are increased with large infants and by instrumental delivery, particularly forceps.
- *Reduced collagen*—abnormal collagen metabolism, for example in Ehlers-Danlos syndrome, can predispose to prolapse. More commonly the reduction in collagen seen after the menopause predisposes to prolapse.
- *Chronic elevation of intra-abdominal pressure*—due, for example, to obesity or a chronic cough.
- *Iatrogenic*—hysterectomy is associated with subsequent prolapse (5% in 15 years). The incidence is even greater when the initial indication was for prolapse symptoms. Ensuring approximation of the ligaments at the time of surgery may reduce it.

VAGINAL WALL PROLAPSE

- A prolapse of the lowest third of the anterior vaginal wall involves the urethra and is, therefore, termed a *urethrocele*.
- In the upper two thirds the bladder is involved and it is, therefore, a *cystocele*.
- A prolapse of the pouch of Douglas is an *enterocele* because the hernial sac contains gut or omentum.
- A prolapse of the posterior vaginal wall brings the rectum with it and is, therefore, a *rectocele*. (This is not to be confused with prolapse of the rectal mucosa through the anus.)

SYMPTOMS AND SIGNS

The commonest symptoms are:

- General
  - a feeling of 'something coming down'
  - awareness of a lump protruding from the vulva
- Uterine prolapse
  - discomfort and backache
- Cysto-urethrocele
  - Stress incontinence because the urethra lies caudal to the pelvic floor (see p. 272) and not primarily because of loss of the posterior urethro-vesical angle. Note that only 50% of women with stress incontinence have a prolapse.
  - Urinary retention where the urethra is kinked by its descent into the urethrocele.
- Rectocele
  - Difficulty with defecation can occur where the rectum is kinked as it prolapses into the vagina behind the rectocele.

EXAMINATION

- Exclude pelvic masses with a bimanual examination.
- Examination is best carried out with the patient in the left lateral position using a Sims speculum, although the prolapse can sometimes only be demonstrated with the patient standing or on straining.
- The walls should be checked in turn for descent and atrophy.
- If absolutely necessary, a volsellum may be applied to the cervix so that traction will demonstrate the severity of uterine prolapse. This can cause marked discomfort and should be performed gently.

MANAGEMENT

Prevention

- A reduction in prolonged labour and a reduction in the trauma caused by instrumental delivery may reduce subsequent prolapse.
- Encouragement to persist with postnatal pelvic floor exercises has been shown to reduce postnatal urinary incontinence and this is often extrapolated to prolapse.
- Weight loss and other measures to reduce chronic increases in intra-abdominal pressure.
- Appropriate use of hormone replacement therapy in some postmenopausal women may reduce general discomfort, but it will not 'correct' existing prolapse.

TREATMENT

The following are among the features on which appropriate treatment is based:

- severity of symptoms
- extent of the signs—asymptomatic first-degree prolapse does not require treatment

- age, parity and wish for further pregnancies
- patient's sexual activity
- presence of aggravating features—e.g. the results of treatment will be poor unless the obese patient loses weight and the smoker stops smoking
- urinary symptoms (see p. 268)
- other gynaecological problems, e.g. menorrhagia.

Conservative treatment

- *Pelvic floor exercises* will improve the tone of the pelvic floor muscles in the young parous woman but they will not produce much benefit for the woman with significant utero-vaginal prolapse.
- *Vaginal pessaries* may be used for women who decline surgery, who are unfit for surgery or for women in whom surgery is contraindicated (e.g. during pregnancy). Vaginal pessaries are changed 6 monthly and the use of topical oestrogen therapy reduces the risk of vaginal erosion.
  - Ring pessaries fit between the posterior aspect of the symphysis pubis and the posterior fornix of the vagina.
  - Shelf pessaries can be used where correctly sized ring pessaries will not sit in the vagina and/or where the perineum is deficient.

Surgical treatment

Prolapse is not a life-threatening condition but surgery has its morbidity. Surgery will ideally correct prolapse without affecting other areas such as coitus and urinary incontinence.

- *Anterior colporrhaphy* is appropriate for the repair of a cystocele.
- *Posterior colpo-perineorrhaphy* will control a rectocele.

Over the last few years there has been an increasing interest in paravaginal, or fascial, tears as a cause for prolapse. Proponents of this view suggest that anterior wall prolapse can be due to detachment of the lateral vaginal wall support to the arcus tendineus, and, therefore, its repair is required to correct a prolapse. Further work is required.

Vaginal hysterectomy is the procedure of choice for uterine prolapse and is often performed as part of a combined pelvic floor repair. In particular, if an enterocele is present the utero-sacral ligaments can be used to obliterate the hernial sac.

Manchester (Fothergill) repair can be performed where conservation of the uterus is required, but is uncommon now.

Burch colposuspension can be performed where there is concurrent stress incontinence, and it will correct a cystocele but may predispose to an enterocele.

Recurrent prolapse and vault prolapse

The incidence of recurrent prolapse after surgery is around 20%. This may reflect poor surgical technique and/or deficiencies in the underlying tissues.

- *Colpocleisis*—occlusion of the vagina is appropriate for non-sexually active women and has good results. It is simple, can be performed under local anaesthetic, and therefore may be appropriate for elderly women with prolapse.
- Vault prolapse is more common after hysterectomy and can be corrected by one of 2 suspension techniques both of which maintain the integrity of the vagina and for which high success rates (90%) are reported:
  - *sacrospinous fixation* where the vault is fixed to the sacrospinous ligament on one side using a vaginal approach. There is a risk of pudendal nerve injury.
  - *sacrocolpopexy* where the vagina is attached to the sacrum using a non-absorbable mesh run around the pelvic side wall in an abdominal procedure. There is a risk of sacral plexus haemorrhage.

FURTHER READING

Hughes P and Jackson S. The Scientific Basis of Prolapse (1999). The Obstetrician and Gynaecologist; 3: 121–129.

Jackson S and Smith P (1997). Diagnosing and managing genitourinary prolapse. BMJ; 314: 875 80.

Pemberton JH, Swash M and Henry MM. (2002) The Pelvic Floor—Its Function and Disorders. Saunders. London.

Shaw RW, Soutter WP and Stanton S. Gynaecology (2nd edition). 1997. Churchill Livingstone. Edinburgh.

Thakar R, Stanton. (2002) Management of genital prolapse. BMJ; 324: 1258–62

24. Genital tract neoplasia

INTRA-EPITHELIAL NEOPLASIA OF THE VULVA, VAGINA AND CERVIX

Nomenclature and definitions
- *Dyskaryosis*—a cytological term that refers to abnormalities of individual cells such as enlargement and hyperchromasia of the nuclei with uneven chromatin distribution, irregular nuclear membrane and multinucleation. It is graded mild, moderate or severe.
- *Dysplasia*—a histological diagnosis that describes abnormalities of epithelium. It is defined as a lesion in which part of the thickness of the epithelium is replaced by cells showing varying degrees of atypia.
- *Carcinoma-in-situ* refers to lesions in which all or most of the epithelium shows the following features:
  - Loss of stratification and polarity throughout the full thickness of the epithelium
  - Variation in size and shape of cells
  - Increased nuclear/cytoplasmic ratio
  - Frequent bizarre mitoses
  - The basement membrane is intact.

The only difference between dysplasia and carcinoma-in-situ is one of degree. Both these terms have now been replaced by the term **intra-epithelial neoplasia**

VULVAL INTRAEPITHELIAL NEOPLASIA (VIN) (see p. 321)

This term replaces previous confusing descriptive terms for hypertrophic dystrophies with varying degrees of cellular atypia. There are two distinct subgroups.

- Conditions affecting women over 50 years of age who present with discrete lesions:
  - The aetiology is unknown, but they do not seem to be related to human papilloma virus.
  - These are potentially malignant lesions with progression occurring in up to 5% of treated cases. The majority of these

lesions may progress to cancer if neglected, but the progression is slow.
- Conditions affecting younger women presenting with multifocal intraepithelial neoplasia—cervical intraepithelial neoplasia, vaginal intraepithelial neoplasia (VAIN), anal intraepithelial neoplasia (AIN) and VIN—affecting different areas of the lower genital tract.

It is associated with wart virus or human papillomavirus (HPV) infection and is also associated with multiple sexual partners, smoking and immunosuppression (e.g. in renal transplant patients and users of systemic steroids).

As with the more common cervical intraepithelial neoplasia (CIN) VIN is graded into three subsets:

- VIN 1 (mild cellular atypia)
- VIN 2 (moderate cellular atypia)
- VIN 3 (severe cellular atypia including carcinoma-in-situ). In VIN 3 atypical cells occupy the full thickness of the epithelium without any stromal invasion.

It may present as well-defined reddish-brown, moist, papular or plaque-like lesions accompanied by pruritus. Growth is slow but the lesions tend to coalesce and invasive carcinoma will supervene if the lesion is neglected. Colposcopy is often used to define the affected areas.

Histology
- Hyperplasia (acanthosis) and irregular thickening of epidermis
- Distorted rete ridges
- Hyperkeratosis
- Chronic inflammatory cell infiltrate.

NB. *Leukoplakia* is a descriptive term for irregular thickening and whitening of the vulval skin that is seen in several pathological conditions. It should not be used as a diagnostic term.

VAGINAL INTRA-EPITHELIAL NEOPLASIA (VAIN)

VAIN is usually asymptomatic and detected only by cytological and/or colposcopic examination.

Its appearances are as for CIN (see below).

The treatment options for VAIN are:

- Laser vaporisation
- Surgical excision
- Radiation (rarely)
- Intravaginal 5-fluorouracil (rarely).

When VAIN is detected following hysterectomy, management is difficult because the angles of the vagina are difficult to assess by cytology and colposcopy.

Discrete areas of VAIN away from the vaginal vault can be vaporised by laser.

Areas involving the vaginal vault hysterectomy scar are treated by upper vaginectomy.

CERVICAL INTRA-EPITHELIAL NEOPLASIA—(CIN)

Aetiology
CIN and cervical cancer have the same origin.

Approximately 30–50% of cases of CIN will, if left untreated, progress to invasive disease.

Epidemiology
- CIN and cervical cancer are sexually transmitted diseases. Associated characteristics of affected women include number of sexual partners, divorce and sexually transmitted infections. There is a negative association with religious and some cultural factors.
- Although the common denominator appears to be age at first intercourse, the majority of affected women are not promiscuous and should not be stigmatised.
- A male factor is also involved. The wives of men with prostatic or penile cancer have a higher risk of cervical cancer.
- Cervical neoplasia is most common among lower socioeconomic groups.
- Prolonged use of oral contraception (in women who are HPV positive—see p. 248) and cigarette smoking are associated with an increased risk of cervical neoplasia.
- The age-specific prevalence for CIN 1 and CIN 2 is 20–29 years, and for CIN 3 it is 36–39 years.

Biology
- The *transformation zone (TZ)* is a circumferential region of tissue between the vaginal (squamous) and endocervical (columnar) tissue. It is composed of columnar epithelium that has descended on to the ectocervix, although the final border between the columnar and squamous epithelium is usually not finally defined until adult life.
- The columnar epithelium of the TZ undergoes metaplasia to a varying degree to squamous epithelium. This active process exposes the epithelium to neoplastic transformation.
- The precise mutagen involved is not proven but human papillomovirus (HPV) types 16, 18, 31 and 33 are found in over 90% of invasive cervical cancers.

Cytological screening and the prevention of cervical cancer
- The success of cytological screening programmes depends on the percentage of women at risk screened.
- Comprehensive programmes have achieved significant reductions in both the incidence of, and death rate from, cervical cancer. The

remaining unscreened women at risk have a much greater risk of having (and dying from) the disease.

- The number of women screened and the frequency of screening depends on the resources available. One recommended screening policy is as follows:
  - The first smear should be taken at 20 years of age.
  - Thereafter, intervals of 3 to 5 years are adequate.
  - Regular testing can stop from 64 years of age if previous smears have been normal.
- Currently over 80% of women in Britain are screened.
- The incidence of cervical cancer and cancer deaths is beginning to fall.

Cervical smears
The correlation between the level of dyskaryosis in a smear and the grade of CIN is not exact (approx 70% agreement).

Cervical smears are graded by assessment of individual cell morphology and recommendations are made as follows:

- *Inadequate*—insufficient cellular material for assessment. Repeat smear required.
- *Negative*—no abnormal cells seen. Repeat in recommended screening interval (usually 3 or 5 years).
- *Borderline*—minor cellular changes. Repeat in 6 months and refer for colposcopy if persists on 2 or 3 occasions.
- *Mild dyskaryosis*—superficial cell (mild); nuclear abnormalities with abundant cytoplasm and angular cell borders. Repeat smear and refer for colposcopy if persists.
- *Moderate dyskaryosis*—intermediate cell (moderate); nucleus much larger in proportion to the whole cell than normally but occupying less than 50% of the cell. Refer for colposcopy.
- *Severe dyskaryosis*—Parabasal cell (severe); the nucleus occupies more than 50% of the cell. The cell border is round or oval. Refer *urgently* for colposcopy.
- *Severe dyskaryosis, invasive*—severe dyskaryosis plus cells suggestive of invasion. Refer *urgently* for colposcopy.
- *Glandular neoplasia*—atypical columnar type cells suggestive of dysplasia of the endocervical columnar epithelium: cervical glandular intra-epithelial neoplasia (CGIN). Refer for colposcopy.

Histological characteristics of CIN grades
- CIN 1 (mild dysplasia)
  - Upper two-thirds of epithelium exhibits relatively good differentiation
  - Minor nuclear abnormalities
  - Few mitotic figures confined to basal third.
- CIN 2 (moderate dysplasia)
  - Upper half of epithelium is well differentiated
  - Moderate nuclear abnormalities
  - Mitotic figures (some abnormal) present in basal two-thirds.

- CIN 3 (severe dysplasia/carcinoma-in-situ)
  - Maturation confined to superficial one-third of epithelium or absent
  - Nuclear abnormalities marked and throughout full thickness
  - Mitotic figures may be numerous, at all levels and with many abnormal configurations.

Taking and processing of cervical smears

- The proper taking, interpretation and follow-up of cervical smears are fundamental to the whole screening programme.
- The cervix must be inspected carefully. The presence of a suspicious abnormality requires referral urgently for colposcopy irrespective of the smear result.
- Specimens for cervical and/or vaginal cytology are usually taken with a wooden (or plastic) Ayre spatula.
- All smears must be accompanied by adequate information about the patient.

False-negative smears

Those reported as normal in a patient who has a neoplastic lesion of the cervix. This may be due to:

- An error in taking the smear—cervix not properly sampled
- Technical problem—smear too thin, too thick, too bloody, poorly fixed or poorly stained
- Diagnostic failures—misinterpretation by the cytologist
- Lesion so small that very few cells exfoliate

The reported frequency of false-negative smears is between 1.8 and 20%!

False-positive smears

Those in which malignant changes are seen but subsequent full examination of the cervix fails to reveal them.

They may be due to errors in the laboratory, therefore positive smears should be repeated before any surgery is contemplated.

However, the cytologist may be correct and the source of the malignant cells may have remained undetected higher in the cervical canal and then detected at colposcopy or even cone biopsy.

Evaluation of the patient with abnormal cervical cytology

In the majority of patients with CIN the cervix will look quite normal to the naked eye.

No patient with cytological evidence of CIN should be treated without prior colposcopic assessment.

Colposcopy is the detailed examination of the cervix using binocular magnification and bright illumination. The aims of colposcopic examination of the cervix in women with CIN are:

- To demarcate the boundaries of the transformation zone (TZ)
- To rule out invasive disease by directed biopsies
- To confirm/refute the suspicion raised by cytology
- To plan appropriate treatment

Treatment of CIN

Intra-epithelial neoplasia is a localised problem and can be treated satisfactorily by excision or destruction of the abnormal epithelium.

The method used is less important than the assurance that all neoplastic tissue is destroyed or removed. Some suggested methods of treatment are given below.

Loop diathermy excision of TZ
- This can often be carried out as an out-patient.
- A major benefit over destructive methods discussed below is that the area removed is available for histology.
- Because of its ease of use, safety and cheapness it is now the commonest form of treatment.

Cone biopsy
- Traditionally performed with a knife under general anaesthesia, this can be done under local anaesthesia using a modified loop diathermy technique.
- It can provide both firm diagnosis and comprehensive treatment. It is even more effective if colposcopically directed (99% primary cure rate).
- The operation is not without immediate or longer-term hazard such as:
  - Primary or secondary haemorrhage
  - Local infection
  - Cervical stenosis (small cones)
  - Cervical incompetence (large cones).
- Fertility is probably unaffected, but mid-trimester abortion and pre-term delivery may be more common and possibly directly related to the size of the cone removed.
- If the raw area of the cervix is covered by mobilising the remainder of the cervical epithelium, residual CIN in the endocervical crypts may be covered and remain occult.
- Apparent incomplete excision may require further definitive surgery (e.g. another cone biopsy, or hysterectomy) in approximately one third of cases.

Local destruction of the whole TZ
- This can be achieved by carbon dioxide laser, cold coagulation, cryocautery, radical electrocoagulation diathermy, or electrocautery.
- These have the advantage that they are not associated with significant morbidity (including fertility-related problems). In addition, laser, cryocautery and cold coagulation may be

performed as outpatient procedures with or without local anaesthesia.
- The criteria for use of a local destructive technique or diathermy excision are:
  - the patient must be assessed by a competent colposcopist
  - the lesion and the transformation zone are seen in their entirety
  - colposcopically directed biopsies have shown that there is no evidence of invasion
  - there is no cytological or colposcopic evidence of abnormal columnar cells that could suggest an endometrial neoplasm
  - regular cytological and colposcopic follow-up is feasible.

Hysterectomy
- This may be the method of choice for CIN 3 in women who have completed their family, who wish complete assurance of cure, and/or in whom follow-up is likely to be difficult.
- *No patient with an abnormal smear should have a hysterectomy without prior colposcopy* because CIN extends on to the vaginal walls in approximately 4% of women. If a hysterectomy is being performed in the presence of CIN, all the affected epithelium must be excised with the hysterectomy specimen.
- Removal of a cuff of vagina is not necessary if the lesion is confined to the cervix.

INVASIVE TUMOURS OF THE VULVA

- Vulval cancer is a disease of older women. The mean age of affected women is about 60 years, and 75% of cases occur in women aged 50 years or over.
- It forms about 5% of all female genital tract cancers.
- There is an association with nulliparity and cigarette smoking.
- Ninety per cent of malignant vulval neoplasms are squamous, and most develop in association with lichen sclerosus and VIN. Chronic granulomatous diseases of the vulva, e.g. syphilis, granuloma inguinale or lymphogranuloma venereum predispose to vulval cancer.
- Between 15 and 30% of women with vulvar cancer have had, or will develop, intra-epithelial or invasive lesions of the cervix.

Presentation and spread of squamous carcinoma
- An ulcer or papillary lesion may develop after a period of intractable pruritus.
- Continued growth is ultimately accompanied by bleeding, secondary infection and pain.
- Delayed presentation is a major problem.
- The commonest sites are:
  - Labia   70%
  - Clitoris   15%

- Perineum or
  fourchette   5%
- Remainder   10%
  (Labia majora three times as common as labia minora)
- Most squamous cell carcinomas of the vulva are well differentiated.
- The primary route of spread is lymphatic (see Figure 24.1)
  - Spread occurs first to the superficial and deep inguinal and femoral nodes then to the external iliac and obturator nodes.
  - The common iliac and para-aortic nodes are involved in late cases.
  - Contra-lateral involvement is not uncommon in tumours near the midline because of the extensive anastomosis of the lymphatic network.
  - Local growth progressively involves the urethra, vagina, anus and, occasionally, the bladder or rectum.

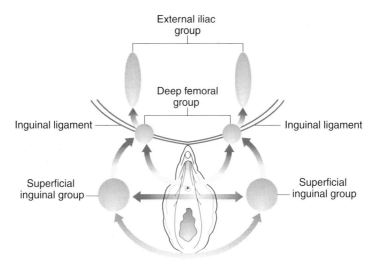

Fig 24.1

Clinical staging of squamous carcinoma
- Clinical staging is unreliable: palpation of inguinal nodes is not a good guide to involvement; palpable enlarged nodes may not be affected by tumour in up to 40% of cases, and lack of enlargement may mask involvement in a similar number.
- Involvement of nodes is an important prognostic sign, as in other malignant tumours.
- The 5-year survival rate in women with squamous carcinoma:
  - Without node involvement   75%
  - With node involvement   40%

- Staging can either use a TNM (Tumour, Nodes, Metastasis) classification or FIGO clinical staging—see boxes below.

Squamous carcinoma of the vulva: TNM classification

Primary tumour (T)

T1	Tumour confined to the vulva <2 cm in diameter
T2	Tumour confined to the vulva >2 cm in diameter
T3	Tumour of any size with adjacent spread to the urethra and/or vagina, and/or anus
T4	Tumour of any size infiltrating the bladder (including the upper part of the urethra) mucosa, and/or the rectal mucosa and/or fixed to the bone

Regional lymph nodes (N)

N0	No nodes palpable
N1	Nodes palpable in either groin, not enlarged, mobile (not clinically suspicious of neoplasm)
N2	Nodes palpable in either one or both groins, enlarged, firm and mobile (clinically suspicious of neoplasm)
N3	Fixed or ulcerated nodes

Distant metastases (M)

M0	No clinical metastases
M1a	Palpable deep pelvic lymph nodes
M1b	Other distant metastases

Squamous carcinoma of the vulva: FIGO clinical staging

Stage I	Lesions 2 cm or less confined to the vulva or perineum. No lymph node metastases
Stage Ia	As above with stromal invasion no greater than 1 mm
Stage Ib	Stromal invasion >1 mm
Stage II	Lesions confined to the vulva and/or perineum with a diameter >2 cm and no lymph node metastases
Stage III	Lesions of any size extending to the lower urethra, vagina or anus and/or unilateral node metastases
Stage IVa	Lesions invading upper urethra, bladder, rectum or pelvic bone with or without bilateral positive groin nodes regardless of extent of primary
Stage IVb	Any distant metastases including pelvic lymph nodes

---

Treatment of invasive squamous cell carcinoma of vulva

RCOG recommendations (see Further reading)

These include the following:

- Health care professionals should be aware of the risk markers for and precursors of vulval cancer (see above).

- Women with these conditions should be made aware of the risks.
- Care is best provided in Cancer Centres by Multidisciplinary Teams.
  - They should develop local protocols to encourage prompt and early referral.
- Women should be seen within 2 weeks of referral and definitive treatment commenced no later than 6 weeks following diagnosis.
- Radical treatment should not (with rare exceptions) be undertaken without prior biopsy confirmation of malignancy.
- Excisional biopsies must include a zone of normal tissue at least 1 cm in width and depth.
- An individualised approach employing a range of treatments is advocated for all cases with advanced disease (see below).

Most of the above principles apply to all gynaecological malignancies.

Surgical treatment
- The potential for groin node disease should be addressed in all but stage Ia squamous cancers, verrucous tumours and basal cell carcinomas.
- FIGO stage I and II lateralised lesions only require ipsilateral lymphadenectomy in the first instance. Contralateral lymphadenectomy may be required if ipsilateral nodes are positive.
- The standard treatment for other vulval cancers is radical vulvectomy and bilateral lymphadenectomy (but not routinely of the pelvic nodes).
- Three separate incisions are used to remove the tumour and the groin lymph nodes.
- Primary closure of the wound can usually be obtained by undermining the skin flaps but tension on the suture lines at the closure junction is almost inevitable. Rotational skin flaps improve healing and cosmetic results.
- The major postoperative complications are wound infection, wound breakdown and lymphocyst collection in the groins. Late complications involve tumour recurrence (about 10%), chronic lymphoedema and profound psychosexual disturbance.

The 5-year survival rate of women treated surgically is 75% with no node involvement, and 40% with node involvement.

Radiotherapy
- Radiotherapy is most commonly used as an adjuvant (planned extra) treatment for the groins in patients with positive groin lymph nodes.
- Vulval cancer is susceptible to radiotherapy but normal vulval skin is exquisitely sensitive resulting in severe side-effects such as moist desquamation, ulceration and fibrosis. This can often prevent full treatment.
- Pre-operative irradiation may reduce the size of primary lesion and make operation possible.

Treatment of advanced lesions is difficult and accompanied by a poor prognosis.

Basal cell carcinoma
- Usually occurs on the labia majora beginning as a small nodule which becomes ulcerated centrally (rodent ulcer).
- Lymphatics are not involved and local excision is usually adequate.
- The co-existence of an invasive squamous carcinoma within the lesions must be excluded.

Melanoma
- Arise from pigmented naevi. Prophylactic excision of pigmented vulvar naevi is recommended because they are usually symptomless even after they have become malignant.
- Treatment is by wide local excision and removal of any affected nodes because more radical procedures did not improve recurrence rates or survival.
- Prognosis is poor, less than 10% 5-year survival if nodes are positive

Sarcoma
- This is a rare lesion. The mean age of patients with sarcoma is about 40 years.
- Treatment is by extensive local excision but the benefit of lymphadenectomy is unclear.
- Distant recurrence is common.

Bartholin's gland tumours
- These are rare lesions which may be adenocarcinoma (45%), squamous carcinoma (40%), sarcoma (5%), melanoma (1%) or undifferentiated (the remainder).
- Diagnosis is usually late because of the deep site of origin and the tumours may present with ulceration of the vulva and vagina.
- Treatment is by extensive local excision accompanied by inguinal and pelvic lymphadenectomy.
- The 5-year survival rate is probably under 10%.

CARCINOMA OF THE VAGINA

Primary malignant tumours of the vagina are rare, and an invasive lesion is more likely to be due to secondary spread.

Squamous cell carcinoma
- This is the commonest histological type and accounts for 1–2% of all gynaecological malignancies.
- Most occur between the ages of 55 and 70 years with a peak incidence of about 65 years.
- The commonest presenting symptoms are vaginal discharge, and bleeding as a result of ulceration of the tumour. The most frequent site is the posterior vaginal wall.

Carcinoma of the vagina: FIGO staging	
Stage 0	Intra-epithelial carcinoma
Stage I	Limited to vaginal wall
Stage II	Outside the vagina but not to pelvic side walls
Stage III	To the pelvic side walls and/or symphysis pubis
Stage IV	Extension beyond the true pelvis or involving the bladder or rectum.

The lesions are usually moderately undifferentiated.

Tumours in the lower third of the vagina spread to the inguinal nodes like carcinoma of the vulva (p. 290). In the upper vagina, spread is similar to that of carcinoma of the cervix (p. 295).

Treatment
Radiotherapy is the treatment of choice except if the lesion is at the introitus, when radical surgery may be possible. Five-year survival rates are: Stage I 85%; Stage II 55%; Stage III 30%; Stage IV <10%.

Adenocarcinoma
- This rare tumour is most often found in association with vaginal adenosis in young women with a history of intrauterine exposure to diethyl stilboestrol (DES), an ineffective treatment previously used to treat recurrent miscarriage.
- The most frequent histological type is a clear cell adenocarcinoma, and the commonest site is the upper third of the vagina.
- Spread is by local extension and by the lymphatics and bloodstream.

Staging
As for squamous carcinoma of the cervix.

Treatment
- Radical hysterectomy, vaginectomy and pelvic lymphadenectomy is preferred.
- Radiotherapy can be used if expert surgery is not available, or in young women with small lesions (because the remainder of the vagina, adjacent structures and ovarian function can be preserved).

  Five-year survival rates are: Stage I 80%; Stage II < 20%; Stages III and IV none.

Secondary vaginal tumours
- Metastatic carcinoma of the vagina is commoner than a primary cancer.
- It occurs frequently in carcinoma of the cervix, sometimes after carcinoma of the endometrium and occasionally in carcinoma of the ovary or choriocarcinoma. It may rarely follow hypernephroma or carcinoma of the colon or rectum.

CARCINOMA OF THE CERVIX

- Cervical cancer is second to ovarian as the commonest malignant tumour of the genital tract, comprising 30% of the total.
- Despite an overall fall in incidence, particularly among older women, the peak age is still 50 to 59 years.
- However, in the past two decades the incidence has doubled in women under 40 years, and the mortality has almost trebled in women under 34 years of age.
- This worrying rise may have halted in well-screened populations. The epidemiology is as for CIN.
- 75% of the tumours are squamous, approximately 15% are adenosquamous and 10% are adenocarcinoma. Adenocarcinomas are becoming relatively more common.

Squamous carcinoma

Histology
- Cell characteristics:
  - Loss of stratification
  - Various degrees of immaturity and lack of differentiation
  - Pleomorphism of cells and nuclei
  - Hyperchromatic nuclei
  - Abundant and atypical mitoses
  - Giant cell formation
- Architecture:
  - The malignant epithelium has broken through the basement membrane
  - Lymphocyte and polymorph infiltration of stroma. The more immature and undifferentiated the tumour the more malignant it is (and more radiosensitive).

Spread
- Early spread occurs by local infiltration.
- Upward spread into the body of the uterus is uncommon, and forward spread into the bladder occurs late. Obstruction of the ureters is common (many deaths occur due to uraemia).
- Lymphatic spread first involves a primary group of nodes:

• Parametrial	• Hypogastric
• Vesico-vaginal	• Obturator
• Recto-vaginal	• External iliac.

and then a secondary group of nodes:

• Sacral	• Vaginal (deep and superficial)
• Common iliac	• Para-aortic.

- Even in clinically assessed stage Ib disease pelvic lymph nodes will be affected in about 15% of patients.

Clinical features
- Cervical cancer may be asymptomatic (even to a late stage) and be detected by routine cervical smear or examination.

- Intermenstrual, postmenopausal or postcoital bleeding are the commonest presenting symptoms. Vaginal discharge is less frequent and a later development.
- Pain occurs only in the very late stages.
  On examination the cervix may:
  - Appear normal (e.g. intra-epithelial or endocervical)
  - Be hard with a granular 'erosion' which bleeds to touch
  - Be ulcerated.
- Moderately advanced growths may be exophytic (polypoid), infiltrative or ulcerative.

Management

A multi-disciplinary team approach involving close co-operation between a gynaecologist, radiotherapist, histopathologist and specialist nursing staff is vital.

- Check full blood count, urea, and electrolytes
- Carry out chest X-ray and excretion urography (IVP), or ultrasound scan of urinary tract. A bone survey for metastasis is not routine. The value of lymphangiography remains controversial.
- Carry out pelvic examination (vaginal and rectal) under anaesthesia to assess the extent of the disease. This is the definitive staging, which allows planning and comparison of treatment results.

Proceed to:

- Cervical biopsy for histology
- Cystoscopy—looking for bullous oedema which suggests involvement of the underlying muscle.

(The first insertion of caesium can be carried out at this time if necessary—see p. 298.)

Treatment of stage Ia1 (micro-invasive) carcinoma of the cervix

Working definition

A micro-invasive lesion is one in which the carcinoma invades the stroma in one or more places to a depth of 3 mm or less below the basement membrane and in which lymphatics and blood vessels cannot be seen to be involved.

The following qualifications are necessary:

- It is not possible to examine the whole specimen histologically in every case.
- It is difficult to distinguish extensive gland or cleft involvement from stromal invasion.
- If clumps of tumour cells can be seen in vascular spaces, even if invasion is minimal, lymph nodes are involved in up to 25% of cases.

Carcinoma of cervix: FIGO clinical staging

Stage 0	Intra-epithelial neoplasia (p. 285)
Stage I	Invasive carcinoma confined to the cervix
Stage Ia1	No lesion visible at clinical examination, and stromal invasion is less than 3 mm (micro-invasion)
Stage Ia2	Stromal invasion between 3 and 5 mm with maximum lateral spread of 7 mm
Stage Ib	All other stage I lesions
Stage Ib1	Clinical lesions no greater than 4 cm in size
Stage Ib2	Clinical lesions >4 cm in size
Stage II	The carcinoma extends beyond the cervix but not to the pelvic side wall; and/or the upper two-thirds of the vagina are involved
Stage IIa	No parametrial involvement
Stage IIb	Obvious parametrial involvement
Stage III	The carcinoma extends to the pelvic side wall and/or the lower one-third of the vagina is involved. Presence of hydronephrosis or non-functioning kidney
Stage IIIa	No extension to the pelvic wall but involvement of the lower third of vagina
Stage IIIb	Extension to the pelvic wall or hydronephrosis or non-functioning kidney
Stage IV	The carcinoma extends beyond the true pelvis or involves the bladder or rectum (bullous oedema is excluded)
Stage IVa	Spread of tumour onto adjacent pelvic organs
Stage IVb	Spread to distant organs

Treatment

- Conservative therapy by cone biopsy can be considered in young women who are anxious to retain fertility. *Close cytological and colposcopic follow-up is vital.*
- Simple hysterectomy should be used:
  - For older women or in those whose family is complete
  - When the pathologist is uncertain of the diagnosis of micro-invasion.
  A cuff of vagina should be taken if the transformation zone extends on to the vagina.
- Radical therapy (as for stage Ib) may be best for those with clumps of tumour cells in vascular spaces, and certainly if stromal invasion is more than 3 mm (stage Ia2)

The cure rate should be close to 100%.

Treatment of stage Ib and IIa carcinoma of the cervix
The choice is between radical (Wertheim's) hysterectomy and radiotherapy.

Radical hysterectomy
- The lesion most suitable for treatment by radical hysterectomy is one which is confined to the cervix or with only minimal extension beyond it, particularly in the younger patient.
- The procedure involves removal of the uterus, cervix, parametria, upper one-third to one-half of the vagina and as many pelvic lymph nodes as possible.
- It is now thought unnecessary to sacrifice ovaries routinely; this is an advantage, particularly in younger women.

Advantages of surgery
- The tumour is removed which patients find psychologically reassuring.
- Treatment is less prolonged.
- The ovaries need not be removed in young patients with early disease.
- Early and late complications of radiotherapy are avoided.
- Infection is no bar to treatment (unlike radiotherapy).
- Potential radio-resistance is overcome.
- More prognostic information is available.
- Follow-up examination and radiological monitoring is easier.
- Local recurrence is treatable with radiotherapy.

Disadvantages of surgery
- Only selected patients benefit from it.
- Bladder dysfunction is common.
- The vagina is shortened.

Complications of surgery
- *Immediate and short-term*: anaesthetic problems, haemorrhage, shock, sepsis, thrombo-embolism.
- *Long-term*: urinary retention, ureteric and rectal fistulae; lymphocyst—a collection of lymph on the pelvic side wall.

Radiotherapy
- The tumour itself and any paracervical spread are attacked using intrauterine and intravaginal caesium-137.
- The pelvic lymph nodes and their lymphatics are dealt with mainly by external irradiation.
- The aim is to deliver 60–75 Grey at point A (2 cm lateral to the midline; 2 cm above the lateral fornix in the same sagittal plane as the uterus). Point B (5 cm from the midline at the same level and the same place) receives only 25% of the dosage according to the inverse square law.
- External irradiation (preferably by linear accelerator) should deliver 50–70 Grey to the pelvic side walls.
- There is considerable variation in individual policies and regimes but the overall aims are the same.

Complications of radiotherapy

- Vaginal stenosis may develop in up to 85% of irradiation patients. This can be minimised by regular sexual intercourse or the use of vaginal dilators. Dyspareunia is common.
- Radiation induced menopause is inevitable. This can be managed by topical or systemic oestrogen replacement.
- Urinary tract injuries may occur. Some frequency and dysuria is inevitable. Bladder ulcers can be difficult to cure. Vesico-vaginal fistulae occur rarely and usually some 3–8 months after treatment.
- Uretero-vaginal fistulae are more liable to occur when radiotherapy and surgery are combined. Surgical correction of fistulae is difficult; urinary diversion is usually required.
- Intestinal complications may arise, varying from diarrhoea to rectal fistulae.
- Local recurrence is difficult to treat. Chemotherapy is ineffective but selected patients can be saved by extensive surgery (pelvic exenteration).
- Follow-up is difficult due to the fibrosis induced in the pelvis by radiotherapy.
- Occasionally radiotherapy causes secondary cancers many years later.

Combined radiotherapy and surgery

- Radiotherapy was formerly given pre-operatively but this is rarely done now because there is no demonstrable benefit and it alters the histological appearances of the specimen.
- Adjuvant (planned additional) radiotherapy is given postoperatively if more than two lymph nodes are involved or if the excision margins of the tumour are incomplete.

Note: if invasive carcinoma is diagnosed as a result of cone biopsy, definitive treatment should, if possible, be deferred for 6 weeks to allow healing to occur. Otherwise the complications of radiotherapy and/or surgery are increased.

Chemotherapy

Combination chemotherapy (e.g. cisplatin, methotrexate, bleomycin) is given to fit patients with proven systemic disease. Tumour partial response is common and survival is lengthened. Cure is uncommon. Chemotherapy is used as palliation (e.g. to relieve pain due to tumour pressing on nerve roots).

Results of treatment

- Whatever the method used to treat carcinoma of the cervix, the 5-year survival rates are comparable at:
  - Stage Ib: 85–90%
  - Stage IIa: 70–75%: (if lymph nodes are positive, survival drops to 50–60%.)

- The results of surgery improve and its complications lessen with the expertise of the surgeon. This condition is probably best fulfilled by sub-specialists in regional cancer centres.
- To ensure the best treatment for each patient the following *minimum* criteria must be met:
  - There must be close co-operation between the surgical and radiotherapeutic teams.
  - Any surgery should be carried out by, or under the guidance of, a gynaecologist adequately trained in radical surgery and able to cope with any contingency.
  - Close follow-up and audit of outcomes is essential.

Treatment of stages IIb to IV carcinoma of the cervix
- The treatment of choice is radiotherapy.
- Pelvic exenteration is applicable when radiotherapy is unlikely to be effective or when the tumour has not regressed following radiotherapy.
  - *Anterior exenteration*—bladder removed in conjunction with radical hysterectomy and lymphadenectomy
  - *Posterior exenteration*—rectum removed
  - *Total exenteration*—both bladder and rectum removed.

These operations are justified only if there is some expectation of useful life as a result. They should only be carried out in specialised centres, usually with a team approach involving a urologist or colorectal surgeon as appropriate. Complications are common. These operations are not applicable if extra-pelvic metastases are present.

- A terminal colostomy and ileal conduit are to be preferred to a 'wet' colostomy.
- Five-year survival rates are as follows: Stage IIb 50–60%; Stage III 30–35%; Stage IV <10%.

Recurrent carcinoma of the cervix
- If the tumour recurs it usually does so within 18 months of treatment. The main sites are:
  - deep pelvis: 35%
  - distant spread: 30%
  - lateral pelvis: 15%
  - bladder or rectum: 10%
  - central pelvis: 10%
- The most frequent signs and symptoms are:
  - renewed vaginal bleeding
  - pain
  - weight loss
  - evidence of urinary tract obstruction.
- If radiotherapy has not been used, or was incomplete, then further treatment is possible.
- Occasionally exenteration can be carried out.

- Palliation is usually all that can be offered.
- For relief of pain in advanced cancer see p. 316.
- The ultimate causes of death, in order of frequency, are uraemia, cachexia, severe haemorrhage, complications of treatment and, rarely, remote metastases to vital organs.

Adenocarcinoma of the cervix
- These tumours are rare but they tend to grow and spread as squamous carcinoma.
- Treatment is as for squamous carcinoma. They respond equally to radiotherapy or surgery.

TUMOURS OF THE BODY OF THE UTERUS AND FALLOPIAN TUBES

ENDOMETRIAL POLYP (ADENOMA)

- These polyps are usually multiple before the menopause and may be a component of endometrial hyperplasia. After the menopause they are usually single (or few in number). They tend to recur.
- Most are symptomless but they may be associated with:
  - Menorrhagia
  - Intermenstrual bleeding
  - Postcoital bleeding
  - Postmenopausal bleeding
- They are easily removed by small ovum forceps and curettage. Hysteroscopy is of value because a polyp may elude curettage. They can be resected under direct vision.
- All polyps should be sent for histology to exclude malignant change.

UTERINE FIBROIDS

- A leiomyoma is a well circumscribed benign uterine tumour derived mainly from smooth muscle but containing some fibrous connective tissue elements.
- It is the commonest tumour of the female genital tract, being present in at least 20% of women over the age of 35. The peak age incidence of symptoms is between 35 and 45 years.
- In Caucasian, but not Black, women they are associated with nulliparity or relative infertility.
- Growth may be related to oestrogen stimulation.

Sites of origin
- Intramural—within uterine wall
- Subserous—projecting from the peritoneal surface of the uterus
- Intraligamentary—between the layers of the broad ligament
- Submucous—indenting the uterine cavity
- Cervical.

Submucous fibroids may become polypoidal and subserous ones pedunculated. Pedunculated fibroids may lose their uterine attachment and gain a secondary blood supply (parasitic fibroid).

Gross characteristics
- They may be small, medium-sized or large, and are usually multiple.
- They are usually firm, but can be soft and cystic if degeneration has taken place.
- They are white and characteristically whorled in appearance.
- There is a false capsule of compressed uterine muscle which allows easy enucleation (cf. adenomyosis).

Histology
Groups and bundles of smooth muscle fibres are interlaced in twists and whorls. The fibrous component becomes more marked as the tumour enlarges.

Clinical features
- The majority are symptomless.
- Increased menstrual loss is usually caused by submucous fibroids. Intermenstrual bleeding may be due to a fibroid polyp with an ulcerated tip. (Note: Atypical menstrual symptoms may be due to a concurrent but separate pathology).
- Pressure effects may give rise to bladder symptoms and interfere with venous return.
- Abdominal swelling may be noted.
- Pain is not a common symptom unless the fibroid has become complicated (see below).
- There is a rare association with polycythaemia

Differential diagnosis
- It must include all causes of pelvic swellings.
- It is not always easy to discern clinically between a solid ovarian tumour and a pedunculated fibroid (ultrasound scanning is useful).
- The difference between a fibroid and an adenomyoma may not be apparent until surgical removal is attempted.

Potential effects of fibroids on pregnancy
- Subfertility
- Miscarriage and pre-term labour
- Malpresentations
- Obstructed labour (rare)
- Third stage problems
- Delayed involution postpartum.

Complications of fibroids
- *Torsion of pedicle*
- *Haemorrhage*

- *Infection*—usually at the tip of a fibroid polyp
- *Hyaline degeneration*—present to some degree in most moderate to large-sized fibroids. The tumour may be painful, enlarged and soft. Cystic degeneration follows.
- *Red degeneration (necrobiosis)*—occurs typically during pregnancy and is due to infarction of the centre of the tumour during mid-pregnancy. Characteristically the fibroid suddenly enlarges and is painful and tender. It can be mistaken for placental abruption or any acute abdominal emergency. It is treated conservatively during pregnancy.
- *Calcification*—usually seen postmenopausally and/or in pedunculated fibroids
- *Malignant change* (leiomyosarcoma—see p. 306) occurs in under 0.5% of cases. The fibroid may grow suddenly and be painful and tender. It is difficult to differentiate clinically from other degenerative changes.

Treatment
Conservative management is appropriate:

- when the tumours are small, the diagnosis is certain and there are no symptoms
- during pregnancy
- near the menopause when there are no symptoms and the tumour is not enlarging.

The short term use (no more than 6 months) of LHRH analogues needs to be studied further. They reduce the size of fibroids which may be of benefit in:

- those with contraindications to surgery
- as an adjunct to surgery if fibroids are large.

Unfortunately fibroids generally re-grow to their original size 3–4 months after stopping treatment.

Bilateral uterine artery embolisation (UAE) is currently being evaluated as a treatment for uterine fibroids. Over 8000 cases have been undertaken world-wide. However two deaths have been reported following the procedure from overwhelming sepsis. UAE should not be used in the presence of large pedunculated subserous fibroids.

- *Surgery* is indicated if:
  - The fibroids are causing symptoms or are growing rapidly. They are larger than a size corresponding to a 16-week pregnancy
  - The diagnosis is in doubt
  - They are likely to complicate a future pregnancy
- *Hysterectomy* is the definitive treatment.
- *Myomectomy* is indicated for those women who are subfertile, want more children or refuse to undergo hysterectomy.
- It may be possible to resect small submucous fibroids endoscopically.

Rupture of a myomectomy scar during subsequent pregnancy or labour is very rare, and vaginal delivery is often possible.

(Any fibroids found at caesarean section should usually be left undisturbed because of the risk of haemorrhage).

ENDOMETRIAL CARCINOMA

- This tumour comprises 25–30% of all gynaecological malignancies.
- The incidence is low before 40 years of age (4%), rises sharply until 55 years and then falls slightly. A greater proportion of women with endometrial carcinoma are postmenopausal than in carcinoma of the cervix. However, 25% of cases are premenopausal.
- Nulliparous women are 2–3 times more likely to develop it than are parous women, although half the women with the disease will have had one or more pregnancies.
- There is no relationship with social class.
- There is an association with gross obesity, polycystic ovary syndrome, and possibly diabetes mellitus.

Pathology
- Usually adenocarcinoma, but there may be benign squamous elements (adenoacanthoma) or malignant squamous elements (adenosquamous).
- It may be diffuse or circumscribed.

Histology
- In most cases the diagnosis is clear-cut due to the disordered architecture, atypical glands, and abnormal activity and characteristics of the cells.
- Benign cystic glandular hyperplasia is not liable to become malignant, but atypical hyperplasia is, and removal of the uterus is recommended.
- Spread is direct within the endometrium and, to a lesser degree, into the myometrium.
- Penetration to the serosa is uncommon.
- Lymphatic spread is along the ovarian vessels to the para-aortic nodes or through the myometrium and cervix to the pelvic nodes.

Clinical features
- Irregular vaginal bleeding—intermenstrual or postmenopausal.
- Watery vaginal discharge may be present in postmenopausal women.
- Abdominal and pelvic examination are unremarkable, except in late cases.

Population screening
- There is no certain method for screening the population at risk.

- Outpatient endometrial sampling (using a Pipelle sampler or similar device) is useful but not foolproof.
- Transvaginal ultrasound to measure endometrial thickness is non-invasive and generally accurate (thickness greater than 5 mm in postmenopausal women is abnormal), particularly if combined with endometrial sampling.

Initial management

- *Hysteroscopy and biopsy* should be carried out if this condition is suspected clinically or if the above tests are suspicious or unsatisfactory.
- *Pre-operative evaluation* is as for carcinoma of the cervix (p. 296). Transvaginal ultrasound, MRI or CT scan may also be useful.
- *Pre-operative radiotherapy* does not improve the prognosis and makes histological grading of the tumour more difficult.
- *Total abdominal hysterectomy and bilateral salpingo-oophorectomy* is the operation of choice. Careful surgical staging is necessary including:
  - aspiration of peritoneal fluid or peritoneal washings
  - palpation and inspection of all peritoneal structures
  - palpation with biopsy of pelvic and para-aortic lymph nodes.

The role of extensive node dissection (as for cancer of the cervix) is controversial. At the time of writing it is being evaluated in a

Endometrial carcinoma: FIGO staging

Staging is surgical

Stage 0	Atypical hyperplasia suspicious of malignancy
Stage I	Carcinoma confined to the body of the uterus
Stage Ia	Tumour limited to the endometrium
Stage Ib	Invasion to < half myometrium
Stage Ic	Invasion to > half myometrium but not reaching serosa
Stage II	Carcinoma involving the body and cervix
Stage IIa	Endocervical gland involvement only
Stage IIb	Cervical stroma involvement
Stage III	Carcinoma outside the uterus but not outside the true pelvis
Stage IIIa	Tumour invades serosa and/or adnexa and/or positive peritoneal cytology
Stage IIIb	Metastases to pelvic and or para—aortic nodes
Stage IV	Carcinoma involving the bladder or rectal mucosa (IVa) or outside the true pelvis (IVb).

Stage I is further subdivided according to the histology:

Grade 1	Well differentiated tumour
Grade 2	Differentiated tumour but with partly solid areas
Grade 3	Undifferentiated tumour or predominantly solid

multicentre randomised trial of lymphadenectomy and adjuvant external beam radiotherapy (The ASTEC trial—*A Study in the Treatment of Endometrial Cancer*).

Further management
- Low risk patients (i.e. stage Ia and Ib with G1 or G2 tumours—see information box) usually require no further therapy.
- Some surgeons perform radical hysterectomy (as carcinoma of cervix) for stage II disease.
- Adjuvant radiotherapy is indicated in patients at high risk of recurrence, although there is great variation in their selection.
- Results from cytotoxic therapy are disappointing.
- Recurrent disease can be treated with progestogens and/or radiotherapy. Pelvic exenteration is occasionally possible and a solitary vaginal vault lesion may be excisable.

Prognosis
The 5-year survival rate is:

Stage I: 80–85% (Grade 1 90%, Grade 3 65%)
Stage II: 55–60% (80% in best centres)
Stage III: 35–40% (60% in best centres)
Stage IV: <10% (15% in best centres)

SARCOMA OF THE UTERUS

These are rare tumours. Malignant degeneration in a leiomyoma accounts for half of them, but they may arise from normal myometrium or endometrial stroma.

Leiomyosarcoma
- Most patients are between 40 and 60 years of age.
- The commonest symptoms are abnormal vaginal bleeding and abdominal pain.
- A uterine mass is frequently palpable.
- Lymphatic spread is not common.
- Treatment is by total hysterectomy and bilateral salpingo-oophorectomy. Radiotherapy is relatively ineffective.

Endometrial sarcoma
- Most patients are between 50 and 70 years of age.
- Signs, symptoms and treatment are the same as for leiomyosarcoma.

Sarcoma botryoides
- A rare tumour probably of mixed mesodermal origin usually occurring in children (any lesion in this age group should arouse suspicion).
- It is polypoidal, either single or multiple.

- Staging is as for carcinoma.
- Treatment combines chemotherapy with radiotherapy and then radical surgery (extended hysterectomy and vaginectomy).

Prognosis
The 5-year survival rate is about 45% for stage I disease and 30% in stage II.

CARCINOMA OF THE FALLOPIAN TUBE

- Primary tumours of the fallopian tube are exceedingly rare (0.3% of genital tract cancers).
- They tend to occur in women aged 40–60 years.
- The histology is papillary adenocarcinoma.
- The majority of patients will have had a watery vaginal discharge, and some will complain of abdominal pain. An abdominal mass may be palpable, but very few patients have all of these clinical features.
- Treatment is by total hysterectomy and bilateral salpingo-oophorectomy. External radiotherapy is applied afterwards, and chemotherapy can be used in some late cases.
- Five-year survival rates are between 5 and 25%, reflecting the lateness of diagnosis in most cases.

CONDITIONS OF THE OVARY

NON-NEOPLASTIC DISTENSION CYSTS
Follicular cyst(s) ('cystic ovary')
- Due to enlargement of one or more follicles which fail to rupture.
- They are seldom more than 5 cm in diameter except when due to overdosage with clomiphene or HMG (see p. 236).
- Often associated with:
  - Anovulatory cycles
  - Fertility drugs as above
  - Polycystic ovary syndrome (p. 213).
- The majority are symptomless.
- Pain (usually mild but sometimes severe) is due to rupture of or haemorrhage into the cyst. (If unilateral pain is accompanied by slight menstrual disturbance an ectopic pregnancy must be excluded.)

Management
- If ovarian enlargement estimated at 4–6 cm is found at pelvic examination carry out pelvic ultrasound.
- If the presumed diagnosis is a 'cystic ovary' rather than a neoplasm no immediate action is necessary.
- Re-examine in 2 weeks; a follicular cyst will usually have disappeared.

- If the cyst is unchanged or larger, further investigation (e.g. laparoscopy) is warranted.
- If discovered or confirmed by laparoscopy, the cysts can be aspirated. Laparotomy is not necessary.
- Send the fluid for cytology and check CA 125 level to definitely exclude neoplasia.
- Treat any underlying condition.

Theca-lutein cysts
- A corpus luteum becomes cystic and persists in a functional state for longer than normal; or the granulosa and theca cells of a follicular cyst become luteinised.
- Characteristically, short periods of amenorrhoea are followed by heavier than usual uterine bleeding.
- The endometrium is secretory.
- Haemorrhage from even a normal corpus luteum can mimic ectopic pregnancy closely.
- Multiple and sometimes moderately large theca-lutein cysts are associated with trophoblast tumours. This is due to hCG stimulation.

Management
- Spontaneous resolution is usual.
- If a laparotomy is performed because of a mistaken diagnosis of ectopic pregnancy interfere with the ovary as little as possible.

Endometriomatous (chocolate) cysts
Due to ovarian endometriosis (see p. 223).

OVARIAN NEOPLASMS
- The incidence tends to rise with age but there is an increase in benign tumours in the fifth decade (40–49 years) and in malignant tumours from 50 years of age onwards.
- There is an association between ovarian cancer and:
  - Nulliparity
  - Social class (mortality in class I twice that in class V).
  - Breast cancer—50% excess of ovarian cancer has been suggested if breast cancer is (or has been) present. This may be due to a genetic risk related to inheritance of the *BRCA1* gene. Such families may account for 1–5% of ovarian cancer cases.
  - Endometrial cancer—this relates mainly to endometrioid ovarian tumour and thecal cysts (see below)
- Oral contraceptives have the same protective effect as pregnancy. There may also be a protective effect associated with mumps virus.
- Ovarian tumours comprise 35% of all gynaecological malignancies. Although it is the sixth commonest in incidence, the ovary is the fourth commonest site for fatal malignant disease in the female, after breast, colon and lung.

Histological types and derivation

Three types of cells give rise to the vast majority of primary ovarian tumours:

- surface epithelium (mesothelium)
- germ cells
- gonadal stroma (sex cord stromal).

They may sometimes be mixed.

Surface epithelial tumours

These tumours mimic tissues derived from the Müllerian or paramesonephric duct. They comprise serous papillary, mucinous, endometroid and clear cell tumours, Brenner tumours and fibromas.

Serous papillary tumours

- *Benign:* serous cystadenoma
- *Malignant:* serous cystadenocarcinoma
- They account for about 10% of ovarian neoplasms, and are bilateral in about 50% of cases.
- Usually unilocular with a smooth outer surface. The internal papillae may sprout through the capsule giving an impression of malignancy. The lining cells are cuboidal or columnar, resembling the epithelium of the endosalpinx.

Mucinous tumours

- *Benign:* mucinous cystadenoma
- *Malignant:* mucinous cystadenocarcinoma
- They form 30–40% of ovarian neoplasms, and are often large, unilateral multilocular cysts.
- Loculi are lined by tall mucus-secreting columnar cells. They may be found along with a Brenner tumour (see below).
- If the cyst ruptures the mucus-secreting cells may implant on the peritoneum and produce the rare but chronic *pseudomyxoma peritonei.*

Endometrioid tumours

- These solid tumours frequently contain elements of both serous and mucinous tumours.
- There is a definite association with endometrial carcinoma, perhaps as a result of simultaneous neoplasia in tissue of common embryonic origin.

Clear cell ('mesonephroid') tumours

This may be a variant for the endometrial tumour because they often co-exist.

Brenner tumour

- Unilateral and usually benign.

- Cords of squamous or transitional cells surround a central core lined by columnar epithelium. The fibrous tissue element closely resembles that found in a fibroma.

Fibroma
- Often moderately large, hard and lobulated with a glistening surface.
- Bilateral in about 10% of cases.
- The main interest of this rare tumour is its association with ascites and pleural effusion (usually right-sided) known as Meigs' syndrome.

Germ cell tumours

Teratomas
These arise from embryonic structures.

- *Benign* (mature tissues): dermoid cyst
- *Malignant* (immature tissues): teratocarcinoma
- Dermoid cysts are the commonest ovarian tumours in young women.

They are:

- usually symptomless, but torsion or rupture may produce signs and symptoms of an acute abdomen.
- bilateral in about 10% of case and seldom larger than 12 cm in diameter.
- lined by stratified squamous epithelium with its usual cutaneous elements—hair, sebaceous and sweat glands. Teeth, neural tissue, cartilage, alimentary and respiratory epithelium and even active thyroid tissue (*struma ovarii*) may be present.
- Solid teratomas are usually malignant. The degree of malignancy and prognosis is related to the maturity of the component tissues.
- True malignant change (usually squamous carcinoma) can develop in any of the tissue types found in a mature dermoid.

Extra-embryonic germ cell tumours
Choriocarcinoma and yolk sac (endodermal sinus) tumours:

- These tumours produce pregnancy-associated plasma proteins, e.g.
  - choriocarcinoma: hCG (and human placental lactogen (hPL) to a lesser extent)
  - yolk sac: AFP.
- These can be used as tumour markers in diagnosis and follow-up after treatment.
- Malignant germ cell tumours have in the past had a bad prognosis. Intensive chemotherapy is now producing better results.

Disgerminoma
- It is a very rare tumour arising mostly between 20 and 30 years of age. It is often wrongly termed dysgerminoma.
- It arises from undifferentiated germ cells and is the counterpart of the seminoma in males.

- It can usually be dealt with by conservative surgery and is very radiosensitive.
- The preferred modern treatment is combination chemotherapy so that fertility can be preserved.

Gonadal stromal tumours

The stromal cells retain a potential for differentiation into any of the cells or tissues arising from the mesenchyme of the gonad (i.e. granulosa, theca, Leydig and Sertoli cells).

These rare tumours may therefore secrete any or all of the ovarian steroids.

They tend to be classified according to morphology:

- *Granulosa–theca cell group* (which may produce oestrogen)
  - Granulosa-cell tumour—not infrequently malignant but usually of low grade
  - Thecoma—fibroma
- *Sertoli–Leydig cell group* (which may secrete androgens)
  - Sertoli–Leydig cell tumour (androblastoma, arrhenoblastoma)
  - Sertoli-cell tumour
  - Leydig-cell tumour (hilus or lipoid cell tumour)
- *Mixed*—elements of granulosa cell tumour and arrhenoblastoma present (gynandroblastoma).

Feminising (oestrogen-producing) tumours cause:

- Precocious puberty before the menarche
- Cystic glandular hyperplasia in menstruating women
- Postmenopausal bleeding in older women.

There is an association with endometrial carcinoma.

Masculinising (androgen-producing) tumours will initially result in defeminisation, including secondary amenorrhoea then hirsutes, enlargement of the clitoris and deepening of the voice.

Secondary ovarian tumours

- Signs or symptoms referable to the breast, stomach, large bowel and uterus must be sought.
- The rare Krukenberg tumour usually results from simultaneous primary tumours in the gastrointestinal tract (particularly stomach) or breast and both ovaries.
- The histology is characterised by clumps of mucus-secreting epithelial cells in stroma.
- The mucin compresses the nuclei of each cell to one pole producing 'signet-ring cells'.

CLINICAL FEATURES OF OVARIAN TUMOURS

- The peak age incidence is between 40 and 60 years with the exception of teratomas and gonadal stromal tumour which occur at any age.

- Ovarian tumours rarely give rise to specific symptoms early in their course.
- The commonest presenting features are vague gastrointestinal upset (usually dyspepsia) or increasing abdominal girth, usually ascribed to 'middle age spread' by patients and medical attendants. This means that:
  - They are often found accidentally
  - If they are malignant the disease has commonly spread outside the ovary before the diagnosis is made
  - Abdominal swelling may be present but ignored by the patient.
  - Menstrual function is not usually affected (except by the rare gonadal stromal tumours).

Differential diagnosis
Ovarian tumours must be distinguished from a whole variety of pelvic and abdominal swellings. Among the most common are a full bladder or rectum; corpus luteum; intrauterine pregnancy; uterine fibroids; and hydrosalpinx.

Aids to diagnosis
- Ultrasound
- Laparoscopy
- Tumour markers—e.g. CA 125. (hCG and AFP in the rare germ cell tumours.)

CLINICAL FEATURES IN MALIGNANT VERSUS BENIGN TUMOURS

- *Age*—tumours in childhood are frequently malignant. In older women the risk of malignancy is proportional to age; 45% of tumours removed from women aged 45 years or over are malignant.
- *Pain and tenderness*—benign tumours are never painful unless complicated (see below). A sudden severe pain suggests torsion or rupture. Dull aching pain may suggest malignancy. Sacral nerve root pain is strongly suggestive of malignancy.
- *Rapidity of growth*—suggests malignancy.
- *Number of tumours*—75% of malignant tumours are bilateral, and 15% of benign tumours are bilateral.
- *Consistency of tumours*—solid, nodular and irregular growths are more likely to be malignant.
- *Fixation* is suggestive of malignancy, but not necessarily so.
- *Ascites* is usually a sign of peritoneal metastasis (especially if the fluid is bloodstained). Remember the possibility of Meigs' syndrome (see above).
- *Oedema* of the legs and vulva or evidence of venous obstruction are suggestive of malignancy.
- *Metastatic deposits*—Remote metastases are not common, but in advanced disease supraclavicular nodes may become enlarged. The pouch of Douglas may contain irregular deposits which can be felt

on bi-manual examination. The majority of patients with ovarian cancer present with advanced disease.

Complications of ovarian cysts
- *Torsion.* Acute or subacute pain may be accompanied by mild shock. The lower abdomen is tender with guarding and rigidity. Pelvic examination reveals a tender adnexal mass. Laparotomy is indicated and removal of the ovary usually necessary.
- *Rupture.* The signs and symptoms will vary. The contents of chocolate (endometriotic) and dermoid cysts are extremely irritant and, therefore, may cause severe symptoms.
- *Haemorrhage* into or from cyst. The signs and symptoms will vary according to the degree of haemorrhage.
- *Infection.* This is an uncommon complication of ovarian tumours.
- *Malignant change.* This occurs mostly in serous and mucinous cystadenoma. New symptoms are not produced. It is commonly assumed that all malignant ovarian tumours develop from benign cysts; there is little evidence that this happens frequently.

OVARIAN CANCER SCREENING
- Ovarian cancer kills about 4000 women per year in England and Wales.
- The population risk is 1 in 70 with a rise in incidence after 40 years of age.
  - Women with one affected relative may have some increase in lifetime risk
  - Two or more first or second-degree relatives affected suggests a genetic predisposition (i.e. they may carry the *BRCA1* or *BRCA2* gene). Their lifetime risk of developing ovarian cancer may be up to 50%. Women in this group are also at more risk of breast, endometrial or colorectal cancer.
- The best available screening strategy combines vaginal examination, vaginal ultrasound (carried out by experienced personnel) and serum CA125 levels.
- The problems with current screening methods are:
  - despite a relatively high sensitivity and specificity, the low prevalence of the disease means that the positive predictive value is only 10%; i.e. 10 women would require laparoscopy or laparotomy for every 1 cancer detected
  - interval cancers occur as frequently as those detected; therefore screening would need to be carried out at least yearly
  - there is no evidence that screening reduces mortality probably because it cannot detect the cancer early enough
- *On current evidence there is no justification for screening women at low or even moderate risk* but this is currently being evaluated by the United Kingdom Collaborative Trial of Ovarian Cancer screening Study (UKCTOCS).

- Screening is probably justified in women with a strong family history (see above). Some opt for prophylactic oophorectomy with HRT around age 40 years.
- The protective effects of oral contraceptive use (see p. 248) should be borne in mind when counselling young women at high risk of ovarian cancer.

MANAGEMENT OF 'BENIGN' OVARIAN TUMOURS

- Laparoscopy or laparotomy (particularly if suspicion of malignancy) must be undertaken in the presence of any ovarian swelling >5 cm diameter, particularly if it is continuing to enlarge.
- A combination of the following features found at operation may indicate a higher risk of malignancy:
  - The tumour is totally or partly solid
  - Bilateral tumours
  - There is fungation through the capsule (not merely papillary growths)
  - Large vessels on the tumour surface
  - Blood-stained ascites
  - Invasion of or adhesion to surrounding structures
  - Metastatic deposits.
- If there is real doubt, a frozen section should be asked for.
- In tumours known or thought to be benign, the treatment depends on the age and parity of the patient.
- In young women who wish to conserve reproductive capacity, enucleation of the cyst (cystectomy) is carried out.
- Larger cysts may demand removal of the ovary.
- In older women past child-bearing, it is customary to remove both ovaries and the uterus.
- If the cyst is unilateral consider biopsy of the other ovary to exclude an occult tumour.

MANAGEMENT OF EARLY CARCINOMA OF THE OVARY

- All the commoner malignant tumours are considered together because the stage and histological grading of the malignancy are more important prognostic indicators than the type of tumour.
- A midline or paramedian incision is required for full examination of the abdomen, particularly the diaphragm.
- Accurate staging is vital.

Technique of staging
The following should be inspected and biopsied if involvement is likely or suspected:

- Peritoneal washings for cytology
- Parietal peritoneum
- Omentum

- Uterus and other ovary
- Bladder
- Pelvic peritoneum—biopsy if ovary is adherent
- Bowel and its mesentery
- Lymph nodes—para-aortic and pelvic; biopsy if possible
- Liver—surface and substance
- Diaphragm—both leaves.

Carcinoma of ovary: FIGO clinical staging	
Stage I	Growth limited to the ovaries
Stage Ia	Only one ovary involved; no ascites (sub-groups: capsule not ruptured; capsule ruptured)
Stage Ib	Both ovaries involved; no ascites (sub-groups as above)
Stage Ic	One or both ovaries involved plus ascites or with malignant cells in peritoneal washing (sub-groups as above)
Stage IIa	Extension/metastases to uterus/tubes
Stage IIb	Extension to other pelvic tissues
Stage IIc	As IIa/b with ascites or positive peritoneal washing
Stage III	Growth involving one or both ovaries with intraperitoneal metastasis
Stage IV	Growth involving one or both ovaries with distant metastasis

Surgery (and adjuvant therapy?) in early disease

- The treatment of choice for stage I carcinoma of the ovary is bilateral salpingo-oophorectomy, hysterectomy and omentectomy.
- Simple oophorectomy may be indicated for younger women with stage Ia disease (and favourable histology) who wish to preserve their reproductive capacity and who fully understand the risks of later recurrence.
- Adjuvant therapy is not indicated for stage I disease unless:
  - The tumour is poorly differentiated
  - Ascites was present
  - The cyst was ruptured.
- Single-agent chemotherapy is the preferred adjuvant but external beam radiotherapy may be used.

MANAGEMENT OF ADVANCED OVARIAN CARCINOMA

- Every attempt should be made to remove all macroscopic tumour.
- Single-agent chemotherapy is, in general, as effective as multiple-agent treatment.
  - An alkylating agent (such chlorambucil, melphelan or cyclophosphamide) or cis-platinum/carboplatin can be used.
  - Initial results using paclitaxel are encouraging.
- 80% of tumours respond to chemotherapy.

- Although complete remissions are possible, the long term outlook with advanced disease is poor.

Survival rates for primary ovarian carcinoma
Stage Ia 85%; Stage Ib–IIa 40%; Stage IIb 25%; Stage IIc–III: 15%; Stage IV <5%.

Second-look operations after 12 months?
- A policy of 'second-look operation', whether by laparotomy or laparoscopy, has not been shown to improve the survival of the patient.
- It may be justified with informed patient consent in chemotherapy trials.

Secondary 'debulking' operations
Patients who have chemotherapy to reduce the volume of cancer in the abdomen may benefit from a second operation to remove residual disease before further chemotherapy.

PAIN RELIEF IN ADVANCED MALIGNANT DISEASE

Pain is an unpleasant sensation arising from stimulation of specific nerve endings, transmitted through more or less specific central nervous pathways to higher centres in the brain mainly located in areas which subserve emotion.

Pain, emotion and personality are, therefore, inextricably linked.

Principles
Aim to keep the patient both free of pain and fully alert.

Assessment
- Treatment varies according to the cause of the pain.
- The malignant disease may not be the cause of the pain.
- Some patients require a combination of drug and non-drug measures (e.g. radiation for bone pain, nerve blocks for nerve compression pain).

CHOICE OF ANALGESICS

- Establish a simple, practical analgesic 'league table' e.g.:
  - non-narcotic—aspirin (alternative: paracetamol)
  - weak narcotic—codeine (alternative: dihydrocodeine, d-propoxyphene)
  - strong narcotic—morphine (alternative: papaveretum, diamorphine)
- Analgesics should be given regularly to *prevent* pain: 'as required' medication is unacceptable.

- Doses should be determined on an individual basis; the correct dose is that which gives relief for at least 4 hours.
- Relief of pain should be assessed in relation to comfort achieved:
  - during the night
  - in the daytime at rest
  - on movement.

FURTHER READING

Coppleson M, Monaghan JM, Morrow CP, Tattersall MH 1991 Gynecologic Oncology, 2nd edn, Churchill Livingstone, Edinburgh

Edmonds DK 1999 Dewhurst's Textbook of Obstetrics and Gynaecology for Postgraduates, 6th edn, Blackwell Scientific, Oxford

Jacobs IJ, Shepherd JH, Oram DH, et al. 2002 Ovarian Cancer. Oxford University Press, Oxford

Luesley DM 1999 Cancer and Pre-cancer of the Vulva. Matthew Arnold, London

Luesley DM, Barrasso R 1998 Cancer and Pre-cancer of the Cervix. Matthew Arnold, London

RCOG 1999 Clinical Recommendations for the Management of Vulval Cancer. RCOG Publications, London

Shafi MI, Luesley DM, Jordan JA 2000 Handbook of Gynaecological Oncology. Churchill Livingstone, Edinburgh

Shaw RW, Soutter WP, Stanton S 1997 Gynaecology, 2nd edn. Churchill Livingstone, Edinburgh

25. Other conditions of the lower genital tract

Intense vulval itching may have a variety of causes (see below).

Intrinsic skin disease
- Non-neoplastic epithelial disorders
  - Lichen sclerosis
  - Squamous cell hyperplasia
- Vulval/Vaginal intraepithelial neoplasia
- Allergic or irritant dermatitis
- Atrophic changes (menopausal).

Infection
- Fungal (candida, tinea cruris)
- Parasitic infestation (scabies, threadworm)
- Viral (herpes, wart virus)
- Sexually transmitted diseases (STDs,–e.g. gonorrhoea, trichomoniasis).

Malignancy
- Melanoma
- Bartholin's gland tumours
- Sarcoma.

General
- Hypothyroidism
- Uraemia.

NON-NEOPLASTIC EPITHELIAL DISORDERS OF THE VULVA

Vulval atrophy is normal in elderly women and is symptomless. No treatment is necessary.

The term 'non-neoplastic epithelial disorders of skin and mucosa of the vulva' has replaced the term 'vulval dystrophies'. They comprise a group of different conditions characterised by disorders of epithelial growth and maturation.

- The characteristic symptom is pruritus.
- Areas of abnormality can appear red, white or pigmented. They may be raised, warty or flat.
- The correct diagnosis can often be made clinically after careful consideration of the age of the patient, the appearance of the lesion, the condition of the skin elsewhere.
- If there is doubt about the diagnosis or suspicion of malignancy, biopsy is mandatory. Those with abnormal and disordered epithelial activity (cellular atypia) are sometimes pre-malignant.

LICHEN SCLEROSUS

A thinning condition of the vulva that is associated with paradoxically increased cell turnover.

- It is of unknown (possibly auto-immune) aetiology. There is an association with some other autoimmune conditions such as achlorhydria and primary biliary cirrhosis.
- Clinically, there may be dyspareunia or vulval pain in addition to pruritus.
- Although traditionally considered to be benign it can be found adjacent to about 30% of vulval cancers. It may itself progress to cancer in about 3% of cases.
- It mainly occurs in older women but can be found in all age groups.
- The commonest sites are the vulva and peri-anal area but extra-genital lesions may develop. It begins with small, irregular, flat-topped, white papules often having a central keratotic plug. The patches become atrophic and coalesce. The skin is paper-thin and may break down. The introitus may shrink causing dyspareunia.
- It involves non-genital skin in 20% of affected women.

Histology
- Atrophic thinning of the epidermis with hyperkeratosis
- Absence of dermal papillae and elastic tissue
- Hyaline replacement of the collagen fibres
- Lymphocytic infiltration of deep layers.

Management
- Patients with typical appearances of lichen sclerosus need not have biopsies, but those with areas in which there is any question of malignancy should have several widely spaced biopsies of vulval skin.
- Aqueous cream may be effective and sedatives at night may help with itching.
- Severe hyperkeratosis that is causing fissuring of the skin can be softened by 2% salicylic acid ointment.
- Pruritus responds to a short, sharp course of potent fluorinated steroids (e.g. Dermovate applied twice daily for 1–2 months). Once

controlled, long-term use of a mild steroid cream with an anti-fungal (e.g. Trimovate), may be needed.

- 2% Testosterone cream is no more effective than simple emollients.
- Vulvectomy or local excision of lesions should be reserved for those cases in which VIN coexists with higher risk of carcinoma or the patient suffers intractable symptoms. The condition can recur after vulvectomy and even skin grafting of the site. Laser therapy, cryosurgery and topical therapy with 5-fluorouracil have also been suggested.
- Lesions that initially respond to topical steroids and then stop should prompt further investigation to exclude malignancy. There are differences in opinion for follow up: annual or clinically based are both acceptable.
- There are support groups available.

SQUAMOUS CELL HYPERPLASIA

Formerly hyperplastic dystrophy without atypia. Thickening of the epithelium without identifiable cause and without cellular abnormalities: of low pre-malignant potential.

Management
As for lichen sclerosus

MANAGEMENT OF NON-NEOPLASTIC EPITHELIAL DISORDERS OF VULVA

Exclude or treat:

- deficiencies of iron, riboflavin, vitamin B_{12} and folic acid
- generalised dermatoses
- diabetes mellitus
- achlorhydria
- fungal infections
- allergies (clothing, cosmetics, toilet preparations).

PAGET'S DISEASE

Atypical glandular cell growth is known as Paget's disease with a 30% chance of underlying adenocarcinoma.

Paget's disease requires wide excision because histological abnormalities spread beyond the edge of the clinically affected areas and recurrence is common.

INFECTION

See section below on vaginal discharge. Infections with *C. albicans* and *T. vaginalis* form up to 90% of pruritic vaginal discharges.

NEOPLASTIC CONDITIONS OF THE VAGINA AND VULVA

Vulval Intraepithelial Neoplasia (VIN) see p. 283

The definitive treatment is wide local excision that may require total removal of the vulva in widespread disease.

Where possible reconstructive plastic surgery should be used (rotational skin flaps or split skin grafts).

The factors to be considered in planning treatment are:

- Certainty of the diagnosis. On the one hand the lesion may not in fact be neoplastic and on the other there may be areas of invasion which have been overlooked
- Age of the patient and her sexual activity. The effect of complete vulvectomy on a young woman can be devastating
- Size and location of the lesion
- Health of the rest of the vulva, e.g. the presence of infection or chronic epithelial dystrophy
- Ease of long-term follow-up. Local excision demands follow-up.

Miscellaneous Malignant Conditions

Among the other malignant conditions that may present with pruritus vulvae are basal cell carcinoma, melanoma, sarcoma and Bartholin's gland tumours. These are discussed more fully on p. 293.

VAGINAL DISCHARGE

PHYSIOLOGICAL CAUSES

- The vaginal fluid is a transudate through the epithelium along with desquamated cells, some polymorphs, and bacterial flora, predominantly large Gram-positive bacilli (lactobacilli).
- Contributions to the fluid also come from the cervical mucus and secretions of Skene's and Bartholin's glands. The vaginal fluid is highly acidic due to the lactic acid from the lactobacilli and glycogen from the desquamated cells.
- The acid pH of the vagina and its normal bacterial flora are among the factors that provide natural defence mechanisms for the lower genital tract.
- Among the factors that impair the defence mechanisms are:
  - age—infection more liable to occur during childhood and after the menopause

- menstrual cycle—the alkalinity of the secretions around menses makes infection more likely
- pregnancy and the puerperium—a rise in pH encourages infection. Trauma at delivery with reduction in acidity by lochia and contamination with potentially pathogenic bowel flora makes the puerperium a time of particular susceptibility
- oestrogen-containing oral contraceptives increase the pH of vaginal fluid
- foreign bodies—objects such as beads or cotton wool in children or forgotten tampons in adults act as a focus for infection
- an IUD may produce a vaginal discharge due to chronic irritation of the endometrium.

Cervical ectropion
- An ectropion is an area of columnar epithelium that has (or seems to have) extended beyond its normal boundaries. *The term 'cervical erosion' is a misnomer and should be abandoned.*
- A cervical ectropion may therefore arise:
  - congenitally—the squamo-columnar junction lies on what should be the ectocervix
  - secondary to oestrogen-containing oral contraceptives
  - as a result of delivery—the squamo-columnar junction is normally sited but the parous cervix is patulous. (Note: the bivalve speculum may open the closed parous cervix and falsely give an impression of ectropion.)
- Vaginal discharge may be augmented by an increased secretion of mucus from a cervical ectropion.
- It is not to be confused with chronic cervicitis (see p. 326).

INFECTIONS
Candida albicans
Clinical features
- Intense pruritus and soreness that may worsen in the evening and at night
- Thick, white discharge (like curdled milk or cottage cheese) adherent to the vaginal skin
- Erythema of the vagina and labia minora which may extend peri-anally and onto the thighs
- The fungus is often carried in the gastrointestinal tract and/or the mouth
- The vagina is frequently infected via the perineum but minor trauma (e.g. intercourse) facilitates infection.

Predisposing factors
- Pregnancy—candidal vaginitis is the commonest of all infections in

pregnancy. Between 15 and 20% of pregnant women may be affected
- Menstrual cycle—growth of *Candida* is promoted at the end of the luteal phase
- Medical disorders such as diabetes mellitus (marked increase) and iron deficiency anaemia
- Drugs—oestrogen-containing oral contraceptives; broad-spectrum antibiotics; corticosteroids; immunosuppressive agents
- Clothing—e.g. occlusive tights.

Diagnosis
- Clinical features—examine the vagina directly
- Microscopy of the discharge suspended in a drop of normal saline—mycelial filaments and spores will be visible
- Culture on glucose agar of swabs obtained in Stuart's transport medium.

Treatment
- Fungicidal drugs, e.g. nystatin or one of the imidazoles vaginally or fluconazole orally; effectiveness is >80%. Recurrent candidiasis is a difficult management problem, but either treatment with clotrimazole pessaries monthly after menstruation or oral fluconazole both seem to be useful.
- Genital hygiene—daily washing with bland soap and water is all that is necessary.
- Clothing—avoidance of close-fitting tights; washing of underwear at >80°C.

Trichomonas vaginalis
- This is a flagellated protozoon.
- It is usually sexually transmitted, and may mask the presence (and the spread) of gonococcal infections.
- Cervical cytology can be highly abnormal in the presence of *T. vaginalis*. The cervical smear must be repeated after adequate treatment of the infection.

Clinical features
- Itching and/or burning sensation with dyspareunia.
- Frothy vaginal discharge (pH 5–6) that may be white, green or brownish. The 'typical' appearance is due to gaseous fermentation by a commensal aerogenic *streptococcus.*
- Some vulval oedema and congestion. Erythema is less marked than in *Candida* infections.
- The vaginal skin is reddish-purple, perhaps with dark-red spots seen best at colposcopy.

Diagnosis
- Clinical features—examine the vagina directly; the vaginal pH is alkaline (pH 5–6)

- Microscopy of the discharge suspended in a drop of normal saline—motile flagellated protozoa are seen (about the same size as a polymorph leukocyte)
- Culture of swabs collected in Bushby's brown transport medium.

Treatment
Metronidazole for both partners.

Gonococcal infections
See p. 265.

Chlamydia trachomatis
See p. 265.

Bacterial vaginosis
Bacterial vaginosis (BV) is a complex alteration in the vaginal flora with an overgrowth of anaerobic bacteria such as *Gardnerella vaginalis*. It is accompanied by a reduction in concentration of lactobacilli. It is not truly an infection but simply abnormal colonisation.

- It has a prevalence of around 15% in antenatal clinics in the UK, the majority of which are asymptomatic.
- The increased prevalence in women seeking termination of pregnancy (nearly 30%) supports sexually transmission though not exclusively so.

Clinical features
- The characteristic symptom is an offensive 'fishy' vaginal discharge due to amines produced by the organisms, which can be very distressing.
- Inflammation or irritation are not common.
- *Gardnerella vaginalis* is also found in over 20% of healthy, symptomless women.
- Bacterial vaginosis, perhaps as a co-infection with *Ureaplasma urealyticum* and *Mycoplasma hominis*, may be associated with chorio-amnionitis and pre-term labour.

Diagnosis
- A drop of 10% potassium hydroxide added to a sample of the discharge on a glass slide releases the fishy odour.
- Microscopy of a wet film shows the motile *Mobiluncus* species.

Treatment
- Asymptomatic BV does not require treatment.
- Where treatment is merited then metronidazole or clindamycin can be used.
- The colonisation tends to recur, particularly around the time of menstruation and repeated courses of antibiotics are often needed.

OTHER CAUSES OF VAGINAL DISCHARGE

These include:

- Tumours
  - Cervical or intra-uterine polyp
  - Pedunculated fibroid
  - Cervical cancer
- Sexual problems
  - Psychosexual upset
  - Sexual abuse (in girls)
- Miscellaneous
  - Vaginal foreign body
  - Postmenopausal vaginitis.

BENIGN CONDITIONS OF THE VAGINA AND CERVIX

GAERTNER DUCT CYSTS

- These arise from the mesonephric (Wolffian) duct and, therefore, occur antero-laterally in the vagina.
- They may be single or multiple and of varied size.
- Histology shows a single layer of cuboidal epithelium.
- Treatment is by excision or marsupialisation.

VAGINAL INCLUSION CYSTS

Usually small and often multiple, resulting from inversion of small fragments of vaginal skin after delivery or vaginal surgery.

ENDOMETRIOSIS

See p. 222.

CONDYLOMATA ACUMINATA (genital warts)

- Caused by papova (DNA) virus, they are sexually transmitted and, therefore, may be accompanied by other STDs.
- They grow larger in pregnancy and tend to regress after delivery.
- Treatment is by podophyllin (avoid in pregnancy), saturated trichloracetic acid or electrocautery. Severe cases can be destroyed by laser (under GA). More recently, Imiquimod, an immunomodulator, has been shown to be as effective as other treatments, but less invasive and with less relapses—see Further reading.

PAPILLOMAS OF VAGINA AND CERVIX

- Cervical papillomas are more common than vaginal.

- Clinically, they can be difficult to differentiate from genital warts.
- They derive from the squamous epithelium with various degrees of keratinisation. The stalk is of fibrous connective tissue.
- They need to be removed surgically and sent for histological examination because of their malignant potential.

OTHER (RARE) BENIGN TUMOURS

E.g. fibroleiomyoma

CHRONIC CERVICITIS

- This is characterised by a hypertrophied, spongy cervix, in parous women presenting with seemingly purulent vaginal discharge.

FURTHER READING

Butcher J 1999 ABC of sexual health: female sexual problems II: sexual pain and sexual fears. British Medical Journal. 318(7176): 110–2

Gilson RJ. Mindel A 2001 Recent advances: Sexually transmitted infections British Medical Journal 322(7295): 1160–4

Powell JJ, Wojnarowska F 1999 Lichen sclerosus. Lancet 353(9166): 1777–83

Shaw RW, Soutter WP and Stanton S 1997 Gynaecology, 2nd edn. Churchill Livingstone, London

Sobel JD 2000 Bacterial vaginosis. Annual Review of Medicine 51: 349–56

26. Gynaecological surgery

PRE-OPERATIVE ASSESSMENT

The correct operation must be carried out for the correct reasons. If the management suggested in outpatients is found not to be appropriate at the time of admission it must be altered accordingly or deferred for further investigation as appropriate.

The purpose of the pre-operative assessment is to optimise the pre-operative condition of the patient. It has three main components:

- Detection of unrecognised medical conditions.
- Understand how medical conditions can affect the outcome of surgery and/or anaesthesia.
- Optimise medical condition, seeking expert help where required.

General issues

- Women who smoke should be advised to stop several weeks before the proposed operation.
- For women on the combined pill give advice about alternative contraception. (see p. 250)

Outpatient assessment should include:

- General physical examination, including breasts, cardiac and respiratory status and BP to determine anaesthetic fitness.
- Haemoglobin level and blood group estimation.
- ECG and chest X-ray, urea and electrolyte estimation in hypertensive women.

Anaemia (haemoglobin <10 g/dl) should be investigated and corrected before admission.

Among those who require particularly careful assessment are women:

- with medical disorders such as cardiac disease, hypertension, diabetes mellitus or other endocrine disorders. *Note*: they often co-exist.
- who abuse alcohol and drugs
- on treatment that may affect their response to anaesthesia or surgery, for example:
  - antihypertensive drugs (particularly β-blocking agents)
  - anticoagulants

- systemic corticosteroids, which can potentially delay healing and, with chronic therapy, need to be increased to cover the 'stress' of surgery.
- who are morbidly obese (e.g. BMI >39/m^2); this is a significant risk factor in post-operative morbidity and mortality.

The 1999 NCEPOD report (see Callum et al in Further reading) identified the elderly as a particularly at risk group and extra care should be taken with their assessment.

Blood should be sent in good time to allow grouping and saving of serum or cross-matching depending on the extent of the surgery involved.

PRE-OPERATIVE SELECTION FOR DAY-CASE SURGERY

Each unit must have *pre-operative selection guidelines* for day-case surgery, such as the following:

- The patient should be fit and healthy or, at most, have *mild* systemic disturbance from the condition to be treated or other pathology.
- Any patient taking long-term medication must be carefully assessed and discussed with the anaesthetist.
- Patients who are morbidly obese or who have imperfectly controlled diabetes mellitus, chronic respiratory or cardiovascular disease are *not* suitable for day-case treatment.
- Although all patients should be judged on physiological rather than chronological age, treatment of a woman >60 years of age as a day case needs to be considered carefully.
- Day-case treatment is inappropriate if the proposed surgery has a significant risk of causing severe post-operative pain and/or haemorrhage.
- If general anaesthesia is to be used (or may be required), no solid food should be taken for 6 hours or clear fluid for 3 hours pre-operatively.
- The operation should not normally exceed 60 minutes' duration.

The patient should be seen by the surgeon before discharge when an explanation of the surgery can be given.

- She should not be discharged until she is fully recovered, awake and with stable vital signs.
- Control of nausea and pain must be adequate.
- She must be accompanied home by a responsible adult.

MINIMAL ACCESS GYNAECOLOGICAL SURGERY (MAGS)

Advantages

Among the *suggested benefits* are:

- less post-operative pain
- shorter hospital stay
- fewer wound-related complications
- more rapid recovery
- lower incidence of post-operative respiratory complications and ileus.

Disadvantages
These include:

- increased operation time
- greater risk of iatrogenic complications (related to experience of the surgeon).

Principles
- MAGS and 'day-case' surgery are not synonymous. Full pre-operative assessment is required and *short-cuts must be avoided*.
- MAGS requires some different skills compared with open surgery. These must be learned and the 'learning curve' varies among individual surgeons.
  - All surgeons should be skilled at traditional open operative techniques before embarking on MAGS procedures.
  - An experienced colleague should supervise the first few cases of a surgeon undertaking a technique new to him or her ('proctoring').
  - *Some gynaecological surgeons may not have the aptitude to perform MAGS safely and effectively.*
- MAGS involves risk that must not be underestimated.
- Those carrying out MAGS must adhere to basic surgical principles of open procedures, for example:
  - meticulous haemostasis is required.
  - surgical specimens should be available to the pathologist for diagnosis, particularly if malignant disease is suspected.

LAPAROSCOPIC SURGERY

Laparoscopy may not be tolerated by 'high risk' patients and there should be a low threshold to convert to an open approach where there are problems (see NCEPOD in Further reading).

Stratification of levels of training required for laparoscopic procedures
The RCOG has produced guidelines for training in laparoscopy and hysteroscopy (see Further reading). They can be summarised as follows:
- *Level 1*—diagnostic laparoscopy
- *Level 2*—minor procedures including sterilisation
- *Level 3*—more extensive procedures requiring additional training, e.g. laparasocopically assisted vaginal/sub-total hysterectomy (LAVH); salpingostomy, salpingectomy/salpingo-oophorectomy or ovarian cystectomy

- *Level 4*—extensive endoscopic procedures requiring subspecialist or advanced/tertiary level skills, e.g. myomectomy, pelvic lymphadenectomy, procedures for incontinence.

For *Levels 1–3* the trainee's performance should be supervised by a trained endoscopist until confirmed competent. *Level 4* procedures are the province of those nationally/internationally recognised in the field of MAGS.

Note: Not all procedures listed have been shown to be superior or safer than their 'open' alternatives. More better-designed trials are still required especially for the more advanced techniques.

Complications of laparoscopic surgery

The non-lethal complication rate is reported as up to 1% for diagnostic laparosocopy and 5% for more advanced procedures (up to 18% of LAVH in one series). These figures can be related to:

- Mode of access in which the Verres needle or trocars may damage abdominal wall or major intra-abdominal blood vessels, bowel or bladder
- Performance of the operation—particularly risk of damage to ureter, bladder, rectum or pelvic blood vessels
- Anaesthetic problems, e.g. due to production of a CO_2 pneumo-peritoneum or prolonged maintenance of lithotomy position.

HYSTEROSCOPIC SURGERY

- The basic principles of hysteroscopy are different from laparoscopy and must be learned separately. Outpatient hysteroscopy is becoming the gold standard for endometrial assessment for abnormal menstrual bleeding.
- The RCOG guidelines also stratify hysteroscopic procedures by levels of training from *level 1* for simple and diagnostic procedures to *level 3* for more complex procedures (e.g. division/resection of a uterine septum).

Complications of hysteroscopic surgery

The complication rate rises with the level of the procedure being about 1/1000 for diagnostic procedures.

Intra-operative	Early post-operative	Late post-operative
Uterine perforation	Infection	Recurrence of symptoms
Intra-abdominal injury	Secondary haemorrhage	
Fluid overload	Haematometra	
Haemorrhage	Cyclical pain	
Gas embolism	Treatment failure	

PERI-OPERATIVE COMPLICATIONS

See NCEPOD report in Further reading.

Where major or minimal-access surgery is carried out:

- Essential services such as recovery rooms, high dependency and intensive therapy units must be ready and available.
- Proper equipment and qualified specialist staff must be available at all times.
- Any surgeon or anaesthetist must be competent to deal with the immediate hazards which may occur during an operation, such as haemorrhage or cardiac failure.

Where complications arise perioperatively (e.g. bowel damage), good practice would include:

- Stop operation and call senior, appropriately qualified, help.
- Consider first aid measures (e.g. antibiotics and local packing).
- Repair defect.
- Close wound appropriately including drains, etc.
- Apply appropriate post-operative care.
- Explain procedure to patient post operatively.

POST-OPERATIVE COMPLICATIONS

THROMBOEMBOLISM (TE)

Deep vein thrombosis (DVT) and TE are important perioperative complications in gynaecological surgery.

- DVT is detected in about 12% of women undergoing abdominal hysterectomy. It is likely that many go undetected in all types of surgery.
- TE is associated with 20% of perioperative deaths after hysterectomy.
- In the majority of patients dying from pulmonary embolism the preceding thrombosis had not been detected.

Risk Markers for TE

Patient-associated factors	Disease-associated factors
• Increasing age • Obesity	• Abdomino-pelvic surgery • Malignancy, especially pelvic, abdominal, metastatic—(accounts for 35% of cases)
• Severe varicose veins	• Infection

Patient-associated factors	Disease-associated factors
• Immobility (bed rest >4 days) or paralysis	• Polycythaemia, paraproteinaemia, paroxysmal nocturnal haemoglobinuria
• Pregnancy or puerperium	• Nephrotic syndrome
• Previous TE	• Inflammatory bowel disease
• 'Thrombophilia'*	• Cardiac failure or recent MI

*e.g. deficiency of protein C, protein S, or antithrombin III; Factor V Leiden or other activated protein C resistance; anti-phospholipid syndrome and lupus inhibitor

Prophylaxis against TE

Prophylaxis reduces the risk of fatal and non-fatal TE. Methods are listed in the box below.

Prophylaxis against TE	
Mechanical methods	e.g. graduated elastic compression stockings or intermittent pneumatic compression
Pharmacological methods	Low-dose subcutaneous heparin will prevent 60–70% of DVTs and fatal PE; low m.w. heparins may be more effective in high risk patients. (caution required with spinal/epidural anaesthesia) Warfarin can be given as peri-operative low dose (1 mg daily) but this needs further evaluation, or at full dose post-operatively in high risk patients; keep INR* at 2.0–2.5. Dextran 70 is not so effective in preventing DVT. Anti-platelet agents (e.g. aspirin) are of limited efficacy

*INR—International Normalised Ratio of the prothrombin time

Contraindications to heparin include:

- hepatic or renal failure
- peptic ulcer or oesophageal varices
- previous hypersensitivity to heparin
- severe hypertension
- thrombocytopenia
- von Willebrand's disease.

The RCOG (see Further reading) suggest the following guidelines for prophylaxis. These need to be regularly reviewed in the light of evidence and experience.

- **Low risk**—*early mobilisation and hydration required*
  - Minor surgery (<30 min); no other risk markers
  - Major surgery (>30 min); age <40 years and no other risk markers.
- **Moderate risk**—*consider one of a variety of prophylactic measures available*
  - Minor surgery (<30 min) in women with a personal or family history of TE or thrombophilia.
  - Major surgery (>30 min)
  - Extended laparoscopic surgery
  - Obesity (>80 kg or BMI >30/m²)
  - Severe varicose veins
  - Current infection
  - Immobility for >4 days before surgery
  - Major current illness (see risk markers above).
- **High risk**—Use heparin prophylaxis (with leg stockings)
  - A total of three or more moderate risk markers above
  - Major abdominal or pelvic surgery for malignant disease
  - Major surgery (>30 min) in women with a personal or family history of TE or thrombophilia *or* paralysis or immobilisation of lower limbs.

Management of suspected or established thromboembolism

- The symptoms and signs of pulmonary embolism (PE) can be missed, and there should be a low threshold for investigation where thromboembolism is suspected.
- Treatment should be started where there is sufficient clinical suspicion to warrant investigation.
- Arrange venography for DVT and a ventilation perfusion isotope lung scan if PE is suspected.
- Chest X-ray; ECG; and blood gases may help to identify/exclude other causes.
- If TE is confirmed it may be appropriate to screen for thrombophilia—if present seek advice of haematologist.

Treatment

- The aim is to prevent extension of existing thrombus and prevent further complications.
- Low molecular weight heparins are now licensed for the treatment of established thromboembolism.
- Acute treatment is with calcium heparin intravenously for at least 48 hours.
- Treatment should be continued for at least 3 months, usually with either low molecular weight heparins or warfarin—the correct dosage maintains the INR at 2.0–2.5.

POST-OPERATIVE SEPSIS

Generalised causes of post-operative pyrexia:

- Pulmonary atelectasis
- Chest infection—typically *Strep. pneumoniae*
- Urinary Tract infection—typically *E. coli*

WOUND INFECTION

Prevention
- Adequate surgical preparation for both surgeon and wound
- Meticulous haemostasis and minimum operating times with an open wound
- Prophylactic antibiotics (particularly for vaginal surgery)— metronidazole +/– cephalosporins, ideally prior to surgery.

Masks and adhesive drapes have not been shown to reduce infection rates.

Treatment
- *Staph. aureus, E. coli, Strep. pyogenes* and other anaerobic streptococci are the most common pathogens in wound infections after gynaecological surgery.
- Most will respond to antibiotics and conservative treatment.
- Pus collections, including infected vault haematomas will need to be drained.

VAULT-HAEMATOMA

This is a common complication of hysterectomy ocurring in:

- 25% of women after vaginal hysterectomy
- 31% after LAVH
- 5–10% after abdominal hysterectomy.

To prevent this there should be optimal haemostasis during surgery and pelvic drainage is advised.

WOUND HAEMATOMA AND DEHISCENCE

- A transverse suprapubic incision should be used when possible but is not appropriate for management of ovarian cancer.
- Aseptic technique is vital.
- Haemostasis and closure techniques are important.
- A non-absorbable or polyglycolic acid suture is preferred for closure of the rectus sheath.
- Drainage must be adequate.
- The risk is increased slightly if low-dose heparin is being used as prophylaxis against TE.

URINARY TRACT COMPLICATIONS

The incidence of *urinary infection* can be reduced by reducing the frequency of urethral catheterisation i.e. using an indwelling catheter overnight post operatively.

If continuous bladder drainage is necessary post-operatively a suprapubic catheter reduces urinary tract infection and bladder function can be assessed whilst in situ.

Injuries to the urinary tract
These are preventable, but if they occur prompt recognition at the time and appropriate remedial action are required.

- Ureteric Injury complicates 0.5–2.5% of gynaecological procedures. There is a higher risk for oncology procedures.
- Bladder perforation complicates 1% of gynaecological procedures.
- Voiding disorders can complicate gynaecological procedures, particularly where there is damage to the pelvic nerve plexus and after incontinence procedures.

BOWEL INJURY

Bowel injuries are uncommon (0.3%), but the incidence increases with previous surgery and laparoscopic surgery.

Exploration by open laparotomy may be required, and a defunctioning colostomy for large bowel injuries.

FURTHER READING

Callum KG, Gray AJ, Martin IC and Sherry KM 1999 Extremes of age: the Report of the National Confidential Enquiry into Perioperative Deaths. London. www.ncepod.org.uk
RCOG 1994 Training in gynaecological endoscopic surgery. RCOG, London
RCOG 1995 Working Party on Prophylaxis against Thromboembolism in Gynaecology and Obstetrics Report. RCOG, London
Read M, James M 2002 Immediate postoperative complications following gynaecological surgery. The Obstetrician and Gynaecologist. 4(1): 29–35
Shaw RW, Soutter WP, Stanton S 1997 Gynaecology, 2nd edn. Churchill Livingstone, London

Index

incontinence, 274
Parity, and perinatal mortality, 177
Partogram, 137–138
Parturition see Labour
Parvovirus B19, 111
Patau's syndrome (trisomy 13), 36–37
Pearl index, 244
Pelvic arthropathy, in pregnancy,
    100–101
Pelvic floor exercises, 273
    for vaginal prolapse, 281
Pelvic inflammatory disease (PID),
    264–267
    and menorrhagia, 218
Pelvis
    cephalo-pelvic disproportion, 154
    childbirth effects, on muscles and
        nerves, 187
    normal diameters, 153–154
Peptic ulcer, in pregnancy, 91
Perinatal morbidity, 178
Perinatal mortality
    definitions, 175
    in developing countries, 183–184
    factors influencing, 176–178
    pathology, 178–180
    rates of, 175–176
Perineal pain, 187
Perineal tears, 162
Peripheral oedema, in pre-
    eclampsia, 63
Phaeochromocytoma, in pregnancy,
    86
Phenylketonuria (PKU), 41, 190
Phenytoin, teratogenicity, 84
Phyto-oestrogens, 260
Pinta, 116
Pituitary gland
    and female fertility, 228–229
    in pregnancy, 14
Placenta accreta, 125, 170
Placenta percreta, 125
Placenta praevia, 125–127
Placental site trophoblastic tumour
    (PSST), 27
Plasma osmolality, in pregnancy, 15
Plasma volume
    and pre-eclampsia, 69
    in pregnancy, 12
Platelet disorders, in pregnancy,
    98–99
Polycystic ovary syndrome (PCOS),
    213–216
    and recurrent miscarriage, 20

Polyhydramnios, 129–130
Polyps, endometrial, 301
Position of fetus
    occipito-posterior position,
        157–158
    see also Presentation
Postcoital contraception, 253
Postmenopausal bleeding (PMB), 263
Postmortem examination, of fetus,
    50
Postpartum blues, 103
Postpartum haemorrhage, 168–170
    secondary, 186–187
Postpartum thyroiditis, 90
Post-term pregnancy, 134
Prazosin, for gestational
    hypertension, 67, 68t
Pre-conception care, 5–6
Pre-eclampsia (PET), 59–60
    development of, mechanisms, 61
    fluid balance, 69
    long-term outcomes, 70
    management, 66
    maternal mortality from, 65
    maternal pathology, 62–63
        central nervous system, 64–65
        HELLP syndrome, 64
    predisposing factors, 60–61
    prevention, 62
Pregnancy
    antenatal care see Antenatal care
    antepartum haemorrhage, 125–129
    cardiovascular disorders see
        Cardiovascular disorders of
        pregnancy
    central nervous system disorders,
        83–85
    drug abuse in, 123–124
    drug prescribing, 122–123
    early pregnancy, problems in
        clinic procedures, 16
        ectopic pregnancy, 21–25
        gestational trophoblastic
            disease (GTD), 25–29
        miscarriage, 16–18
        recurrent miscarriage, 18–20
    ectopic see Ectopic pregnancy
    emergency procedures, 171–173
    endocrine disorders in, 85–90
    gastrointestinal disorders, 91, 93
    haematological system see
        Haematological system
    liver disease, 91–93
    maternal adaptation to, 11–15